Third Edition

Guide to Medical Billing

Sharon E. Brown, Esq.

Lori Tyler, MS
President/Owner Innova, Inc.

PEARSON

Boston   Columbus   Indianapolis   New York   San Francisco   Upper Saddle River
Amsterdam   Cape Town   Dubai   London   Madrid   Milan   Munich   Paris   Montreal   Toronto
Delhi   Mexico City   São Paulo   Sydney   Hong Kong   Seoul   Singapore   Taipei   Tokyo

Publisher: Julie Levin Alexander
Publisher's Assistant: Regina Bruno
Editor-in-Chief: Mark Cohen
Executive Editor: Joan Gill
Associate Editor: Bronwen Glowacki
Editorial Assistant: Stephanie Kiel
Director of Marketing: David Gesell
Marketing Manager: Katrin Beacom
Marketing Specialist: Michael Sirinides
Marketing Assistant: Crystal Gonzalez
Managing Production Editor: Patrick Walsh
Production Liaison: Julie Boddorf

Production Editor: Karen Jones
Senior Media Editor: Amy Peltier
Media Project Manager: Lorena Cerisano
Manufacturing Manager: Lisa McDowell
Creative Director: Jayne Conte
Senior Art Director: Maria Guglielmo
Interior Designer: Ilze Lemesis
Cover Designer: Ilze Lemesis
Composition: Aptara®, Inc.
Printing and Binding: Courier/Kendallville
Cover Printer: Lehigh-Phoenix Color/Hagerstown

All photographs/illustrations not credited on page, under or adjacent to the visual were photographed/rendered on assignment and are property of Pearson Education.

Library of Congress Cataloging-in-Publication Data
Brown, Sharon E.
  Guide to medical billing/Sharon E. Brown, Lori Tyler.—3rd ed.
  p.; cm.
  Rev. ed. of: Guide to medical billing and coding. 2nd ed. c2007.
  Includes bibliographical references and index.
  ISBN-13: 978-0-13-504137-6
  ISBN-10: 0-13-504137-6
  I. Tyler, Lori.   II. Guide to medical billing and coding.   III. Title.
  [DNLM: 1. Practice Management—economics.   2. Forms and Records Control.   3. Patient Credit and Collection.
  4. Reimbursement Mechanisms. W 80]
  LCClassification no assigned
  651.5′04261—dc23
                                                                      2011045327

10 9 8 7 6 5 4 3 2 1

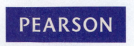

ISBN 13: 978-0-13-504137-6
ISBN 10:   0-13-504137-6

Disclaimer

This text is a guide to the medical billing field. Decisions should not be based solely on information within this guide. Decisions impacting the practice of medical billing must be based on individual circumstances including legal/ethical considerations, local conditions, and payer policies.

The information contained in this text is based on experience and research. However, in the complex, rapidly changing medical environment, this information may not always prove correct. Data used are widely variable and can change at any time. Readers should follow current coding regulations outlined by official coding organizations.

Any five-digit numeric Current Procedural Terminology, 2011 standard edition (CPT®) codes, services, and descriptions, instructions, and/or guidelines are copyright 2011 (or such other date of publication of CPT® as defined in the federal copyright laws). American Medical Association. All Rights Reserved.

CPT® is a listing of descriptive terms and five-digit numeric identifying codes and modifiers for reporting medical services performed by physicians. This presentation includes only CPT® descriptive terms, numeric identifying codes, and modifiers for reporting medical services and procedures. The most current CPT® is available from the American Medical Association. No fee schedules, basic unit values, relative value goods conversion factors, or scales or components thereof are included in CPT®.

The American Medical Association assumes no responsibility for the consequences attributable or related to any use or interpretation of any information or views contained in or not contained in this publication.

The publisher and author do not accept responsibility for any adverse outcome from undetected errors, opinion, and analysis contained in this text that may prove inaccurate or the reader's misunderstanding of an extremely complex topic. All names used in this book are completely fictitious. Any resemblance to persons or to companies, current or no longer existing, is purely coincidental.

Brief Contents

Contents

Introduction

Medical billing is the study of medical billing procedures from the time a patient walks into the office to the moment the patient walks out, as well as the final billing and reconciliation of the patient's account.

Medical billing is one of the fastest-growing employment opportunities in the United States today. Insurance companies, medical offices, hospitals, and other health care providers are in great need of trained personnel to create and bill medical claims.

The most important ingredient to success is the desire to learn, without which the learning process is ineffective. The desire to learn can lead to a rewarding career in the medical billing field.

Text Features

Special features of the text, such as learning objectives, key terms and definitions, critical thinking questions, and end-of-chapter exercises, enhance understanding and retention of the material.

Learning Objectives. Each chapter begins with a bulleted list of learning objectives to help focus the students on the most pertinent topics, key skills, and concepts covered in that chapter.

Key Terms and Definitions. Key terms are listed at the beginning of the chapter and defined within the text. Key terms are bolded and defined when initially introduced, thus allowing for quick identification. This structural element allows the students to read the term in context to the related material. In addition, the students can remain focused on reading the material without having to stop and refer to a glossary for a definition.

Critical Thinking Questions. Critical thinking questions are scattered throughout the chapters. The nature of the questions are meant to challenge the reader into thinking about what they are learning and to use reasoning to answer the posed questions.

Chapter Activities. These in-text activities allow the students to immediately practice concepts as they are learned. They are professional practice exercises that will prepare the students for real-life job duties.

Suggestion for Online Research. Provides students' suggestions of conducting further research using online tools for various topics discussed.

Practice Pitfalls. This special feature provides the students with a professional insider's point of view. These practice pitfalls provide additional information for professional success and ideas, shortcuts, good habits to follow in the office, as well as bad work habits, the outcomes of sloppy work, and common mistakes that the students can avoid.

Summaries. Each chapter ends with a bulleted list of key concepts. These summaries are useful study tools that enable the students to assess their level of knowledge and are also useful as a quick study reference.

End-of-Chapter Exercises

Review Questions. Located at the end of the chapter, these help to reinforce key concepts. Answering questions without looking back at the chapter will help students determine if they have grasped the principles within the chapter or if there is a need for further study. The questions also serve to prepare students for examinations. Additional end-of-chapter activities provide students the opportunity to put their knowledge into practice. These hands-on exercises help to ensure competence in medical billing. Answers are contained in the instructor materials for this course.

Pedagogy. *Guide to Medical Billing* will aid students in learning the skills necessary to become a successful medical biller. The material is designed to be comprehensive yet user friendly. The text follows a logical learning format by beginning with a broad base of information and then, step by step, follows the course for learning the specific medical biller job duties.

Organization of the Text

Guide to Medical Billing provides students with all the theoretical knowledge and practical skills needed to achieve success as a medical biller. The text introduces students to the medical practice, before proceeding to the more in-depth procedures and practices of the medical office and hospital. All aspects of medical billing are covered. Content includes a variety of subjects, such as International Classification of Disease (ICD-9-CM and ICD-10-CM) coding, Current Procedural Terminology (CPT) coding, stress and time management, the CMS-1500 form and medical procedures, the UB-04 form and hospital procedures, as well as basic office functions and communications.

Ancillary and Program Material

Guide to Medical Billing Instructor Resource Guide. This all-inclusive combined performance evaluator and curriculum gives the instructors the necessary tools to both run and manage a medical billing program as well as assess the student's progress at critical points in the program. The Instructor Resource Guide includes the following components:

- Daily Lesson Plans
- PowerPoints
- Test Banks

About the Author

For twenty years, Lori Tyler was directly involved in two- and four-year colleges, holding various positions including faculty member, program director, and dean. Courses she taught included medical billing, medical coding, law and ethics, medical office management, medical terminology, and medical office computer software. Prior to working in education Lori worked in health care for ten years. Her passion for education and wanting the best materials made available for both faculty and students led her to the publishing industry. In addition to providing consulting and workshops to education facilities through the development of her own company, Lori has been successful at authoring various educational materials, including six textbooks and handling the job of Developmental Editor for materials published through Pearson Education.

Review Acknowledgment

Many people have contributed to the development and success of *Guide to Medical Billing*. We extend our thanks and deep appreciation to the many students and classroom instructors who have provided us with helpful suggestions for this edition of the text.

We would like to express our thanks to the following individuals:

Robin Berenson, EdD, JCTC, American Public University System, Charles Town, WV; Susan DeGirolamo, AAH, RMA, NCPT, NCICS, CMHT, Pennsylvania Institute of Technology, Philadelphia, PA; Regina Glenn, MS, RHIA, CCS, Davenport University, Grand Rapids, MI; Stevan Hidalgo, MS, RHIA, Health Information and Credentialing Manager, University Hospital, Denver, CO; Robert D. Linville, MBA/HCM, Oklahoma State University, Oklahoma City, OK; Fannie Sue Martin, CPC, YTI Career Institute, Mechanicsburg, PA; Deborah McGichen, BS Education, All-State Career, Baltimore, MD; Lorraine Papazian-Boyce, MS, CPC, Instructor, Colorado Technical University Online Consultant, Vancouver, WA; Letitia Patterson, MPA, CPC, CCS-P, Rasmussen Online, Chicago, IL; Simone Thomas, MHSc, MHL, CCS, Medical Coding and Billing Professor, Miami Dade College, Miami FL.

A special thanks to Lorraine Papazian-Boyce for her knowledge related to ICD-10-CM.

SECTION
MEDICAL PRACTICE ADMINISTRATION

1

Introduction to Medical Billing

Key Words and Concepts you will learn in this chapter:

Health Maintenance Organizations (HMOs)

Job stress

Provider

After completion of this chapter you should be able to:

State the job responsibilities of a medical biller.

List the different types of health care settings.

Identify the symptoms of stress.

Explain methods to deal with stress.

As a medical biller, it is your responsibility to properly bill for services received by patients. One of the vital functions of the medical biller is to bill and collect the revenue that is generated by patient care and is crucial to the cash flow in the medical office. As such, the medical biller is an integral part of the medical team. The biller's contribution is essential to running the medical office.

Medical billers may complete claim forms, correspond with patients, manage office supplies, and handle minor accounting for the office (Figure 1-1 ●). The scope of a medical biller's duties often depends on the size of the office. Larger offices may have multiple personnel responsible for running the office, setting appointments, and handling the clients. Smaller offices may assign more of these duties to a medical biller/receptionist.

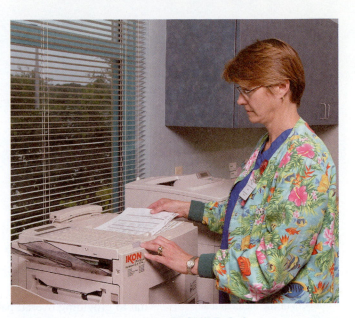

FIGURE 1-1

Medical biller handling various tasks

The purpose of this textbook is to provide an introduction to the tasks that an entry-level medical biller would perform. Throughout the text, readers are provided an opportunity to answer critical-thinking questions related to the field of medical billing and to perform general billing and coding activities. For purposes of this textbook, the fictional main provider of service used throughout for illustrative purposes is Paul Provider, M.D., 5858 Peppermint Place, Anytown, USA 12345. Other providers of service will be used as well.

Although many offices are moving toward, or have already transferred over to, the electronic medical record, it is important to know how to perform medical office billing tasks manually. This knowledge is particularly useful if the technology is not in working order. Although some electronic methods are discussed in this book, the focus of this text is on the manual methods of medical billing. To learn electronic methods of medical billing, an additional course using a medical billing software program is required. Advanced coding and reimbursement skills require further studies beyond what is provided in this text.

▶ **CRITICAL THINKING QUESTION:** What do you hope to get out of the course in which this book is being used, and what do you feel will be important for you to learn about medical billing?

Job Roles and Duties

Medical billers play diverse roles in the medical office. The most common duties associated with medical billing include the following:

- Billing insurance carriers for services performed
- Billing patients for any amounts not covered by the insurance carrier
- Performing basic accounting for the practice, including tracking incoming and outgoing cash flow
- Handling collections on overdue accounts
- Greeting patients

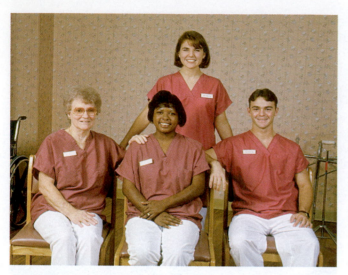

FIGURE 1-2

Members of the medical team

© Michal Heron/Pearson Education

- Answering the office phones
- Scheduling appointments for patients
- Maintaining and updating patient files, filing, and retrieving files when needed
- Ordering general office supplies
- Keeping current on software programs used in the office for billing, correspondence, and accounting

In addition to the job title of Medical Biller, other titles given to individuals who are employed in health care settings as billers include Hospital Biller and Patient Account Manager.

The Medical Team

In any medical office, a number of people work together to provide complete health care to the patient. Although the physician may be the main provider, without the ancillary staff it would be difficult for the office to function. Each member of the team is vital to providing overall patient care (Figure 1-2 ●). In a medical office setting the members of the team typically include the provider; clinical staff, including the medical assistant; and front office staff, including the receptionist, medical biller, and office manager.

Medical assistants not only assist the provider with patient care but also handle some minor procedures themselves. For example, they are often responsible for sterilization of equipment, room preparation, setting up the patient, and administering injections.

The medical biller and receptionist have important duties. The medical biller follows up on unpaid services and negotiates with insurance companies for payment. The receptionist greets the patient, checks the patient in, and then prepares the patient's chart. When the patient is ready to leave, the receptionist can set a new appointment and/or present a bill for services rendered (Figure 1-3 ●).

The office manager supervises the staff and handles the day-to-day operations of the medical office. The office manager may be responsible for scheduling staff, handling payroll, and managing office expenses.

In a hospital setting, the same levels of patient care exist with some minor differences. The doctors usually provide the direction of care by giving verbal or written orders to the nursing staff. The nurses and other medical personnel provide most of the direct patient care. The billing department is often separate from the other departments and handles patient billing and revenue collection. In a hospital setting, there are many departments, administrative offices, and reception areas.

Regardless of the number of departments a medical provider has, each department is a necessary part of the whole operation. Without any one department, the facility could easily cease to exist.

FIGURE 1-3

Medical biller collecting money from a patient for received medical services

© Michal Heron/Pearson Education

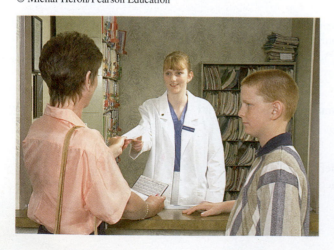

Employment Opportunities for Medical Billers

There are several places medical billers can work, depending on their experience and their preferences. The most common places include those listed here.

Provider's Office

Many individuals who provide health care are called **providers**. These include medical doctors, dentists, optometrists, chiropractors, physical therapists, and so on. A medical biller may work in many areas in a provider's office. In addition to handling the billing, a medical biller may perform all other front office duties, such as greeting clients and handling patient intake, and often will be responsible for scheduling patient appointments and maintaining patient files.

Billing Company

Some medical billers work for independent billing companies. These companies perform billing tasks for small and large health care settings. For medical doctors, billing companies often perform the billing for a number of doctors, each of whom may have only a small practice and no need for a full-time medical biller. If the provider only sees ten or fifteen patients a day, performing the billing for those patients may take only an hour. Having a full-time medical biller would probably not be cost-effective. Other providers that medical billing companies work with include those that don't maintain traditional offices, such as emergency room doctors, anesthesiologists, radiologists, and ambulance companies.

The medical billing company creates the claims and often handles patient accounting. The billers enter any information regarding payments received onto the account and then bill the patient for any balance remaining. Some billing companies have the capacity to transmit information directly to the provider's computer, allowing the provider's office to have current account information on their patients.

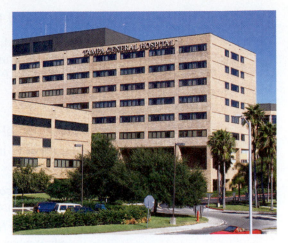

FIGURE 1-4

The hospital setting

Hospital

Hospitals need billers who can make sure that every item the patient uses is accounted for and billed. In a hospital setting (Figure 1-4 ●), billers have little contact with the patients. The only exceptions occur when a patient or family member of a patient comes to the billing office to make a payment, or phones to inquire about an account. Most often, face-to-face contact happens when a portion of the fee is payable before services are rendered.

Health Maintenance Organization

Health Maintenance Organizations (HMOs) are groups that provide services in exchange for premiums. An example of an HMO service is Kaiser Permanente. Kaiser is one of the nation's largest not-for-profit health plans and serves more than 8.6 million members. Unlike traditional insurance companies, HMOs that operate like Kaiser Permanente act as both the insurance carrier and the service provider. However, there are always times when an HMO facility sees a patient who is not one of its members. This usually occurs during a medical emergency when the patient is transferred to the nearest facility. If a patient is treated at an HMO facility but is not a member of that HMO, the HMO facility will bill the patient's insurance carrier for the services provided.

An HMO facility also may have to bill another insurance carrier when a patient with a work-related injury sees his or her regular HMO provider for treatment. Because most workers are covered by workers' compensation insurance, the HMO will bill the workers' compensation carrier for the services.

FIGURE 1-5

A skilled nursing facility

Durable Medical Equipment Provider

Companies that supply durable medical equipment (e.g., a wheelchair) for patient use outside the hospital sometimes have billers on staff, although some companies may rely on patients to file their own insurance claims. However, equipment providers are realizing that it can be a worthwhile marketing tool to file insurance claims for patients.

Other Care Facilities

Other types of facilities also need medical billers on staff. These include nursing homes, convalescent homes, hospices, rehabilitation centers, and any other place that provides medical services.

Individual providers may specialize in any specialty, such as general practice, cardiology, pediatric medicine, and so on. Medical billers are needed and may find employment at all of these facilities (Figure 1-5 ●).

▶ **CRITICAL THINKING QUESTION:** When considering all of the facilities where you might be able to work in the health care field, what area interests you the most and why?

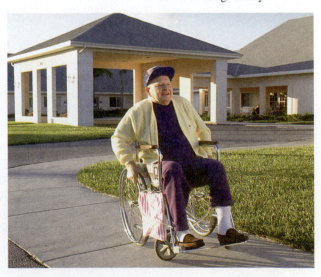

Basic Skill Requirements of the Medical Biller

Successful medical billers have mastered certain basic skills and knowledge, including oral and written communication; basic anatomy and physiology; medical terminology; ICD-9-CM, HCPCS, and CPT coding; math; computers; critical reading and comprehension; and attention to detail.

Interpersonal Skills

The following interpersonal skills will help you get along harmoniously with others in the workplace.

Place the company ahead of yourself. Give your absolute best at work. Establish a reputation that shows people they can rely on you to do good work on time.

Be willing to admit when you are wrong. People want to be able to trust others. If you admit when you are wrong, your honesty and humility about the error will be appreciated and will lead to better relationships.

Speak well of others whenever possible. Remember to praise people for a job well done, both to them and to their superiors.

Show an interest in what others say. Take the time to listen to others. If you cannot spare the time, politely find words to postpone the conversation—for example, "Unfortunately I am under a deadline. What if we discuss this further over lunch?" Be sure to set a time and date for lunch and mark it on the calendar to ensure this will be accomplished.

Give credit where credit is due. If someone else helps you with a project, even in a small way, do not take the credit for his or her work. Be sure that the superiors know who actually did the work. If you try to take credit for work that someone else has done, this will not only hurt the person who did the work but will hurt the organization and your potential for developing trusting relationships.

Compromise. Sometimes you may disagree with a co-worker. In such cases, a compromise can work wonders toward keeping the relationship intact and resolving the conflict. Compromise is not about winning or losing. It is about creating a win–win situation where others don't feel discredited for their opinions.

Provide solutions and take responsibility. If you are asked to help with a project, do your best work. Go the extra mile in finding solutions for a problem, then allow the responsible person to turn in the project and take the deserved credit. If that individual takes credit for your work, do not contest it since you may not know that they gave you credit at another time. If you start insisting that you helped, you will appear to lack confidence in others and yourself.

Introduce yourself to new people. The office environment will often change quickly. Taking the time to learn the names of those you work with lets them know that they are important to you. Take the time to accomplish this by walking around and interacting with your staff.

Build networks. If a task is new or very advanced, be willing to defer the work to someone more experienced than you. Also be willing to explore new tasks. The more knowledgeable you are about your workplace and the more you can multitask or cross-cover, the more valuable you become to your employer. Talk to people during lunch hours or break times about matters that are not work related. Get to know your colleagues a little better, and let them get to know you.

Smile and be positive. Positive people are more pleasant to be around. No one wants to spend time with someone who brings out the worst in everyone. Maintain a positive attitude. If you are positive, it makes other people positive as well.

Try to keep your personal problems to yourself. Constantly discussing personal problems at work can make others feel uncomfortable and will often strain your relationships, as others may be reluctant to engage in conversation with you.

Avoid gossiping. If someone passes information on to you, do not share it with others unless you are specifically asked to do so.

Actions to Avoid

You should avoid several actions on the job. These include:

- Having loud phone conversations.
- Neglecting to say please and thank you.
- Talking behind someone's back.
- Asking someone else to tell a lie or to be dishonest.
- Asking someone, especially a subordinate, to do an errand that is not work related.
- Telling offensive jokes or making sexist or politically incorrect comments.
- Complaining about another person.
- Being condescending toward others.
- Spending personal time on the Internet.

ACTIVITY #1

Rating Your Interpersonal Skills

Directions: Rate yourself on each of the qualities listed below, and then answer the following questions.

1 = Never, 2 = Almost Never, 3 = Sometimes, 4 = Almost Always, 5 = Always

Do you:

Embrace innovation?	1	2	3	4	5
Take the initiative?	1	2	3	4	5
Consider all aspects that you are responsible for?	1	2	3	4	5
Strive for *knowledge* recognition rather than *social* recognition?	1	2	3	4	5
Take pride in the quality of your work?	1	2	3	4	5
Like to learn new skills?	1	2	3	4	5
Align yourself with powerful people?	1	2	3	4	5
Have high morale?	1	2	3	4	5

Are you:

Willing to learn and do someone else's job?	1	2	3	4	5
Logical, not emotional?	1	2	3	4	5
Self-confident?	1	2	3	4	5
Willing to take on more than your responsibilities?	1	2	3	4	5

1. For which assets did you circle a 5? _____

_____

2. For which assets did you circle a 4? _____

_____

3. For which assets did you circle a 1, 2, or 3? _____

_____

4. What can you do to improve each of those assets for which you ranked yourself 1, 2, or 3?

_____

_____

_____

Stress

Job stress is defined as the harmful physical and emotional responses that occur when the requirements of the job do not match the capabilities, resources, or needs of the worker. Often people will say, "A little bit of stress is good for you." However, this often depends on your definition of stress, as well as on how much is "a little bit." What people often mean is that a challenge can be good for you.

Challenges energize us psychologically and physically and help motivate us to learn new skills. When challenges are met, we feel relaxed and satisfied. Thus, challenge can be an important ingredient for healthy and productive work.

Although challenges can be good for us, stress is not. Stress causes negative physiological reactions, such as an increase in adrenaline and heart rate, without the physical ability to expend and use the adrenaline.

Symptoms of Stress

Stress can cause a variety of symptoms that can inhibit your ability to function properly, both at work and in your daily life. The following are the most common symptoms of stress:

- Headaches
- Anxiety
- High blood pressure
- Trouble falling asleep or other sleep disturbances
- Difficulty concentrating
- Short temper
- Upset stomach
- Job dissatisfaction
- Low morale
- Hyperventilation
- Clenching or grinding of the teeth

Pent-up stress also can cause emotional outbursts, ranging from intense anger to tears and self-pity. Chronic stress can cause problems in relationships, heart problems, and may weaken the immune system.

Handling Stress

Although stress is a part of everyday life, it is important to deal with stress appropriately so it does not accumulate and become overwhelming. Handling stress is an important part of being able to function in the working world.

Quick stress relievers include the following:

- Exercising vigorously
- Getting a massage
- Breathing deeply and slowly
- Getting more sleep
- Skipping extra caffeine in items such as coffee, cola, and chocolate
- Eating properly and regularly

FIGURE 1-6

Laughing together can be a great stress reliever.

© Michal Heron/Pearson Education

Other means of accomplishing a stress-free state may take a bit longer but can be more effective. These include the following:

Finding the humor in life. Learn to laugh at the mistakes you make and things that go wrong. Laughter is a great stress reliever (Figure 1-6 ●).

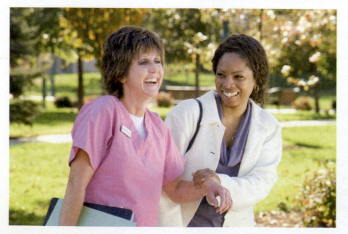

Creating a new attitude. Try to see each problem as a challenge. Think of it as a chance for you to go up against an imaginary adversary and come out victorious by conquering the problem. By changing your attitude toward problems, you can create an aura of excitement, thus giving yourself the energy to tackle and handle problems.

Giving yourself opportunities to relax. You should spend at least half an hour every day doing something that helps to relax your body and mind. This can be reading a book, exercising, socializing with friends, or anything else that helps you work off stress and relax. Remember, these should be activities that give you pleasure, not those that give you stress of a different nature.

Creating a stress barrier. Do not bring your family or life problems to work, and do not take your work problems home with you. Establishing a routine that provides a break between the two environments can help. Some people create this barrier by having a long commute home; others will take a few minutes after arriving home to relax before tackling home activities; and others will stop off on the way home to do something else. These types of habits can help you keep the troubles of work and home from interfering with each other.

Making a "To Do" list. We often get overwhelmed thinking of all the things we need to accomplish, and sometimes everything we think of leads to something else. There is only so much that one can accomplish in a day. To accomplish as much as possible, prioritizing tasks and breaking them down into smaller pieces can be helpful. It is important to celebrate when tasks are successfully completed.

Also remember to do one thing at a time. Multitasking does not mean doing everything at once. Performing the items on your list one at a time allows you to concentrate on each item and be more productive, which gives you the opportunity to complete them more efficiently.

Asking others not to disturb you. If you have a time-sensitive project or a fast-approaching deadline, ask to not be disturbed. Hang a sign on your desk with the words "Please Do Not Disturb, Important Deadline Looming." In some companies, notifying others that you do not want to be disturbed can be easily accomplished by closing your door.

Ask the receptionist to hold your calls, or, if you have voice mail, switch to a greeting that informs people that you are working on a very important project. Include in your message when you will be available, and ask callers to leave a message or call you back later.

Other people are busy, too, and they understand the need to buckle down and focus on a project. Most people are more than willing to respect your request.

ACTIVITY #2

Online Research: The Impact of Stress

Directions: Conduct online research regarding the impact of stress and how stress can be managed. Put together a short presentation on the information that you discovered in your research. Be prepared to discuss your findings with your classmates.

Pre-Vacation Work Planning

Taking a vacation can be great for you but stressful for your co-workers. Taking a vacation means the rest of the staff is left with one less person to do the work.

Although many people think only of themselves when planning a vacation, good medical billers also think of their organization. Following are some guidelines to use when planning a vacation.

Take your vacation during the company's slow period. Nearly all companies have one or two seasons that are busier than others. Schedule your vacation around these times so that you are there when you are most needed. Co-workers, and especially your bosses, will appreciate your thoughtfulness. Some people may think that scheduling a vacation during the busy time will reveal how valuable they are. Unfortunately, this will give the negative impression that the individual is only thinking of himself and not of the company and will outweigh any thoughts of how important the person's skills are.

Before leaving, be sure that your desk is in order. All paperwork and folders should be filed appropriately. This allows anyone who needs something to find it while you are away. All work with a due date before your vacation should be completed and turned in. Sometimes, this means working through lunch or working harder to make sure everything is accomplished. Others can get a negative impression of you if you leave without completing assignments or without properly filing items so others can find them. If important tasks are pending and must be dealt with during your absence, be sure to leave detailed notes with your supervisor or the person covering your desk.

Let others know two weeks in advance that you are leaving. This gives your supervisors and others enough advance notice for any projects that need your input for completion.

Leave a contact number with a trusted co-worker for emergencies. Providing a number where you can be reached in case of emergency shows those in your office that you care. A brief comment, such as "So-and-so knows how to reach me if it is an emergency," should be enough to let people know how you can be contacted.

Enjoy your vacation. Ignore what is happening at work. Give your mind and body a break. This will allow you to come back and face work with a fresh outlook because you will be more rested, refreshed, and ready to take on new challenges.

Certification Programs for Medical Billers

Currently, no state or federal certification or licensing is required for medical billers. However, more and more employers are requesting or requiring certification of their medical billing and coding applicants. In addition, certification offers increased job security, income, prestige, advancement, recognition, and professional affiliation.

There are several different certification programs:

American Academy of Professional Coders (AAPC)

2840 South 3850 West, Suite B

Salt Lake City, UT 84120

Phone: 800-626-2633

Website: www.aapc.com

Certifications offered include Certified Professional Coder (CPC), Certified Professional Coder–Hospital Outpatient, and Certified Professional Coder–Payer (CPC-P)

American Health Information Management Association (AHIMA)

100 Sycamore Avenue, Suite M

Modesto, CA 95354

Phone: 800-335-5535

Website: www.ahima.org

Certifications offered: Certified Coding Associate (CCA), Certified Coding Specialist (CCS), or Certified Coding Specialist-Physician (CCS-P)

Professional Association of Health Care Office Management (PAHCOM)

1576 Bella Cruz Drive, Suite 360

Lady Lake, FL 32159

Phone: 800-451-9311

Website: www.pahcom.com

Certification offered: Certified Medical Manager (CMM)

Organizations that provide useful information for medical billers include the following:

Alliance of Claims Assistance Professionals (ACAP) – **www.claims.org; askacap@charter.net**

American Health Information Management Association (AHIMA) – **www.ahima.org**

American Medical Billing Association (AMBA) – **www.ambanet.net/AMBA.htm**

Health Professions Institute (HPI) – **www.hpisum.com**

Medical Association of Billers – **www.physicianswebsites.com**

Medical Coding and Billing – **www.medicalcodingandbilling.com**

National Center for Competency Testing – **www.ncctinc.com**

National Electronic Billers Alliance (NEBA) – **www.nebazone.com/part1.html**

CHAPTER REVIEW

Summary

- Some of the job responsibilities of the medical biller include billing insurance carriers, billing patients, performing basic office accounting, handling collections, scheduling appointments, and handling charts.
- Some of the basic skills and knowledge required of a medical biller include oral and written communication skills; knowledge of anatomy and physiology, medical terminology, and basic math; computer skills; reading and comprehension skills; and excellent organizational skills.
- Interpersonal skills are vital in dealing with co-workers.
- Although stress is part of everyday life, it is important to deal with stress appropriately.

Review Questions

Directions: Answer the following questions without looking back at the material covered in this chapter. Write your answers in the space provided.

1. List three job responsibilities of the medical biller.

   _____

   _____

2. List six symptoms of stress.

   _____

   _____

   _____

   _____

   _____

   _____

3. List five stress relievers.

   _____

   _____

   _____

   _____

   _____

4. List six types of health care settings.

   _____

   _____

   _____

   _____

   _____

   _____

5. (True or False?) Do not compromise when you have a disagreement with a co-worker, as it only proves that you are wrong and makes you look bad. _____

6. List the four things to consider before taking a vacation.

_____

_____

7. (True or False?) An HMO facility may have to bill another insurance carrier when a patient with a work-related injury sees his regular HMO provider for treatment. _____

8. List six actions that should be avoided on the job.

_____

_____

_____

_____

_____

_____

9. What are other job titles for the medical biller?

_____

_____

10. Explain the difference between traditional insurance and HMOs.

_____

_____

_____

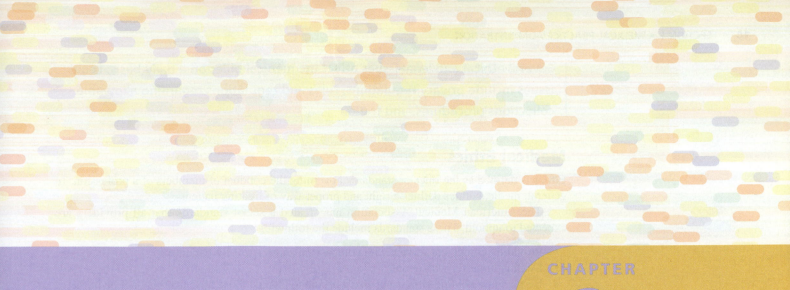

Ethical and Legal Issues of Medical Billing

After completion of this chapter you should be able to:

Discuss the two main issues covered by HIPAA exceptions to the HIPAA privacy guidelines.

Explain what disclaimers are and how to use them appropriately.

List and describe the instances in which the patient should be notified and the patient chart notated.

Describe the most common causes of fraud.

Key Words and Concepts you will learn in this chapter:

Abuse

Audits

Bonding

Claims audit

Embezzlement

Errors and omissions insurance

External audit

External auditor

Fraud

Health Insurance Portability and Accountability Act (HIPAA)

Internal audit

Legal damages

Medicare abuse

Medicare fraud

Respondeat superior

Subpoena

Subpoena duces tecum

Several ethical and legal issues affect the medical biller on a daily basis. Legal issues include privacy regulations, rules and regulations regarding allowable collections procedures, and fraud.

Medical Ethics

Ethics is defined as the rules or standards governing the conduct of members of a profession. In general, medical ethics defines a right and proper way of treating patients.

The American Medical Association has created a set of standards that all providers are expected to uphold. These standards include the following:

- Providing competent service with compassion and respect for patients
- Dealing honestly with people
- Being a law-abiding citizen but also working to change those laws that may not be in the best interest of the patient
- Respecting the rights of others
- Continuing to study and upgrade skills with the latest in medical advancement
- Providing emergency medical treatment to anyone who is in need
- Working to improve the community

Although the medical biller has not sworn an oath to uphold these principles, he or she should realize that the provider for whom he or she works upholds this oath. As an adjunct to the provider, the medical biller also should do his or her best to uphold these standards and to assist the provider in doing so.

Among other things, ethics guidelines include the following:

1. Not making critical remarks about your provider, another provider, or any treatment given or not given.
2. If you discover that a patient is being treated by more than one provider for the same ailment, notify your provider immediately. It is not only unethical for two providers to treat a patient for the same condition, but it also can be dangerous. Prescription overdose or complications between treatment plans could result if one provider is unaware of treatment given by another provider.
3. Respecting the dignity of others. This includes calling patients and co-workers by their appropriate title and last name (e.g., Dr. Smith, Mrs. Hall); not using slang terms in reference to someone (e.g., honey, dear, sweetie); making no references to race, religion, creed, color, sex, or ethnic origin unless it is medically necessary for the treatment of the patient; and refraining from touching a patient or co-worker unless it is medically necessary.
4. Refusing to participate in illegal or unethical acts, or concealing the illegal or unethical acts of others.

▶ **CRITICAL THINKING QUESTION:** As a health care professional, what ethical standards do you think you should be held to?

FIGURE 2-1

The physician and clinical staff member discussing a patient's information in a closed office setting

© Pat Watson

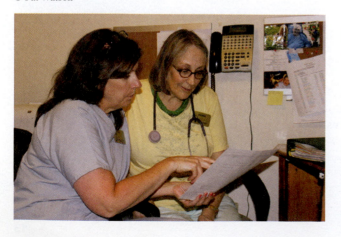

Legal Issues Related to Privacy

The very nature of health care requires a great deal of personal information to be gathered and maintained about many individuals. Therefore, the needs of the company must be carefully weighed against the person's right to privacy so as to avoid unwarranted invasions of that right.

In particular, medical information is considered to be privileged and confidential in the context of the provider/patient relationship. Unauthorized disclosure of information may represent a violation of that confidentiality (Figure 2-1 ●).

The confidentiality of medical records has assumed a new importance for several reasons:

1. People are becoming more litigation minded.
2. Health plans reimburse for more sensitive services that were excluded in the past, such as alcohol detoxification, mental health treatment, and AIDS-related illnesses.
3. More employers are self-administering or self-funding their health plan, which means highly personal medical information is, in some instances, routinely handled by fellow employees.
4. New HIPAA regulations require that all personnel involved in the health care process respect the patient's right to privacy and confidentiality.

HIPAA

In 1996, the **Health Insurance Portability and Accountability Act (HIPAA)** was signed into law to set a national standard for electronic transfer of health data. The portability issues refer to persons being covered by insurance when they transfer from one job to another. These issues are most important to the health claims examiner. However, the privacy issues and the health insurance fraud and abuse issues are vitally important for the medical biller to understand.

HIPAA encompasses the following:

1. Portability, or the ability to transfer insurance coverage, and still be covered for preexisting conditions; and
2. Accountability, generally dealing with the patient's right to privacy from the health care provider, health insurer, and any other parties required in the health care process (e.g., billers, clearinghouses, etc.), and the lack of fraud and abuse when dealing with health care (Figure 2-2 ●).

Regarding the Privacy section of HIPAA, the Department of Health and Human Services states the following:

> The privacy requirements limit the release of patient Protected Health Information (PHI) without the patient's knowledge and consent beyond that required for patient care. Personal information of patients must be more securely guarded and more carefully handled when conducting the business of health care.

Most health care entities were required to meet the standards set in the privacy issues section of HIPAA on April 14, 2003. HIPAA calls for severe civil and criminal penalties for noncompliance, including fines up to $25,000 for multiple violations of the same standard in a calendar year; and fines up to $250,000 or imprisonment up to ten years for knowledge of misuse of individually identifiable health information.

● **ONLINE INFORMATION:** For a summary of the HIPAA privacy rule visit www.hhs.gov/ocr/privacy/hipaa/understanding/summary/privacysummary.pdf

▶ **CRITICAL THINKING QUESTION:** As a medical biller, how can you help to ensure patient privacy?

General Rules to Ensure Privacy

There are several general rules for ensuring that privacy guidelines are met:

1. Always obtain an authorization for release of medical information before releasing any information. Most releases routinely signed in the medical practice only authorize the provider to release information necessary to process a patient's claim. Additional authorization should be obtained to release any information to other parties. These releases should state exactly what information is to be released, the dates of any services provided that fall within the release, the person to whom the information may be released, the signature of the patient, the date of the signature, and the date the release expires.
2. Gather only the information that is necessary and relevant for billing or processing the claim.
3. Use only legal and ethical means to collect the information required. Whenever permission is necessary, obtain written authorization from the insured or patient (guardian or parent if the patient is a minor).

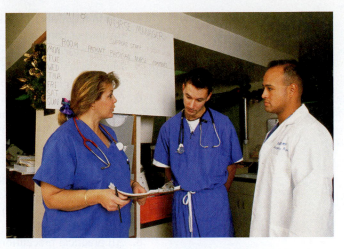

FIGURE 2-2

Every discussion within patient hearing range must be professional in nature.

© Michael Newman/PhotoEdit Inc.

4. When requested, and subject to any applicable legal or ethical prohibition or privilege, the insured or patient concerned should be advised of the nature and general uses to be made of the information.

5. Make every reasonable effort to ensure that the information on which an action is based is accurate, relevant, timely, and complete.

6. On request, the patient or insured should be given the opportunity to correct or clarify the information given by or about him or her, and the file should be amended to the extent that it is fair to both the provider and the patient or insured. Requests for review or clarification of medical information are accepted only from the person from whom the information was obtained.

7. In general, disclosures of information to a third party (other than those described to the insured or patient) should be made only with the written authorization of the patient or insured. This includes disclosure to employers, family members, or former spouses.

8. All practical precautions should be taken to ensure that medical files are physically secure and that access to the use of these files is limited to authorized personnel. This includes not leaving files out, locking up all files, and even turning your computer screen away from where it might be seen by other persons. Security passwords and other security measures also may be required, depending on your office situation.

9. All personnel involved in keeping the medical records should be advised of the need to protect the right of privacy in obtaining required information and the need to treat all individually identifiable information as confidential. Willful abuse of the privacy of any insured or patient by an employee may be cause for dismissal.

10. The disclosure of a diagnosis should never be made to a patient or his or her family. If the patient requests this information, refer the patient to the provider. It is not the place of the biller or coder to tell the patient about the medical information.

11. Unless otherwise instructed, never release any information to an ex-spouse. This includes the patient's address, phone number, when services were rendered and to whom, and other information. The ex-spouse should be instructed to contact the patient directly.

12. Do not leave files, patients' records, or appointment books open on a desk or in an area where they may be seen by others. This includes patients' files or information that may be displayed on a computer screen. The best way to handle this is to be sure that all files are closed or are face down on your desk. Computer screens must be placed in such a way that they cannot be seen by anyone passing by. If necessary, use a screen saver or other unrestricted document that can be clicked on to instantaneously replace the one you are working on.

13. When addressing a patient in the waiting room, use as little information as possible to gain the attention of the patient. Never use full names. For example, you might address the patient as Bob L., or better yet a first name only. If there is more than one patient in the waiting room with the name Bob, you might address the patient as B. Smith, Mrs. Smith, etc. Actually, the more cryptic, the better for maintaining confidentiality.

14. If a minor patient has the legal right to authorize treatment for services, disclosure to the parents, legal guardians of the minor, or to other persons may be a violation of HIPAA or the confidentiality of the Medical Information Privacy and Security Act (MIPSA).

If in doubt as to whether specific information should be released, check with your supervisor before, not after, releasing it.

These guidelines cover some of the basic aspects of HIPAA privacy regulations. For detailed information regarding HIPAA guidelines, complete rules and regulations regarding HIPAA are printed in the *Federal Register*. The *Federal Register* is the daily newspaper of the federal government. For those who are concerned with government actions that affect topics such as health care, financial services, and education, the *Federal Register* is a good source. The *Federal Register* is available in paper, on microfiche, and on the World Wide Web at www.gpoaccess.gov/fr.

Maintaining Confidentiality When Faxing

When faxing items, be aware of sensitive information. All faxes should contain a cover sheet that announces to whom the fax is addressed, who sent it, and that the enclosed information is personal and confidential. Information regarding diagnosis, treatments, sexually transmitted diseases, HIV,

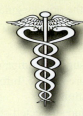

Anne Wager, MD

Quan Lee, MD
8282 Arlington Way
Arlington, WA 12345
360-555-4545

Facsimile transmittal

To: _____   Fax number: _____

From: _____   Date: _____

Re: _____   No. of pages, including cover sheet: _____

___ Urgent   ___ For Review   ___ Please Comment   ___ Please Reply

Comments:

CONFIDENTIAL INFORMATION
The information in this facsimile message and any accompanying documents is confidential. This information is intended for use only by the
individual or entity named above. If you are not the intended recipient of
this information, you are hereby notified that any disclosure, copying, or
distribution of this information is strictly prohibited. Please notify the
sender immediately by telephone. Thank you.

FIGURE 2-3

Sample of HIPAA compliant fax cover sheet

drug or alcohol abuse, or financial information should never be faxed. Figure 2-3 ● provides an example of a HIPAA-compliant fax cover sheet.

When faxing other information, consider asking the receiving party for a code number (e.g., the patient's ID number or birth date), then black out all pertinent information about the patient and replace it with the code number. Although faxing information is necessary in certain circumstances, such as an emergency or if a patient is scheduled for an unexpected procedure on the same day, when possible avoid faxing information and use regular or certified mail. If faxing, it is always a good practice to call first and have someone waiting for the fax. When verifying that someone will be waiting, you can verify the fax number to ensure that the information is going to the correct place.

Most important, the biller when faxing must follow the rules of HIPAA along with the processes in place in the office.

Exceptions to Privacy Laws

There are a few exceptions to the privacy laws. In the following instances, the privacy guidelines may be considered less stringent, or the patient may be deemed to have waived his or her rights to confidentiality:

1. Less stringent guidelines apply for providers who are employed by insurance companies. Disclosure to their employers of patient records and information is more routine. Information that is shared among co-workers must remain within the organization.
2. Cases of gunshot wounds, stabbings resulting from criminal actions, and suspected child abuse that must be reported to the local police department or child care agency. Some states also require reporting of incidents of spousal abuse.
3. Reports of communicable diseases and some diseases and illnesses of infants and newborns. These are most often used for compiling statistics and attempting to stop the spread of communicable diseases.
4. Information obtained by the Medicare insurance carrier that pertains to a patient may be reported directly to that patient's beneficiary or his representative. The Medicare insurance specialist cannot accept or withhold information received regarding a patient, even if the information is marked "Confidential."
5. If a patient is seen at the request of a third party who is covering the bill (e.g., workers' compensation cases), limited confidentiality is waived and the information may be provided to the person or company ordering the procedures.
6. If records are subpoenaed or a search warrant is issued, records may be turned over to the court or its representatives.

Fraud and Abuse

When providers are inconsistent in conducting sound medical or business practices, **abuse** may be occurring. A common example of abuse is when a payment for items or services is obtained when there is no legal entitlement to that payment and the provider unintentionally (or without knowledge) misrepresents the facts to obtain payment.

Fraud is defined as intentional misrepresentation of a fact with the intent to deprive a person of property or legal rights. Intentional means the individual has knowledge that the misrepresentation is occurring. The most common instance of fraud occurring in the health claims industry is doctors or other service providers billing for goods or services that were not actually provided.

Because of the high incidence of fraud and abuse, all billed services must be documented in the medical record to prove that they were actually provided. The law of documentation states that "If it was not documented, it did not happen." Billing for services not provided is a serious offense and constitutes fraud. If a person is convicted, the penalties are extremely stiff. In addition, both the provider and the medical biller can be held liable for the filing of fraudulent claims.

The most common cases of fraud include the following:

1. Overbilling or billing for services not rendered
2. Altering records or claims to upgrade the service presented (e.g., billing for a high-complexity office visit when the services provided were for a low-complexity visit)
3. Changing dates on services or splitting procedures (e.g., placing different dates on services that were actually performed on the same date, changing the date to make it appear as if treatment were rendered after the surgery follow-up days, rather than during the follow-up days)
4. Unbundling of charges (e.g., listing lab charges as though a number of separate tests were done when several tests were done simultaneously from the same sample)
5. Allowing a patient to use the medical coverage card of another patient, or billing services under an incorrect patient name (e.g., Sally Smith, age twenty-three, not covered under her parents' insurance, is billed as Sandy Smith, her sixteen-year-old sister, who is covered)
6. Allowing, offering, soliciting, or accepting a kickback or return of monies for a referral or for use of a specific product
7. Altering the diagnosis to substantiate procedures performed
8. Billing twice for the same services

9. Billing group services as if they were individual services (e.g., a psychiatrist has several patients in a group session but bills as if each patient was seen individually)
10. Ordering or billing for services that were performed but were not medically necessary
11. Accepting payment in full from insurance carriers (Such practice is considered fraudulent, especially with Medicare, because the insurance is actually paying 100 percent of the services, not the 80 percent or other coinsurance percentage that the insurance carrier contracted with the patient to pay. Such a practice often leads providers to increase their bills to make up the difference and can lead to patients overutilizing services as there is no financial incentive to limit visits. If occasional cases are written off because of hardship, this should be documented in the records, along with an explanation of the hardship circumstances and the reason for dismissal of the debt.)
12. Billing different patients at different rates (e.g., one charge for Medicare patients and a different charge for uninsured patients for the same services)
13. Requiring patients to pay balances in excess of Medicare, Medicaid, or HMO limits (Exceptions would be nonparticipating and/or non-filing providers.)
14. Requiring Medicare patients to pay for services that should be covered by Medicare, thus not being limited by the Medicare-approved amount
15. Failing to refund copayments and deductible charges for Medicare patients whose charges have been deemed by Medicare to be not medically necessary
16. Submitting claims to two or more insurers without disclosing that more than one insurance may cover the charges
17. Billing Medicare or other insurance carriers when bills should be submitted to a third party (e.g., workers' compensation coverage, a third party that may be liable in the case of an accident)

If the provider is engaging in such practices and it can be shown that the biller participated, or even if the provider merely knew about the fraudulent acts and did nothing, the medical biller can be charged as an accomplice, even if he or she personally received no money. As a precautionary measure, having billers initial the claims they create or submit for payment can help to track down the guilty party.

Because a provider is considered ultimately responsible for everything that goes on in his or her practice, the provider may be considered guilty of fraud even if he or she had no knowledge of the crime. The provider may be criminally sentenced or may merely have to reimburse the insurance carrier for all fraudulently submitted claims.

If a person, either a provider or a biller, is found guilty of Medicare or Medicaid fraud, the individual is excluded from ever again participating in the program.

Medicare Fraud and Abuse

It is important to understand the rules and regulations regarding Medicare reimbursement. Penalties are assessed for not complying with these rules. For minor violations, if the provider accepts assignment, the claim may be returned for correction of the problem and may be subject to postpayment review by Medicare. If the provider does not accept Medicare assignment, the provider may be subject to a penalty per claim. Unintentional errors or mistakes that anyone is likely to make do not constitute a charge of fraud. Other violations, or repeated violations, can subject the provider to audits, stiff fines, dismissal from the Medicare program, and—in some cases—criminal penalties and jail sentences.

MEDICARE FRAUD. **Medicare fraud** is the intentional misrepresentation of information that could result in an unauthorized benefit. The regulations are very specific about the activities that are allowed and not allowed under the Medicare rules and regulations. Examples of fraudulent practices include the following:

- Billing for services or supplies not rendered, including billing patients for not showing up to an appointment (because the patient never showed, and no services were actually rendered)
- Altering the diagnosis to justify services
- Altering claim forms to misrepresent or falsify data
- Duplicate billing
- Billing both Medicare and an additional insurance as the primary payer

- Soliciting, offering, or receiving a bribe, kickback, rebate, or finder's fee for any services (This includes fees offered for referring a patient to a specific facility for additional tests or services. It also includes automatically writing off that portion of the bill that is the patient's responsibility, as this is considered a kickback or bribe to induce the patient to obtain services from one provider over another.)
- Unbundling or exploding charges, or billing for multiple services when one procedure code adequately describes the services provided (Many Medicare carriers provide a list of codes that are often unbundled. The computer is set up to look for these codes and automatically pays only the major procedure, denying the additional procedures.)
- Providers who complete certificates of medical necessity or write prescriptions for patients they have not actually seen
- Altering amounts charged for services, dates of services, identity of patients, or misrepresenting the services provided to obtain reimbursement (This includes upcoding of services, e.g., billing for a level IV visit when a level II visit was performed.)
- Altering the code or description of noncovered services to identify them as covered services
- Any collusion between the provider and an additional party (e.g., patient, lawyer, etc.) to misrepresent charges or services to obtain reimbursement
- Altering claims history or medical records to substantiate services that were upcoded or misrepresented
- Using or allowing the use of an incorrect or additional person's Medicare card to obtain coverage for services
- Billing inappropriately for "gang visits" (e.g., heading a group psychotherapy session but billing for each patient as if each had an individual visit)
- Not disclosing or providing false data regarding physician ownership of a clinical laboratory, medical supplier, or other related entity (Physicians are not allowed to refer patients to a lab or medical supplier in which they have a financial interest.)
- Split billing, or billing supplies and services as if they were provided over a series of dates rather than during a single visit
- Collusion with an employee of the insurance carrier to generate false payments
- Repeated violations of Medicare regulations when warning and instruction have been provided

MEDICARE ABUSE. Unlike Medicare fraud, **Medicare abuse** does not require the proof of intent to defraud the Medicare system in order to be assessed. Many times, abuse can appear to be similar to fraud, except that it is not possible to establish that abusive acts were committed knowingly, willfully, and intentionally. Abuse includes any item or procedure that is inconsistent with accepted norms or practices:

- Excessive charges for procedures or supplies, or billing over the limiting charge
- Billing for services that are considered not medically necessary (This includes ordering more tests than necessary for diagnosis or ordering services that are of no great benefit to the patient)
- Billing at different rates for Medicare and for other insurance, unless a lower amount is charged to Medicare in order to comply with fee schedules or limiting charges (There are some exceptions to this rule regarding service fees set by a contractual agreement with a Health Maintenance Organization. This violation includes accepting another insurance carrier's payment as payment in full for services, thus waiving coinsurance amounts. Such a practice results in charging non-Medicare patients 20 percent less than Medicare patients.)
- Improperly billing Medicare when another carrier should be billed, or billing Medicare first when it should be the secondary payer
- Violation of any of the provisions of the Medicare participation agreement
- Unintentional unbundling or upcoding of procedures, or violations of rules

Medicare may accept "I didn't know" as an excuse for a single violation of any of the Medicare rules and regulations. However, repeated abuses, especially after a provider has been warned, will result in the upgrading of a violation from an abuse to intentional fraud.

If the Medicare carrier identifies overpayments or abuses, the carrier may contact the provider and request documentation to substantiate the claims or will simply send a request for repayment of an overpaid amount. Do not ignore letters requesting a refund of overpayment. If the provider disagrees with the request, you should file additional documentation to substantiate the services and request a review. If the provider agrees that there was an overpayment, the Medicare carrier should be reimbursed as soon as possible. Any fines levied by the carrier must also be paid. Because a downgrading of the service provided may result in a lower allowed amount, often reimbursement also must be made to the patient for excessive payment of coinsurance amounts.

Medicare often will audit claims using a peer review panel. This panel is a group of physicians who review documentation regarding the services provided. If they find medical or documentation errors, points will be counted against the provider. When a provider receives a certain number of points, he or she may be subject to forfeiture of his or her license. Because of this, it is important that proper care is rendered and that all evidence supporting the care and the justification of services is fully documented.

Sanctions and Penalties

Different levels of penalties and sanctions have been included in the Medicare provisions. The most common sanctions include the following:

1. *Educational contact or warning.* If Medicare determines that you are improperly billing, you may be contacted and instructed in the proper procedures and necessary steps to rectify the situation. Such a contact may or may not include a formal warning, which is placed in the provider's file.
2. *Recoupment of overpayments.* A letter may be sent requesting repayment of any amounts Medicare determines have been overpaid. If payment is not received (and no review is requested), the carrier may withhold future payments to recoup the losses.
3. *Fines.* Many penalties include the assessment of fines for failure to follow regulations. Fines can vary per incident. Penalties of up to twice the overpayment amount also may be levied. Additional fines may be levied for not repaying overpayments in a timely manner.
4. *Criminal prosecution.* Providers or billers may be criminally prosecuted for fraudulent actions against the Medicare system. Penalties include conviction of a misdemeanor or felony and may include additional fines and even jail time.
5. *Suspension or dismissal from the Medicare program.* Repeated or severe abuses can cause a provider (or a biller) to be excluded from the Medicare program. This sanction may be imposed for a limited time (suspension, often for up to five years) or permanently (dismissal from the Medicare program). In such a case, announcements are made to all patients and in the press that the provider is no longer allowed to accept Medicare patients. If a patient submits a claim after the provider has been dismissed, he or she will be informed that the provider is not allowed to provide Medicare services and that no coverage exists. A provider who is excluded from participating in the Medicare program may also be excluded from participating in Medicaid; the Early Periodic Screening, Diagnosis, and Testing (EPSDT) program; and the Social Services Block Grant (SSBG) program.
6. *Referral to licensing agencies and professional societies.* Extremely severe cases, especially those involving fraud, mismanagement of patient care, improper or unprofessional conduct, or unethical practices, may be referred to a state licensing agency or a professional society for possible revocation of licensure.

If the Medicare carrier determines that a penalty or sanction has not solved the problem, it may proceed to the next level. Because providers are responsible for what happens in their offices, they will be held responsible for abuses and fraudulent actions committed by their employees or contracted independent billing services.

HIPAA and Fraud and Abuse

The new HIPAA fraud statutes have greatly broadened the scope of the federal government for prosecuting fraud and abuse in the health care industry. HIPAA defines four new criminal health care fraud offenses: Health Care Fraud, Theft or Embezzlement in Connection with Health Care, False Statements Relating to Health Care Matters, and Obstruction of Criminal Investigations of Health Care Offenses.

HIPAA now defines a health care benefit program as "any public or private plan or contract, affecting commerce, under which any medical benefit, item, or service is provided to any individual, and includes any individual or entity who is providing a medical benefit, item, or service for which payment may be made under the plan or contract." By including private health benefit plans and any individual or entity, the U.S. Department of Health & Human Services has effectively given itself the right to prosecute anyone involved in the health care industry for fraud or abuse.

The following four sections further define the HIPAA statutes.

Health care fraud (18 USC 1347): Whoever knowingly and willfully executes, or attempts to execute, a scheme or artifact—

1. to defraud any health care benefit program; or
2. to obtain, by means of false or fraudulent pretenses, representations, or promises, any of the money or property owned by, or under the custody or control of, any health care benefit program, in connection with the delivery of or payment for health care benefits, items, or services, shall be fined under this title or imprisoned not more than 10 years, or both. If the violation results in serious bodily injury (as defined in section 1365 of the title), such person shall be fined under this title or imprisoned not more than 20 years, or both; and if the violation results in death, such person shall be fined under this title, or imprisoned for any term of years or for life, or both.

The medical biller needs to keep in mind that if he creates or submits a health claim which he knows to be fraudulent he may be held liable under this portion of the statute.

Theft or embezzlement in connection with health care (18 USC 669):

1. Whoever knowingly and willfully embezzles, steals, or otherwise without authority converts to the use of any person other than the rightful owner, or intentionally misapplies any of the moneys, funds, securities, premiums, credits, property, or other assets of a health care benefit program, shall be fined under this title or imprisoned not more than 10 years, or both; but if the value of such property does not exceed the sum of $100 the defendant shall be fined under this title or imprisoned not more than one year, or both.
2. As used in this section, the term "health care benefit program" has the meaning given such term in section 24 (b) of this title.

Any medical biller that does any of the following: accepts payment on claims which the individual knows to be fraudulent; applies medical payments to the wrong account; takes home office supplies, equipment or other items with the intent to keep; and drafts unauthorized checks to himself or others, may be held liable under this portion of the statute.

False statements relating to health care matters (18 USC 1035):

1. Whoever, in any matter involving a health care benefit program, knowingly and willfully—

a. falsifies, conceals, or covers up by any trick, scheme, or device a material fact; or

b. makes any materially false, fictitious, or fraudulent statements or representations, or makes or uses any materially false writing or document knowing the same to contain any materially false, fictitious, or fraudulent statement or entry, in connection with the delivery of or payment for health care benefits, items, or services, shall be fined under this title or imprisoned not more than five years, or both.

2. As used in this section, the term "health care benefit program" has the meaning given such term in section 24 (b) of this title.

A medical biller who creates false claims and/or claim documents, alters and/or falsifies claim information, lies about claims situations, or does not come forward to disclose fraudulent situations that the person is aware of, may be held liable under this portion of the statute.

Obstruction of criminal investigations of health care offenses (18 USC 1518):

1. Whoever willfully prevents, obstructs, misleads, delays or attempts to prevent, obstruct, mislead, or delay the communication of information or records relating to

a violation of a Federal health care offense to a criminal investigator shall be fined under this title or imprisoned not more than 5 years, or both.

2. As used in this section the term "criminal investigator" means any individual duly authorized by a department, agency, or armed force of the United States to conduct or engage in investigations for prosecutions for violations of health care offenses.

Destroying records, not turning over files or documents when asked, lying to investigators, and generally being uncooperative during an investigation may cause a medical biller to be liable under this portion of the statute.

It is important for the medical biller to be aware of these issues. If you discover a possibly fraudulent claim, it is important to bring it to your supervisor's attention as soon as possible. In addition, if an investigation is initiated, you should cooperate fully with the investigators. Not doing so could be construed as hindering their investigation, and this can make you liable for fines and imprisonment up to five years. It is important to note that the statutes are written in such a way that you can be found guilty of hindering an investigation even if that investigation later fails to turn up fraud.

In addition, medical billers need to be cautious about the statements or comments they make regarding a claim, especially written comments that are placed in a file. If those comments turn out to be fraudulent, the medical biller may be held liable.

▶ **CRITICAL THINKING QUESTION:** If you see a co-worker commit an illegal act, such as fraud or embezzlement, what should you do?

Embezzlement

Embezzlement is the fraudulent appropriation of money entrusted to one's care. Embezzlement can be committed by anyone in a firm, including the receptionist, the biller, or the provider. Embezzlement is unfortunately not uncommon, and often undiscovered until it is too late to recover the money. This said, control systems must be in place.

To protect against embezzlement:

1. Accurate records must be kept of all transactions. Be sure to issue a receipt for all amounts received and to accurately record these amounts against the patient's account.
2. Any amounts removed should be notated and a receipt given for them. This is not only true for amounts that may have been taken from the cash drawer to pay for office supplies but also for amounts a provider may remove. Even if the provider is the sole owner of the practice, he or she should never be allowed to take money from the cash drawer without a receipt being issued. Such a practice helps maintain accurate records for financial accounting purposes, and it protects the keeper of the cash drawer from being charged with removing the money.
3. All checks should be immediately stamped For Deposit Only and the account number should be written or stamped on the check. The bank should be given instructions that any check made payable to the practice should never be cashed and that cash should never be given back from a deposit.
4. All monthly bank statements should be matched with the daily and monthly journals for the office. Total deposits should tally with the total of all daily journals. Any discrepancies should be reported immediately to a supervisor.
5. Consider developing a system where duties are separated. This provides a set of checks and balances within an office to guard against embezzlement. For example, have one person open the mail and a different individual deposit the checks received. The person who writes checks should not also be responsible for balancing the checkbook. In a small office a competent employee may be asked to take on a variety of duties, but for the employee's own safety as well as that of the provider, certain overlapping duties should never be performed by one person.
6. If embezzlement is suspected, the proper person should be notified. If a worker knows of embezzlement by a co-worker and says nothing, that worker is guilty of being an accomplice to the crime. Thus, the supervisor should be contacted when a co-worker is suspected of financial wrongdoing.

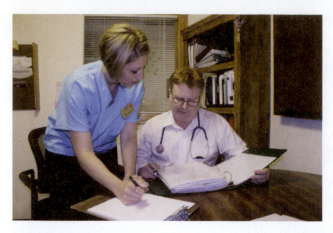

FIGURE 2-4

To avoid possible mistakes when reading a patient's chart, it is important to confirm with the physician when questions arise.

© Pat Watson/Pearson Education

7. A bond (insurance against embezzlement) should be obtained for each member of the practice who deals directly with the practice's receipts. These bonds can be issued on individual persons, on a job position, or for the entire office staff.

8. If you notice poor bookkeeping or inaccurate records that were kept by a previous employee or a current co-worker, it should be brought to the attention of your supervisor or employer. You should then document the problems in writing and ask the supervisor or employer to initial a copy for you to keep. This may provide minimal protection in case the reported problems are found to conceal embezzlement or mismanagement of funds.

As with fraud, a provider is considered ultimately responsible for everything that goes on in his or her practice. If embezzlement is found, the provider may be considered guilty and may be responsible for monies embezzled by their employees.

Employee Bonding and Errors and Omission Insurance

Generally, an employer is liable for harms caused by an employee while that employee is acting within the scope of his or her employment. This is called **respondeat superior**. However, a court of law may find the employee personally responsible for an incident that occurred as a result of an error, omission, or negligent act committed by the employee. A professional liability policy usually covers errors, omissions, or negligent acts, which may arise as an employee carries out the normal or usual duties of employment. **Errors and omissions** comprise part of a professional liability insurance policy in most cases (Figure 2-4 ●). This insurance covers damages caused by mistakes (errors) or damages caused by something an employee failed to do (omissions). A professional liability policy is something the medical biller would secure for herself.

Some employers protect themselves from employee dishonesty by bonding their employees. **Bonding** is the process by which an employer can be indemnified (insured) for the loss of money or other property sustained through dishonest acts of a "bonded" employee. Bonding can cover many types of acts, including larceny, theft, embezzlement, forgery, misappropriation, wrongful abstraction, willful misapplication, or other fraudulent or dishonest acts committed by an employee, alone or in collusion with others.

Claim Audits

Audits are performed to prevent and detect fraud. Fraud means that the provider knew, or reasonably should have known, that a statement or claim submitted was false. A **claims audit** is an analysis of claims payments made to a health care provider to determine whether the claims were allowable and whether the provider was paid the appropriate amount for services rendered. This type of audit usually includes reviewing the medical record to determine if services were documented and medically necessary. An **external auditor** is someone hired by an insurance company or governmental organization such as Medicare or Medicaid to perform an audit.

Medical billing personnel are required by law to cooperate with regulatory audits or investigations consistent with their contracts and applicable law. Audits are performed to ensure compliance with the established reimbursement requirements. A provider may be selected for an audit for a variety of reasons including questionable billing practices, a complaint lodged with a referral or enforcement agency, or random selection.

There are two types of audits: internal audits and external audits. **Internal audits** are considered to be prospective reviews because they are performed before a claim is submitted for payment. **External audits** are considered to be retrospective reviews because they are performed after a claim has been submitted for payment and after the claim has been processed by the insurance carrier.

One type of external audit is the Recovery Audit Contractor (RAC) program performed through the Centers for Medicare & Medicaid Services. This program was created in 2003 by the federal government to detect and correct improper Medicare payments to health care providers. From 2003–2006, through these audits a total of nearly $693.6 million has reportedly been recovered.

The external auditor will complete the audit and then will perform an audit exit with the medical biller or the person overseeing the audit. In addition, the external auditor will issue to the provider an audit report detailing the findings. Penalties for noncompliance with regulations and guidelines include the following:

- Recoupment of funds
- Reporting to a regulatory agency or relevant law enforcement agency
- Terminating or suspending the provider's participation or contract
- Suspending claims for special review
- Imposing certain corrective actions
- Suspending payments for a specified period of time

PRACTICE **PITFALLS**

The following are examples of abusive billing:

- Repeatedly submitting duplicate claims for the same service provided to the same member on the same date
- Billing for services that were not provided
- Repeatedly billing services at a different level or intensity than what was actually provided
- Repeatedly billing for medically unnecessary services
- Repeatedly using diagnosis codes that are not consistent with medical records
- Repeatedly billing certain procedure codes when a global code is more appropriate
- Repeatedly billing certain procedure codes in addition to a global code that reflects those procedures
- Billing for services provided by an individual who is not licensed to provide the service
- Repeatedly failing to follow applicable Medicare and standard industry billing guidelines
- Submitting false or fraudulent information

Subpoenas

Occasionally, the medical records of a patient may be needed in a court action. In such cases a subpoena is issued requesting the records. A **subpoena** is a court order demanding a person to appear at a certain time and place. A **subpoena duces tecum,** or a subpoena for production of evidence, requires the person to produce books, records, papers, or other tangible evidence.

One person in the office should be designated in charge of medical records. This person should also be specifically designated as the only person to accept a subpoena of medical records. The subpoena must be served in person only to that person. It cannot be laid on a desk or sent through the mail. No one else should accept the subpoena in the designee's absence.

A witness fee or mileage amount may be provided to the witness. Any fees payable should be requested at the time the subpoena is served.

If the subpoena is only for the records (i.e., not also for the record keeper), the designee should call the attorney who sent the subpoena and ask if the records can be sent. If so, the records should be sent by certified mail, return receipt requested.

The designee will usually be given a specified amount of time to produce the records. Occasionally, the records will need to be turned over at the time of the subpoena. In all cases, the designee should consult with the provider before turning over the records. If the provider is unavailable, the server should be informed that the records cannot be turned over without proper authorization and that the individual can come back and serve the subpoena directly on the provider. This will

Paul Provider, M.D.
5858 Peppermint Place
Anytown, USA 12345
(765) 555-6768

PATIENT NOTIFICATION OF SUBPOENA

Date:
To:
Address: _____

Dear Ms. Patient and Attorney:

Please note that records pertaining to you are being sought by _____; as shown in the subpoena attached to this Notice.

If you object to us furnishing any part of the records described in this action, you must file papers with the court prior to our release of these records. This subpoena requires that we furnish the records on or by _____ (date).

You or your attorney of record may contact the attorney for the party seeking to examine such records and determine whether they are willing to agree to cancel or limit this subpoena. If no such agreement is reached and you are not already represented by an attorney in this action, **you should consult an attorney to advise you of your rights in this matter.**

If we do not have notification in writing regarding the cancellation or limitation of this subpoena at least 24 hours prior to the above date, we will assume you have no objection to us releasing this information.

Signed: _____   Date: _____

FIGURE 2-5

Subpoena notification

provide time to ensure that the records are complete, accurate, and in good order. All signatures should be verified as identifiable.

If more than one provider works in your office, the subpoena must be served on the record keeper for that provider or on that provider directly. If no one who is authorized to accept the subpoena is present, the situation should be explained to the person serving the subpoena and a time suggested when the person can come back or contact the doctor's attorney. The doctor or the attorney should be notified of the situation.

Once a subpoena has been served, the doctor should check the medical records to ensure that they are accurate and complete. In most cases, the original record must be sent, so pages should be numbered and copies made and kept of everything sent. This provides an opportunity to check for changes in the records and to protect against loss of information if the records are lost. The original file should then be sent out immediately (if delivery by certified mail is allowed) or placed under lock and key to avoid tampering. The day of the trial should be determined, and all orders given by the court should be complied with. No one should be allowed to see the records or tamper with them. The records should be turned over to the appropriate party and documentation obtained indicating that you delivered the records.

Subpoena Notification

If a subpoena is served to request medical records, many offices will notify the patient in writing that the records have been requested. (A sample of a subpoena notification can be seen in Figure 2-5 ●.) This allows the patient's attorney to file papers with the court, if desired, to block the subpoena.

If there is very little time between the date that the subpoena was served and the date that the records have been requested, the letter may be faxed or the patient may be contacted by telephone. In either case, the patient should be informed that he or she does not have the authority to stop the release of the records. The patient's attorney may file a motion with the court to have the subpoena rescinded.

Instances in Which the Patient Should Be Notified and the File Notated

The following sections include situations that may warrant sending a letter to the patient. In each case, the letters are samples and should be modified to fit the individual circumstances.

A copy of any letter sent to the patient should always be placed in the patient's file. The provider may choose to have the patient sign this letter and return it, which serves to acknowledge receipt of the letter and the information it contains. This is a further step to protect the provider against a lawsuit.

If a signature is requested, two copies of the letter should be sent to the patient and a third copy placed in the file. The patient should keep one of the copies and sign the other and return it. If a letter is not returned with a signature within two weeks of it having been mailed, the patient should be called and the situation discussed, then the phone conversation should be documented in the patient's medical file.

Patient Who Fails to Keep an Appointment

Any patient who fails to keep an appointment when his or her condition is serious or needs constant monitoring should be sent a letter regarding the need for treatment or monitoring (Figure 2-6 ●). The patient may not realize the seriousness of his or her condition, and he or she may hold the doctor liable for this lack of knowledge if consequences arise as a result of lack of treatment. Always notate in the file whether a letter has been sent or not.

Patient Left Facility Against Medical Advice

Occasionally, a patient will leave the hospital against medical advice or will refuse to follow the advice given by the doctor. In such cases, the medical practice needs to be protected against lawsuits resulting from the lack of proper treatment.

In the case of a patient who leaves a treatment facility against the doctor's advice, the facility often will ask the patient to sign a form stating that he or she is leaving despite understanding

---

Paul Provider, M.D.
5858 Peppermint Place
Anytown, USA 12345
(765) 555-6768

Date:

Dear. Mr./Ms. Patient:

An appointment was scheduled for you on (date) _____ at _____ a.m./p.m. which you failed to keep. Please be advised that I consider your condition to be serious and in need of further medical treatment and/or monitoring.

Please contact my office for another appointment as soon as possible. If you choose to be treated by another physician, I urge you to seek an appointment with him or her without delay. With your authorization, I would be happy to share any test results or medical records with such a provider.

Two copies of this letter are enclosed. One is for your files. Please sign the second copy and return it to our office in the enclosed envelope.

Please understand my purpose in writing this letter is concern for your overall medical health.

Sincerely,

Paul Provider, M.D.

Patient Signature: _____ Date: _____

FIGURE 2-6
Failed appointment letter

PAUL PROVIDER PATIENT TREATMENT CENTER

STATEMENT OF PATIENT LEAVING AGAINST MEDICAL ADVICE

Date:

     This letter is to certify that I, _____(patient name), am leaving the above-named facility at my own insistence and against the advice of my attending provider and other treatment facility authorities. I understand the dangers of my leaving at this time. This letter hereby releases the facility, its employees and officers and any attending provider from any and all liability which may be caused as a result of my departure.

     This letter may also be construed as an agreement to hold harmless the above facility, its employees and officers and any attending provider from any and all liability which may be caused as a result of my departure.

Patient Signature: _____   Date: _____

Parent/Guardian Signature: _____   Date: _____

Witness: _____   Date: _____

Witness: _____   Date: _____

     If the patient refuses to sign this form, place an X in the space at left, fill out the form, and have it signed by two treatment center personnel. The words SIGNATURE REFUSED should be placed on the line reserved for the patient signature.

FIGURE 2-7

Statement of patient leaving against medical advice

that the doctor advises against it. A patient cannot be restrained from leaving or forced to sign the waiver. If the patient refuses to sign the waiver, a notation should be made on the form about the refusal to sign, and the form should then be signed and dated by two witnesses.

    Most facilities have a standard form to use for this purpose. A copy of such a form can be seen in Figure 2-7 ●.

Refusal to Follow Treatment

Some patients refuse to follow the advice of their provider. This can range from a decision not to give up smoking for improving overall health to a refusal to take the prescribed medication that could save the patient's life.

    In all cases, the practice should be protected as much as possible by having the patient sign a letter. The letter should state the condition of the patient, the medical advice, and the possible consequences of not following the advice (Figure 2-8 ●). Having a signed copy of this letter in the patient's file helps to protect against a lawsuit in which the patient states he or she was not informed of the consequences of not following the medical advice.

Termination of Treatment

It sometimes becomes necessary for a patient to terminate care with a provider. This most often happens at the request of the patient and is often a result of circumstances beyond control (e.g., relocation). To protect the practice, it is best to ask the patient to complete a letter of termination of care (Figure 2-9 ●).

When a Provider Terminates Care

Occasionally, a provider will feel the need to terminate the care of a patient when the patient continually refuses to follow medical advice. Termination of treatment should occur only after the patient has been fully advised of the consequences of not following the prescribed

---

Paul Provider, M.D.
5858 Peppermint Place
Anytown, USA 12345
(765) 555-6768

Date:

Dear Mr./Ms. Patient:

Two weeks ago you were diagnosed with hypertension (high blood pressure). At that time I prescribed a dosage of 500 mg of Diuril (Chlorothiazide) to be taken twice daily. It has come to our attention that you are not taking your medication as prescribed. I strongly urge you to take your medication as prescribed and return to my office for another checkup in two weeks to monitor your condition. If you choose to seek care from another physician, we will be happy to provide him or her with any test results or records.

Please understand that not taking your medication can result in severe damage to your kidneys, heart, circulatory system and other organs. Not getting your hypertension under control can lead to a heart attack, stroke or even death.

Please sign the bottom of this letter and return it in the enclosed envelope to attest that you have read it and are aware of the consequences that may result from not following the medical advice given to you.

Sincerely,

Paul Provider, M.D.

Patient Signature: _____ Date: _____

FIGURE 2-8

Refusal to follow treatment letter

Paul Provider, M.D.
5858 Peppermint Place
Anytown, USA 12345
(765) 555-6768

LETTER CONFIRMING TERMINATION OF TREATMENT

Date:

Dear Mr. /Ms. Patient:

This letter is to confirm our understanding that as of _____(date) you wish to discharge Donald Doctor, M.D. as your provider. We will be sorry to see you go.

Please know that we have enjoyed the opportunity to serve you and will be happy to provide your medical records, with your authorization, to any new provider you choose.

Please sign the bottom of this letter to confirm termination of treatment and return it to our office in the enclosed envelope.

Thank you very much.

Sincerely,

Paul Provider, M.D.

I hereby acknowledge receipt of this letter and agree to termination of treatment on the above date.

Patient Signature: _____ Date: _____

FIGURE 2-9

Letter confirming termination of treatment

Paul Provider, M.D.
5858 Peppermint Place
Anytown, USA 12345
(765) 555-6768

Date:

Dear Mr. /Ms. Patient:

    I find it necessary to terminate any further care of your case due to your repeated refusal to follow medical advice. It is my opinion that your condition requires further treatment or serious consequences may develop. I strongly urge you to seek the care of another provider immediately .

    I would be happy to provide, upon your authorization, any test results or medical records needed by the new provider.

    If you desire, I shall continue to provide your medical care for the next _____ days, until _____. This should give you ample time to secure the services of a new provider.

    Please sign one copy of this letter and return it to our office to acknowledge that you have read and understand this information. The second copy is for your records.

Sincerely,

Paul Provider, M.D.

Patient Signature: _____ Date: _____

FIGURE 2-10

Physician terminating care letter

medical advice (Figure 2-10 ●). A provider may also terminate care if he no longer accepts the insurance of the patient. Sometimes providers have difficulty getting paid from certain insurance carriers and, as a result, may choose to no longer accept patients who carry that specific insurance.

CHAPTER REVIEW

Summary

- The medical biller should be aware of the appropriate legal and ethical issues. These include being aware of the most common causes of fraud as well as understanding HIPAA guidelines.
- Instances or situations in which the patient should be notified and the patient's chart notated include when a patient fails to keep appointments, when a patient leaves a medical facility against medical advice, and when a patient refuses to follow medical advice.

Review Questions

Directions: Answer the following questions without looking back at the material covered in this chapter. Write your answers in the space provided.

1. Medical information is considered to be _____ and _____ in the context of the provider–patient relationship.

2. What are the four reasons why the confidentiality of medical records is more important today than it may have been in the past?

_____

_____

_____

3. List the two main issues HIPAA addresses.

_____

_____

4. What information should be contained in a fax cover sheet?

   a. _____

   b. _____

   c. _____

5. What are the six exceptions to the privacy laws?

_____

_____

_____

_____

_____

_____

6. List six of the most common cases of fraud.

_____

_____

_____

_____

_____

_____

7. Define embezzlement.

_____

_____

8. Define ethics and outline the ethical standards set by the American Medical Association that providers should follow.

_____

_____

_____

_____

9. (True or False?) Willful abuse of the privacy of any insured or patient by the employee may be cause for dismissal. _____

10. Name three instances in which the patient should be notified and a notation made in the patient's chart.

_____

_____

_____

   If you are unable to answer any of these questions, refer back to that section in the chapter, and then fill in the answers.

Activity #1: Word Search

Directions: Find and circle the following words. Words can appear horizontally, vertically, diagonally, forward, or backward.

1. Bonding
2. Claims audit
3. External audit

4. HIPAA
5. Fraud

```
J C Y X J A J F R P N I C H Y Z U Q R N W M B U E I M Z O T
X U C K H Y Z Z I X D O M U P H I N S A Y L Y P S W Q A L C
D C L P K H F M J S D F Z P L O J S Q R D H V V Z B O U V P
X Z R Y Q S B J T K W L I O A K K O S U J V T C I N H A B X
Q U W O A J N Z N W I Z Q T G M I Z Q K R W E P A K K C M L
C S T R A T E K T O X C L O U W A I I C Y S X X M W C J D U
V Y J O P S F E M Z M N L L H K X Y L M N U T U T V X W Q A
T F H K I W I Y S K S W T C H G N K W N G U E X V B N W X I
K F Y A H B H Z Q G V I U M J J W Y J Q X R R S X Z X X Y M
T R D X Z Q K U J T X U E M U E I F G F G R N N N B E K B A
X S T I Y Y L R B F W T C Q G Z M N V T X H A T R L G G B T
A A Y R R W B W V N C Y G W M P F K Y I Y R L V Z K H G Y A
D U H D P I I H H Y M A Z N B T S B T A B R A B Z A Q Z Z R
Q F R A U D G N V X L J F H X R P M Q P Q C U Z W R M D J L
M Q N H H M H D S Q C K B I Z U V I Z F V V D K F A Y D H J
H F W G Y O E P N I N Y R U W Z N L O H U H I H F T N O B T
E W P U H V T K K Y O W U Y I L O I E E S C T R T H T S O C
R Y E P M A X U W I V R P B T U Y I R C V O O Y Y I A N Q G
O I D D Z D C O Y V L L Y B F B L N Z H G A J Z A I Q S L S
Y R B J L A Y J V C D P C D L O F T L I D R R W Z Z K U Z S
F S M T Y I J D Z X Z L Q P U F M U M T H S S E R T S B O J
C O U N V I R T S E A C S G R N B Y Q L T L O Q P Y E W Z W
K K W X N Q A F K I S G R U K V D F B L W P H V U V T Z S A
P R F B F U M V M K V T N F X U U O V I N N S Y H U N P V O
G R B S I W R S V Q O E U I O M F F P N C Y R S K O I Q H L
R Z J Z V K A Q Z Q N W N L D J Z P G V Z R G P Q W E T T F
X L Z C Y U N H T L T V V K O N L W Y G T Z N Y R R M D W W
V N U I D E S T C C P J L O V D O Y T K K T B Q J D K L P K
Q U T I Z L G D Q E D G D J Q W D B Z F X B L J C Q K Q I J
E P T W L D Q E P Q I Q T W R T K G A P K U U J G B Y I E Z
```

Activity #2: Matching Key Terms

Directions: Match the following terms with the proper definition by writing the letter of the correct definition in the space next to the term.

1. _____ Errors and omissions insurance

2. _____ Health Maintenance Organizations (HMOs)

3. _____ Legal damages

4. _____ Respondeat superior

5. _____ Subpoena duces tecum

a. Monetary awards that a plan member may attempt to recover, which are above and beyond the benefits provided by the group plan

b. An employer's liability for harms caused by an employee while that employee is acting within the scope of employment

c. Organizations or companies that provide both the coverage for care and the care itself

d. Requires the person to produce books, records, papers, or other tangible evidence

e. Insurance that covers damages caused by mistakes (errors) or damages caused by something an employee failed to do (omissions)

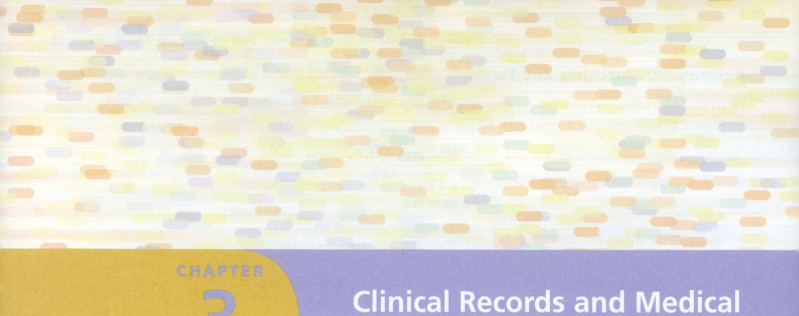

Clinical Records and Medical Documentation

Key Words and Concepts you will learn in this chapter:

Alphabetical filing

Alter

Assignment of Benefits Form

Children's charts

Claim

Electronic prescriptions

Emancipation

Emancipated minor

Encounter Forms

Guarantor

Insurance Coverage Form

Maintaining records

Noncompliance

Patient History Form

Patient Information Sheet

Pediatric charts

Problem-oriented medical record (POMR)

Release of Information Form

Request for Additional Information Form

Signature card

SOAP notes

After completion of this chapter you should be able to:

- Describe how a medical chart is organized.

- Describe how charts for pediatric and emergency patients are different from other medical charts.

- Demonstrate how to file x-rays in a chart.

- Properly file a patient chart.

- List the rules for medical documentation.

- Properly complete a signature card.

- Describe the use of a signature card.

- Explain why and for how long records should be retained.

- Describe the process for storing medical records.

- Describe features available with electronic medical charting.

- Discuss the pros and cons of computerized medical charting.

▌ Properly complete a records transfer request.

▌ Discuss the purpose of a Patient Information Sheet.

▌ Properly complete a Patient Information Sheet with information from a given situation.

▌ Discuss the purpose of the Authorization to Release Information and the Assignment of Benefits forms.

▌ Properly complete an insurance coverage form with information from a given situation.

▌ List the guidelines for facilitating the gathering of information.

Keeping accurate patient charts is essential to running a good medical practice. Without accurate patient charts, the provider may find it difficult to treat the patient's condition properly. In addition, without an accurate chart it can be difficult to bill insurance companies or the patient for treatment that was performed.

Medical charts contain a number of forms. Some of these forms are needed at each visit. Other forms, such as those authorizing treatment, are completed once and merely stored in the patient's file.

Maintaining records means keeping the information in a chart updated and, if using a paper record, filing the chart or recording it in a manner that makes it easy to locate if needed in the future. This chapter covers the general practices in maintaining patient charts both in paper form and electronically. The actual forms found within a patient's chart will be covered in other chapters in this text.

The Paper Medical Chart

In most medical offices, a separate chart is kept on every patient (Figure 3-1 ●). Although this can often necessitate the repetition of some information, it is necessary to ensure compliance with HIPAA rules and to keep the information separate for each patient.

Medical billers often are responsible for creating new patient charts. This means completing or having the patient complete the initial forms and putting them in the charts in the proper order. If the patient has an insurance card or other proof of coverage, a photocopy of this information is included with these forms. Every page in the medical chart must have patient identification information contained on it.

Often the medical biller or receptionist is the first person who sees a new patient. At that time, this individual may ask the patient (or the patient's parent or guardian, in the case of a minor) to complete a number of forms. It helps to have the required forms already placed together on a clipboard so that the patient can complete them easily. These forms then must be placed in the patient's chart in the proper order. If forms are not in the proper order, a lot of time may be spent searching for the right information.

There are many different types of forms used in the medical office, and the style of the forms varies from provider to provider. In addition, a number of companies create and produce medical forms. The actual creation of the chart will therefore differ from provider to provider. Information typically seen in a patient's chart includes the following:

- Acknowledgment of Receipt of HIPAA Privacy Practices Notice
- Patient Information Form
- Examination/Treatment Forms
- Pathology/Laboratory/X-ray Reports

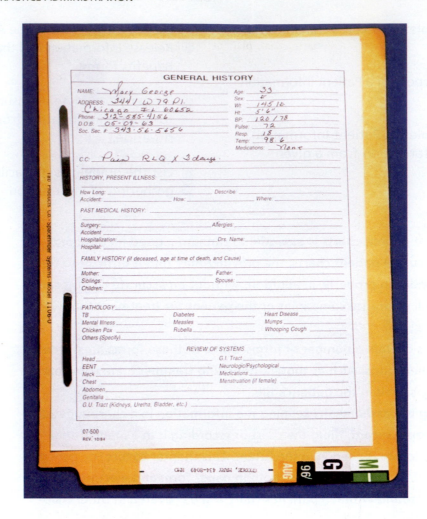

- Operative Reports
- Discharge Summaries
- Billing Forms for previous visits
- Consent Form
- Signature on File
- Forms related to financial arrangements
- Correspondence Log
- Letters to and from provider

During the course of treatment, the provider may add additional forms to the patient chart, such as a History and Physical Form, Progress Notes, or a Medication Flow Sheet for tracking prescribed medicine. If the patient is a child, a pediatric chart would be assembled. (Contents of a pediatric chart are discussed later in this chapter.)

After the patient has become established and has had several visits, lab and x-ray results and consultation reports may be submitted from other providers. These results should be reviewed by the provider or, in some offices, by a nurse. If reviewed by a nurse, abnormal lab, x-ray, or urgent results or requests will be forwarded directly to the provider for an immediate response. After review, these results should be stamped with the date and signed by the provider before they are filed in the patient chart.

Items should be grouped together (e.g., all pathology reports together, followed by all laboratory reports, etc.). They should then be placed in order by date, with the most recent one on top. A specific order allows the provider to find the necessary information quickly and easily.

Items should be placed in the patient's file as soon as they are received from the provider. If a report comes in from an outside entity (e.g., results of tests from an outside lab), the report should be given to the provider immediately with the patient's file. The provider should initial the report to indicate that he has looked at it before the report is placed in the file. Reports should not be placed in a medical record without having first been initialed by the provider.

When preparing a chart for a patient's visit, be sure that the provider has space on the necessary forms for recording the examination, treatment plan, and progress notes. If necessary, add additional forms to the chart. Most medical offices add additional forms on top of the existing forms rather than underneath them. This places the most current information on top where it can be found easily.

Under no circumstance should old information from a chart be removed, no matter how full the chart has become. If additional chart space is needed, create a second volume of the patient's chart. Medical treatment plans can extend over a length of time. At any point in the patient's treatment, the provider may need to refer back to the initial examination or treatment plan to clarify a point about the patient's situation.

Pediatric Charts

Some medical offices use a different type of chart for children. These are called **children's charts** or **pediatric charts**. Pediatric charts may contain additional or different forms. For example, a Children's Medical History form would not include information that is not appropriate for children, such as pregnancy history. A growth chart that records the child's growth is an additional form that would not be found in an adult chart (Figure 3-2 ●).

Pediatric charts also require additional forms such as immunization records to track immunizations, and forms for hearing and vision exams. These records often are needed by a parent to enable them to enroll their child in a public school.

Some medical offices also may use restraints on young children to prevent them from moving and causing themselves injury during medical treatment. Signed documentation regarding the authorization of the parent or guardian for use of these restraints should be obtained.

CRITICAL THINKING QUESTION: How might a patient chart differ if the individual were only being seen on a one-time, emergency basis? Why would the contents of this chart be different?

Charts for Emergency Patients

Some patients come to medical offices on a one-time, emergency basis. This may be someone from out of town who has a medical emergency, someone who needs a procedure done and is unable or unwilling to see their own provider for treatment, or someone seeking a second opinion.

Many medical offices use a separate type of chart for these patients. Because these patients will not be receiving extended treatment, many of the documents in a normal chart, such as callback and telephone records, will not be needed. However, even these patients need to give the provider information regarding their medical history.

The forms that are typically included in an emergency patient record include:

- Registration
- Medical History
- Provider's Notes (or Treatment Plan)
- Release and Consent

Radiology Records

Many offices take radiological films (x-rays) of patients. Unless stored electronically on a CD, x-ray film can be a large item (depending on the body part that has been radiographed). Because of this, x-rays are often stored separately from the patient files.

If not stored digitally, x-rays are often placed in a large envelope and labeled with the name of the patient, the date that the x-ray was taken, and the specific body part shown on the x-ray (e.g., "Right Wrist"). Many offices also label the x-ray itself with this information. In addition, many medical offices include a birth date, an account number, or another identifying number to ensure that the x-rays for two people with similar names are not mixed up.

Once the x-ray has been properly labeled, documentation of the x-ray should be added to the patient chart. By documenting all the x-rays that have been taken in the patient chart, a provider can easily see if an earlier x-ray was taken of a body part that is being treated. This can help to show changes in the patient or in the patient's condition or disease.

X-rays often are kept in a back office and are filed alphabetically by the last name of the patient. It is important to remember not to place other items in the same pocket with the medical

2 to 20 years: Girls
Stature-for-age and Weight-for-age percentiles

NAME _____

RECORD # _____

Mother's Stature _____	Father's Stature _____			
Date	Age	Weight	Stature	BMI*

*To Calculate BMI: Weight (kg) ÷ Stature (cm) ÷ Stature (cm) x 10,000
or Weight (lb) ÷ Stature (in) ÷ Stature (in) x 703

AGE (YEARS)

STATURE

WEIGHT

AGE (YEARS)

Published May 30, 2000 (modified 11/21/00).
SOURCE: Developed by the National Center for Health Statistics in collaboration with
the National Center for Chronic Disease Prevention and Health Promotion (2000).
http://www.cdc.gov/growthcharts

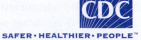

FIGURE 3-2
Sample growth chart

x-rays, as these items may scratch the x-ray. For space reasons, other offices may choose to destroy the film or give it to the patient once the results have been documented.

Some providers also take photographs of a patient to document conditions or situations. These photos may be needed to verify the need for treatment to an insurance carrier or for explanations provided to the patient. These pictures should be labeled and treated in the same manner as the x-rays. However, some medical offices will file pictures directly in the patient chart, as they often are small enough to fit in the chart.

PRACTICE **PITFALLS**

If you are writing on the envelope containing the x-ray film, write on it before placing the x-ray inside. This will prevent damage to the x-ray from pressing on it.

Over time, labels placed on x-rays or charts may lose their adhesion and become loose. Any labels that are beginning to peel away from an x-ray or chart should be reaffixed as soon as possible, or new labels should be applied.

To make labeling easier, some medical offices use x-ray film that has a white covering in one corner for labeling the x-ray. This is put on by the manufacturer and usually solves the problem of missing labels. The information contained on a CD sleeve would be the same as that provided on the outside of an x-ray envelope.

Filing the Paper Chart

Once the chart has been completed, it must be filed so that it can be located easily. Medical offices function in many different ways, thus there are several different filing methods, including numeric, alphanumeric, terminal digit, subject, and alphabetical.

Because of HIPAA regulations, the name of the patient should not appear on the outside of the chart. This is especially true if the charts are kept in a place that is visible to other patients or to anyone entering the office. If at all possible, all patient charts should be placed in a locked room that is inaccessible to anyone who is not authorized to enter. If this is not possible, the outside of charts should contain only information that is considered to be nonpersonal. Thus, charts should be identified with a number rather than with the patient's name. Some medical offices will use an account number that is alphanumeric (a combination of numbers and letters). In such cases, care must be taken to preserve the patient's identity. The letters used should not be those that could indicate the patient's name.

A numeric or alphanumeric filing system often will necessitate use of a master list with the patients' names in alphabetical order. This allows for the correct patient chart to be found quickly and easily.

When creating a new chart for a patient, the chart should be labeled as soon as it is put together. If the practice uses a numeric or alphanumeric filing system, the chart information should be added to the master list immediately.

A master list is often computerized. Even when the list is on the computer, a printed list should always be kept available. This allows access to patient charts when the computer system is down or otherwise in use.

Adding a file to a computerized master list can be done quickly and easily. If the master list is not computerized, or if you are unable to add the information to the master list immediately, you can write the information on the printed master list.

ALPHABETICAL FILING. If a practice keeps its charts in an area that is not accessible or viewable by unauthorized personnel, then an alphabetical filing system may be used. **Alphabetical filing** simply means filing the charts alphabetically by the first letter of the patient's last name. If a patient's last name is hyphenated, then the name should be filed under the first part of the last name. For instance, Robert Doe-Johnson would be filed as "Doe-Johnson, Robert." If a name is compounded, such as Juan Blanco de Paz, then the name would be filed as "Blanco de Paz, Juan."

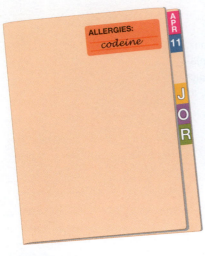

FIGURE 3-3

Chart with color-coded labels

ONLINE INFORMATION: For further rules on filing visit the ARMA International (Association of Records Managers and Administrators) Web site at www.arma.org.

Many medical offices use color-coded tabs for alphabetical filing (Figure 3-3 ●). Depending on the number of patients or files, the color coding may be broken down into the first letter of the last name, or the first two letters of the last name.

Many medical supply companies sell labels with letters in a multitude of colors. It is not uncommon to use nine or ten colors (e.g., A is red, B is orange, C is yellow, D is green, etc.).

By placing the proper label or labels on the outside of the chart, any charts that are out of order can easily be seen. In addition, it is much easier to find a chart because you have only a few, rather than many, to look through.

Each practice has a specific area where the letter should be placed on the outside of the chart. Keeping the letters in the proper area also helps to spot charts that may be out of order.

ACTIVITY #1

Alphabetical Filing

Directions: Using the chart names provided, place the following files in alphabetical order by client name. Use a separate sheet of paper to list your answers.

Patient Name

Sam Samson

Ricky Rodriguez

Gina Garret

Fred Frick

Nick Nap

Tom Tucker

Dana Daniels

Monica Manner

Tina Thomas

Kerri Kane

Jane Varley-Hampden

Jose Morelas de Diego

Brent Edgeworth-Barr

Medical Documentation Rules

Regardless of the type of medical practitioner you work for, there are some important factors to consider when documenting in a medical chart. A patient's chart often will include notations from three or more people within the medical office:

- Medical biller/receptionist
- Medical assistant (or nurse in a hospital)
- Medical provider (provider, surgeon, anesthesiologist, etc.)

Much litigation occurs in the world today. Because there is always the chance that a lawsuit may be filed someday, everyone who touches a medical chart needs to think about what they are writing in it.

The following rules are important to remember when performing medical charting:

Document only in your area of responsibility. Your notations on the chart should be limited to those areas that are your responsibility for the patient. This can include appointment setting,

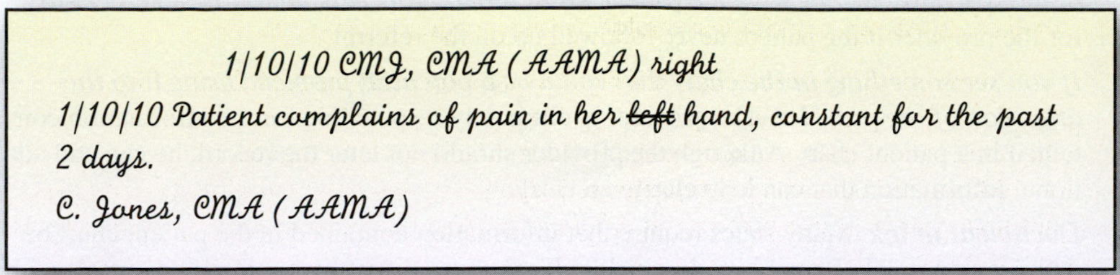

FIGURE 3-4

Sample correction of a charting error

> 1/10/10 *CMJ, CMA (AAMA) right*
>
> 1/10/10 *Patient complains of pain in her ~~left~~ hand, constant for the past 2 days.*
>
> *C. Jones, CMA (AAMA)*

follow-up phone calls, and encounters in the reception area. Under no circumstances should an individual make any notations regarding the patient's treatment, even when asked to do so by the provider, unless the person's training and credentials allow it.

Never use correction fluid on a chart or obscure any writing. Liquid correction fluid or roll-on correction tape that covers over writing on paper should never be used. If a mistake is made, draw a single line through the error in such a way that the original entry can still be read. Then write the correction directly next to the crossed-out entry and initial and date it. The date shows when the change was made and allows for creation of a timeline, if needed (Figure 3-4 ●). If a malpractice lawsuit is ever filed, correction fluid or tape always makes people wonder what was removed. By drawing a single line through the entry, there is no question about what was there before.

Use standard abbreviations and terms. Each office should have a set of standard abbreviations and terms to be used in medical documentation. Using different abbreviations and terms can cause confusion in the records. These confusions can be detrimental to the treatment of a patient, or they can lead to confusion during a lawsuit, which may mean a higher damage award. A chart of standard abbreviations and terms should be available to all office staff.

Do not write in the margins. If most material written in the chart falls within the margins, but one sentence is outside the margins, it can appear as though that sentence was added at a later time and inserted into the available space. If you run out of room, write on the next line. If there is no next line, use an additional form and continue writing on it. Paying for an additional form is much less costly than having a lawyer argue that the material was not on the chart from the beginning.

Never alter the information already entered on a chart. To **alter** means to change or amend (add to) the information contained in a record or chart. If information in a chart has changed or needs to be corrected, the information should be documented on the next available line, with the date of documentation.

Never write information in a patient chart that you do not want the patient to see. Patient charts legally belong to both the patient and the provider. However, the provider is considered to be the legal custodian of the records. Thus, patients are allowed to see their records any time they wish. However, no patient may remove the records from the provider's office.

Document anything the patient says with quotation marks. Juries automatically believe that anything inside quotation marks is a direct quote. Documenting comments made by patients is important and can work to the provider's advantage if the patient later sues. This is especially true when listing the details of a phone call. Without face-to-face contact in which observations can be made, words carry a greater impact.

Take the time to document noncompliance. **Noncompliance** means not following the instructions given by the provider. If the provider has suggested that the patient perform a certain action (e.g., physical therapy exercises twice a day, etc.), ask if the patient is performing such actions during a follow-up call. If the patient indicates not, make sure that this is recorded in the chart. This will protect the provider in case the patient sues. Juries will wonder if the patient's outcome would have been different if the patient had followed the provider's advice.

Be specific when documenting. The more specific you can be, the better. For example, instead of saying "Patient was referred to a specialist," include the name, title, and address of the specialist and for what the patient was referred. This person may be able to testify for the provider if the patient never followed up on the referral.

If you see something in the chart that could be a potential problem, bring it to the attention of the provider. The provider is ultimately responsible for the information contained in a patient chart. Although the provider should not alter the record, he can add additional information that can help clarify an entry.

Document in ink. Many states require that information contained in the patient chart be documented in ink. Pencil is unacceptable. If you have difficulty expressing yourself without reworking the wording, write the information on a piece of scrap paper first, then write it into the patient's chart.

Be sure that any change to a patient's appointment is documented. If the patient calls and says that he or she will be late, be sure it is noted on the patient's chart. If the patient calls to cancel or reschedule the appointment, be sure it is notated. If the patient later sues the provider, documentation can be shown that the patient repeatedly changed or canceled appointments. The argument can then be made that the patient's condition could have been better taken care of if the individual had been compliant with follow-up instructions. Documenting changes to an appointment also can fend off accusations of sloppy documentation if the patient chart no longer matches the appointment book. For example, if the patient postponed an appointment for a week, the chart may have one date and the appointment book a different date.

When documenting an appointment, include the reason for the appointment. If the patient indicates that he or she is having a problem, the details should be notated on both the appointment calendar and the patient's chart. This helps the provider know what to look for and to have a better understanding of how urgently the patient may need care. It also helps to protect the provider if the patient then cancels an appointment.

Make detailed notes of follow-up calls. If the proper follow-up call is not performed, the provider may be considered guilty of "patient abandonment." This can carry a high price tag in the event of a lawsuit. Many providers have the medical biller or receptionist make follow-up calls. This is completely legal. However, if the procedure was extraordinarily difficult or the results were not those anticipated, it might be better if the provider made the follow-up call. This will show more concern for the patient.

Update the patient's medical history at each visit. This is not as complicated as it might sound. Simply ask the patient if there have been any changes to his or her medical history or drug/medication use. If the patient indicates that there have been no changes, note the date on the chart and "No Change in Medical History" (sometimes abbreviated as NCMH).

SOAP Notes

Many medical offices use the **SOAP notes** format to standardize medical evaluation entries made in clinical records. SOAP stands for Subjective, Objective, Assessment, and Plan (Figure 3-5 ●). Medical documentation of patient complaint(s) and treatment must be consistent, concise, and comprehensive. SOAP notes should be organized in a manner that allows the current patient documentation to be found quickly when necessary. The following are the four parts of a SOAP note:

1. The first part of the format is the *Subjective* portion of the SOAP note, which consists of subjective observations. These are symptoms that the patient or the patient's representative verbally expresses. These subjective observations include the patient's descriptions of pain or discomfort, the presence of nausea or dizziness, and a multitude of other descriptions of dysfunction, discomfort, or illness.

2. The next part of the format is the *Objective* observation. These objective observations include conditions that the medical provider actually can see, hear, touch, feel, or smell. Included in objective observations are measurements such as temperature, pulse, respiration, skin color, swelling, and the results of tests.

3. *Assessment* follows the objective observations. Assessment is the diagnosis of the patient's condition. In some cases, the diagnosis may be clear; however, in other cases, an assessment may not be clear and could include several diagnostic possibilities.

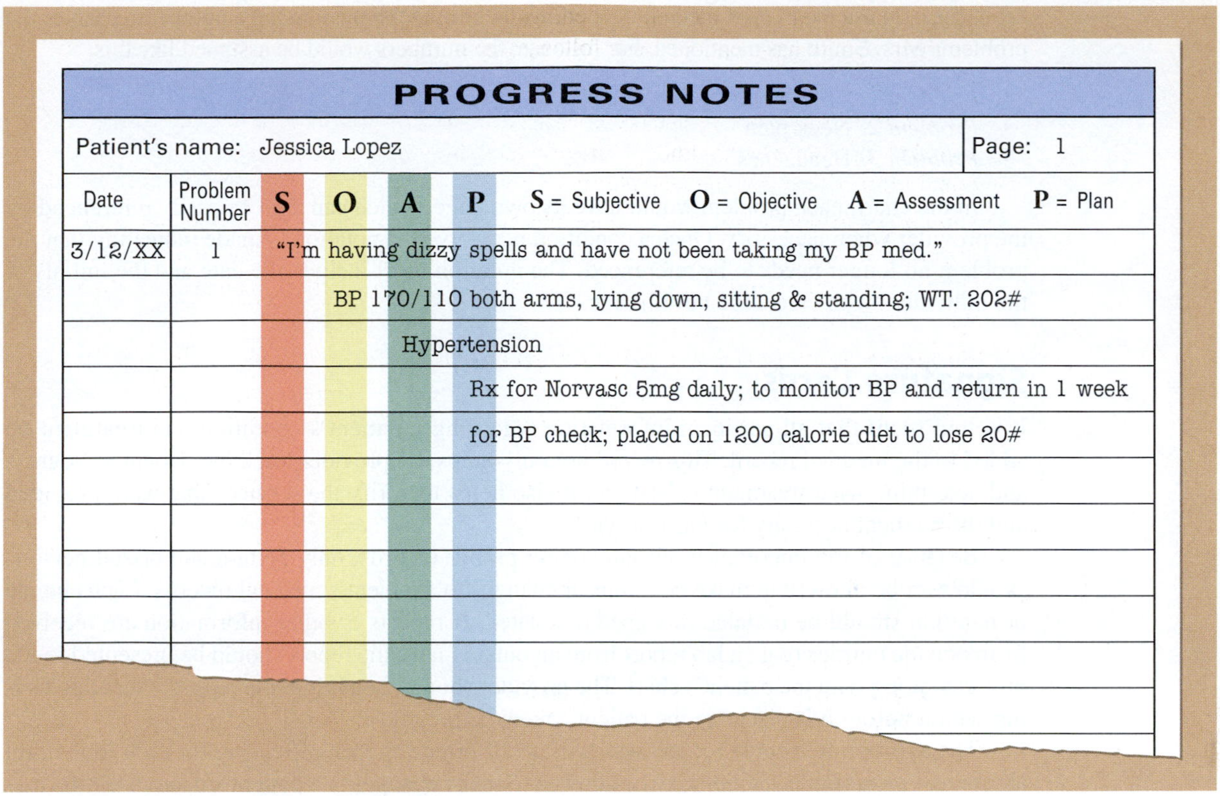

PROGRESS NOTES

Patient's name: Jessica Lopez

Page: 1

Date	Problem Number	**S**	**O**	**A**	**P**	**S** = Subjective **O** = Objective **A** = Assessment **P** = Plan
3/12/XX	1	"I'm having dizzy spells and have not been taking my BP med."				
			BP 170/110 both arms, lying down, sitting & standing; WT. 202#			
				Hypertension		
					Rx for Norvasc 5mg daily; to monitor BP and return in 1 week	
					for BP check; placed on 1200 calorie diet to lose 20#	

FIGURE 3-5

Sample of SOAP note charting

4. The last part of the SOAP note is the *Plan.* The plan may include laboratory tests, x-rays, or medications ordered for the patient; treatments performed; patient referrals; patient disposition, such as being sent home or to the hospital; patient directions for care; and any follow-up directions.

ACTIVITY #2

SOAP Charting

Directions: Read the following scenario and then use the SOAP note format to document the patient's visit. The date of the patient's visit is 5/12/20XX.

On 5/10/20XX, Dirk Stewart had a ganglion cyst removed from his right hand. He is at the office for the surgical site to be examined. His mother called the office yesterday indicating there was some redness around the surgical site.

   On examination, Dr. Timothy James notes redness and drainage from the site. The patient's temperature is taken and is 99.9° F. The patient is placed on oral antibiotics for 10 days. Prior to the patient leaving the office, the mother is given instructions to keep the area clean and dry and to call the office if the condition worsens. The patient is to return in one week for suture removal.

POMR Charting

The **problem-oriented medical record (POMR)** is used to track a patient's medical progress. A number is assigned to each problem the patient has. When the patient comes in for care, the number associated with the condition is referenced. The philosophy behind the use of POMR charting is that charting according to a patient's conditions will decrease the possibility of a provider overlooking previous issues.

   For example, Mrs. Smith is seeing the provider due to her chronic bronchitis. While discussing her condition, Mrs. Smith mentions that her neck has been bothering her lately and that she is having headaches. To use the POMR method of charting, the provider would assign a number to each of the problems Mrs. Smith has mentioned. For instance, the numbers would be assigned like this:

- *Problem 1:* Chronic bronchitis
- *Problem 2:* Neck pain
- *Problem 3:* Headaches

In the chart, each problem would have its own page, which can then be easily referenced by the provider when necessary. Once a condition is resolved, a notation is made indicating that the problem no longer needs to be referenced. The notation must include the date and the initials of the individual who enters the information.

Signature Cards

It is important that all pertinent information regarding a patient's condition and treatment be added to the medical record. This record not only helps the provider track the patient's progress and determine what treatment is best, but it also helps to verify the services that were provided and the medical necessity for those services.

Because of the importance of maintaining proper records, only certain authorized persons should ever be allowed to make notations or changes to a patient's medical records. Each change or notation should be initialed or signed and dated. If reports or other information are received from outside entities (e.g., a lab report from an outside lab), the report should be presented to the provider along with the patient's chart. The provider should then initial the report to indicate having seen it before it is placed in the patient's medical record.

The appropriate people for any task will be different for each office and for each job within an office. For example, a biller may be allowed to make changes to a patient's insurance information or account but not to any medical information. The best way to track those authorized to make notations or changes is by use of signature cards.

A **signature card** shows the person authorized to make changes, the dates of the individual's authorization period, and the scope of the changes he or she is allowed to make (Figure 3-6 ●). These cards should be kept in the billing office.

Paul Provider, M.D.
5858 Peppermint Place
Anytown, USA 12345
(765) 555-6768

SIGNATURE CARD   Date Created _____

A copy of this card shall be maintained on file at all times and updated as needed. The following person is authorized to make notations and/or changes to the patient medical records as indicated.

Name _____ Title _____

Authorized from _____ to _____

Signature: _____ Initials: Printed _____ Signed _____

Scope of authorization (i.e., all records and files, insurance data only, etc.) _____

_____

_____

FIGURE 3-6

Signature card

If changes are to be made to a person's signature card, the old card should be terminated by putting the ending date in the "Authorized from . . . :" space. A new signature card should be completed with the new information. The old signature card should be kept on file. Then, if an auditor or other person is looking through older medical records and needs to know whose signature was authorized and signed on a certain date, the old signature card can be pulled.

Some medical offices choose to have a signature log on file. A signature log contains the information from several signature cards on a single sheet of paper. The disadvantage of signature logs is that some information on a signature log can be outdated, whereas other information is still current. Because several people are listed on a single paper, if one person leaves the practice, then his or her name is no longer valid but the other signatures still are. Such a system makes it much more difficult to track authority. You may need to go through any number of signature logs to find the signature that you are looking for.

Signature cards have the advantage of allowing each authorized person to be listed on a separate card. This can be neater in an office that has a high turnover rate or for whom the job status and authority for notations often changes. The current cards are kept in a card file in front of a divider in alphabetical order by last name. The outdated cards are kept behind the divider in alphabetical order.

Retention of Records

Storing medical charts can become a huge undertaking for a medical practice, especially if it is large and has been in operation for a number of years. However, it is important to maintain patients' medical charts for an extended time.

All records should be kept as long as they are needed or for the period of time state laws require. Because many conditions are linked to previous episodes of care, records may be needed on patients long after they have been treated for a condition. For example, pediatric records may be needed for a twenty-five-year-old pregnant woman to determine if she had measles as a child. For such reasons, many medical offices put their medical records on microfiche, microfilm, or computer files and keep them indefinitely.

The laws regarding records retention vary from state to state; however, many states require medical offices to keep records for several years after the patient has died. This essentially can mean keeping medical records forever, especially if the practice treats a number of young patients.

One of the main reasons for keeping records so long is the way laws are written. Many states allow patients to sue a provider five or even ten years after the patient discovers a problem. If the patient does not discover a problem until thirty years after treatment has ended, the patient still has the right to sue for five more years. In effect, you cannot be certain that a patient will not sue, and that the records will not be needed, until five to ten years after the patient is dead.

Thus, a medical office must maintain a tremendous amount of paperwork. To make it easier, records of patients who are no longer seen by the medical office will often be placed in storage or on microfiche or microfilm.

In addition, federal regulations mandate that records on Medicare and Medicaid patients be retained for at least ten years after treatment. At any time during this ten-year period, the medical practice can be audited and must provide substantiation for all charges and receipts.

For tax purposes, records should be kept for at least seven years after the tax return is filed.

PRACTICE **PITFALLS**

It is better to err on the side of keeping files a little longer than sending them to the shredder as soon as the time limit expires. As luck would have it, you will not need information from the file until after it is shredded.

Storing Medical Records

When storing medical records, it is important to keep them in a manageable order in order to locate the records if you should need them at a later date. This often means creating lists of the items that are included in the storage boxes and properly labeling these boxes.

Box: Medical Charts 1999, A–L	
Adams, Sean	10/01/68
Adams, Sydney	12/14/70
Adams, Thomas	06/05/56
Adamson, Kirk	05/10/63
Alexander, Betty	08/21/35
Alexander, Karen	11/03/60

FIGURE 3-7

Sample master list for box contents

Patient Name	Birth Date	Box
Adams, Amy	03/15/48	Med Charts 2000 A–L
Adams, Sean	10/01/68	Med Charts 1999 A–L
Adams, Sydney	12/14/70	Med Charts 1999 A–L
Adams, Thomas	06/05/56	Med Charts 1999 A–L
Adamson, Kirk	05/10/63	Med Charts 2001 A–L
Alexander, Betty	08/21/35	Med Charts 1999 A–L
Alexander, Karen	11/03/60	Med Charts 1999 A–L

FIGURE 3-8

Sample master storage list for practice

Many companies use numerical or alphabetical labels on their boxes. For example, the labeling on a box might be shown as "Medical Charts, 2009, A–K." This could mean that charts for all patients who terminated care in the year 2009 whose last names began with A–K would be found in this box. However, a master list would still be needed to easily find a chart, as it may be difficult to determine in which year a patient terminated treatment.

Labeling boxes with clearly defined content indicators can allow them to be stored in a logical sequence. This makes these boxes, and the files that they contain, much easier to locate.

Because many patients may have the same or similar names, it is important to create a master list that provides the details needed to locate the correct medical chart. This is often done by listing the name of the box at the top of the master list page (Figure 3-7 ●). The medical charts included in that box are then listed in alphabetical order by the patients' last names. Another piece of identifying information also can be included, such as the patients' birth dates.

If the medical office has been around for a while, there may be a large number of boxes in storage (Figure 3-8 ●). In this case, listing the contents in each box may not be practical. These medical offices often create a single list of all charts that are in storage. This list includes the names of the patients on the charts, the identifying information (e.g., birth dates or account numbers), and the name of the box in which the charts can be found.

Many medical providers use a storage service to help with file management and storage. The medical provider's files are placed in specified storage boxes and then placed in a specific location at the storage company. The storage company usually picks up the boxes to be stored, takes them to the facility, and places them in the designated location.

For medical offices using electronic medical records, there are companies that allow providers to store all information on secure servers in a secure facility, with all HIPAA rules followed.

PRACTICE **PITFALLS**

If a file needs to be retrieved from storage, the storage company is contacted and is told to retrieve the needed box and return it to the medical office. The practice then pulls the file from the box.

Because the storage company often charges for each box brought back or forth, it is important to have a master list that indicates the contents of the boxes in storage. You do not want to spend several days shipping the wrong box back and forth.

Electronic Medical Charting

More often than not, software programs for medical billing are including electronic medical charting. Previous computer programs used by the medical office were often limited to billing software. Those that were considered "high-tech" may have included the opportunity to submit the claims electronically rather than just print them on paper and mail them to the insurance carrier.

However, new software programs include a much wider variety of features. Following are some of the most common features, as well as information about how these features could impact the job of the medical biller.

Patient Identification.   In addition to the standard patient information included in software programs (e.g., name, address, employer, insurance information, etc.), many new programs include the addition of a patient photograph. This photo allows the medical staff to ensure they are with the proper patient before services are rendered. It has the added benefit of decreasing fraud caused by one person seeking treatment under a different person's Medicaid or insurance coverage. In addition, it can increase customer satisfaction as medical staff will be able to recognize more patients.

If this type of software is used in the medical office, it often falls to the medical biller or the receptionist to take a quick snapshot of the patient and download it into the computer program. In addition, the patient's information must be added into the program.

Prescription Control.   Some software programs allow the creation of electronic prescriptions. **Electronic prescriptions** are entered into the provider's computer and then sent electronically to the patient's pharmacy.

Electronic prescriptions have many advantages over paper prescriptions, including the following:

- Prescriptions can be sent immediately, without the patient having to carry a paper prescription to the pharmacist.
- There is no danger of the patient losing the prescription.
- The prescription is typed rather than handwritten, preventing medication error due to a provider's illegible handwriting.
- Fewer errors result from pharmacists entering the prescriptions incorrectly into their computer.
- Provider computers can be tied to the patient's chart, thus alerting the provider if there is a possible complication with a patient's medical condition or other medications. The medical office computers can also be tied to a local pharmacy. This provides for direct delivery and helps prevent fraud.

▶ **CRITICAL THINKING QUESTION:** What would be the use of an office keeping a paper record even though the medical office is utilizing computerized files?

Computerized Files

It is now common practice to utilize electronic health records in the medical office. In addition, the Federal Government is providing physicians monetary awards for switching to electronic health records and billing. This is part of the Patient Protection and Affordable Care Act. The physician is given a specified amount of money for complying with EHR adoption, implementation, and use. The medical office can use computers to keep all patient records, including x-rays, in a computerized file.

The provider is able to display a patient's record from anywhere in the office. This allows the provider to have the patient's records at hand as the patient is being treated. The provider, or other clinical staff members, can make notations in the medical record as the treatment is taking place. This can prevent problems caused by providers having to remember what treatment was provided. Sometimes providers will work on several patients at the same time, so it is easy to become confused regarding which patient had which treatment.

The legality of electronically stored records has yet to be established in the courts. In a written record, it is easier to determine when changes have been made to a document. The handwriting or ink color may be different. This also can occur with the electronic record as once the record is signed it is sealed and changes are viewed as appended items.

Regulations for electronic signatures have been implemented to satisfy the previous laws that required a "written signature" for each entry.

An additional problem with computerized files is the issue of vulnerability. Computers, and the records on them, can be hacked into by outsiders. Allowing this information to be shared with anyone, without the patient's approval, is a violation of HIPAA laws.

To protect against electronic sabotage, a committee (HITEC) has been appointed to create and implement guidelines for implementation of electronic health records, including required security measures for such records.

Because much of the patient information is stored in electronic files, it is important to ensure the privacy and security of these files. This includes making sure that all files require a login and password to access them. Security levels must be in place to ensure that people do not have access to records they do not need to do their job.

Everyone in the office must be made aware of the need to maintain the secrecy of their login name and password. To share this information with anyone, even inadvertently, could be considered a violation of HIPAA regulations.

Record Transfers

At times, it may be necessary for a provider to transfer records or medical information to another provider. This is often the case when a patient is referred to a specialist, moves to another area, or begins treatment with another provider. To avoid legal complications, written permission should be obtained by having the patient sign a Release of Information Form. In this form they may specify what information should be transferred and when the transfer should take place. Often a letter such as the one in Figure 3-9 ● is used.

When transferring records or information, do not send the original record or file. Instead, make a copy of all the information to be transferred. The envelope containing the records should be marked "Personal and Confidential." To ensure privacy and confidentiality, most medical offices will send the information via courier, or via registered mail, return receipt requested. The

---

Paul Provider, M.D.
5858 Peppermint Place
Anytown, USA 12345
(765) 555-6768

I,_____(Patient's Name)_____, request and authorize Paul Provider, M.D., to release the following medical information from the medical records of _____

_____ (myself or patient name) to the provider of the facility listed below.

Information to be released: _____

_____

_____

_____

Dates of treatment: From _____ To _____

Information should be sent to:_____

Person _____

Facility _____

Address _____

Street, City, Zip _____

Phone _____

Date information is to be sent _____

I release you from all legal responsibility or liability that may arise from this authorization.

Signed _____ Date _____

FIGURE 3-9

Sample record transfer form

receipt can specify, if necessary, that the information be delivered only to the person to whom it is addressed (e.g., the provider). This ensures that it is not opened by others in the office and handled carelessly. A cover page should be included that states the information contained in the envelope should be considered confidential and is for the express use of and dissemination to only the person to whom it is addressed.

Be sure that only the information the patient has authorized for transfer is sent. If information that has and has not been authorized is on the same page (e.g., information regarding two separate diagnoses), be sure to cover the unauthorized information and make a copy. If it is not possible to cover the information, make a copy of the record, black out the unauthorized information, and then copy the page again. Blacking out prevents the information from being revealed by holding the page up to the light or by other means.

Under no circumstances should patients be allowed to take their original records, or any information from their records, to another provider as it provides opportunity for the patient to alter, falsify, or remove information from the records. Such actions could put both the patient and the provider at risk. For example, a patient may remove the evidence that a certain drug was prescribed in order to get an additional supply of it. Additionally, the new provider may prescribe a drug that is counteractive or could produce an adverse reaction when mixed with the first drug. Keep in mind that patients do have the right to ask for copies of their records and the provider is obligated to provide these copies.

Medical Documentation Forms

Whether the patient has insurance coverage or will be responsible for self-payment for the services, a **claim** or bill for the services rendered by a provider will be prepared. In the following sections we will walk you through the basic forms needed in a medical chart to properly bill for services provided.

When a patient walks into a provider's office for the first time, a patient file must be established and several forms must be filled out. These forms provide all the information needed to treat and bill the patient. The most commonly used forms include the following:

- Patient Information Sheet
- Release of Information Form
- Assignment of Benefits Form
- Patient History Form

Each form has a distinct purpose and, in one style or another, will be present in nearly every provider's office. However, sometimes two or more items are combined on a single form. This is most often true of the Release of Information Form, the Assignment of Benefits Form, and the Patient Information Sheet.

Filling out these forms is relatively simple, as the information called for is self-explanatory. Let's look at each of the forms in greater detail.

Patient Information Sheet

The **Patient Information Sheet**, also sometimes called the Patient Registration Form, is used to collect general information regarding the patient (Figure 3-10 ●). The medical biller should always ensure that the information obtained on the Patient Information Sheet is complete and accurate, as this information will be used for billing and collection and for notifying family members in case of emergency. For those offices using electronic medical records, patients may be asked to complete the registration information online, or a computer may be set up in the reception room that allows the patient to complete the registration form at the time the patient arrives for an appointment (Figure 3-11 ●). The Patient Information Sheet should be updated periodically to ensure its accuracy.

There are various versions of this form, but they all usually request the following basic information:

- Name: first, middle, and last
- Address and telephone number
- Business address, telephone number, and occupation

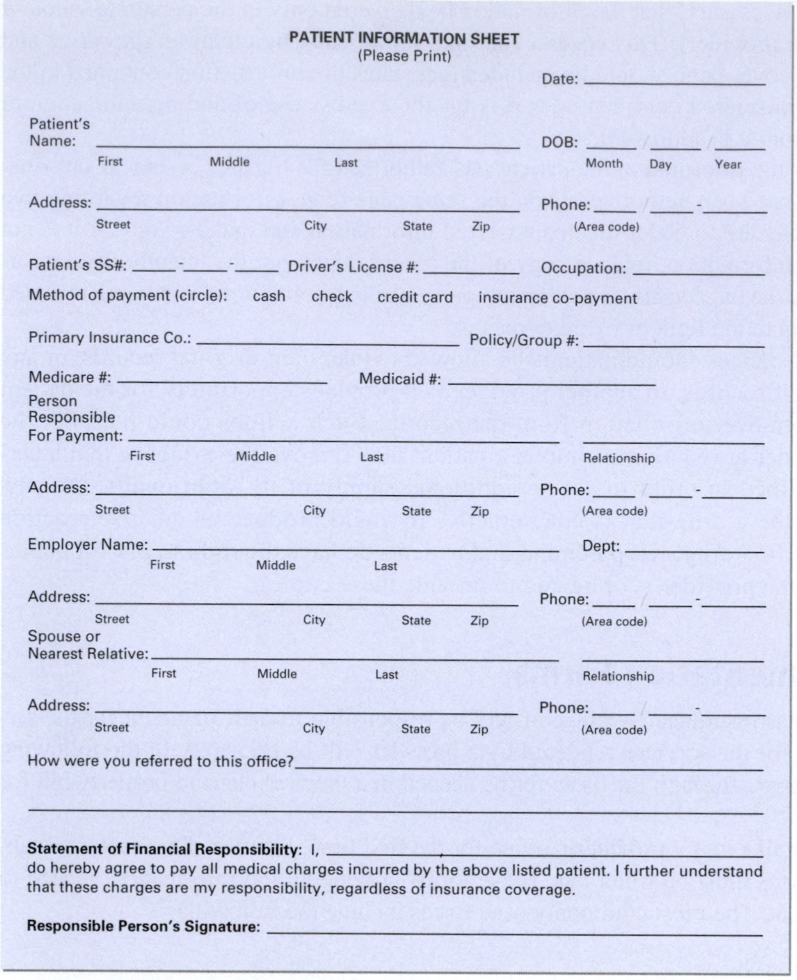

PATIENT INFORMATION SHEET
(Please Print)

Date: ______

Patient's Name: ______ (First, Middle, Last) DOB: ___/___/___ (Month, Day, Year)

Address: ______ (Street, City, State, Zip) Phone: ___/___-___ (Area code)

Patient's SS#: ___-___-___ Driver's License #: ______ Occupation: ______

Method of payment (circle): cash check credit card insurance co-payment

Primary Insurance Co.: ______ Policy/Group #: ______

Medicare #: ______ Medicaid #: ______

Person Responsible For Payment: ______ (First, Middle, Last) ______ (Relationship)

Address: ______ (Street, City, State, Zip) Phone: ___/___-___ (Area code)

Employer Name: ______ (First, Middle, Last) Dept: ______

Address: ______ (Street, City, State, Zip) Phone: ___/___-___ (Area code)

Spouse or Nearest Relative: ______ (First, Middle, Last) ______ (Relationship)

Address: ______ (Street, City, State, Zip) Phone: ___/___-___ (Area code)

How were you referred to this office? ______

Statement of Financial Responsibility: I, ______ do hereby agree to pay all medical charges incurred by the above listed patient. I further understand that these charges are my responsibility, regardless of insurance coverage.

Responsible Person's Signature: ______

FIGURE 3-10

Patient Information Sheet

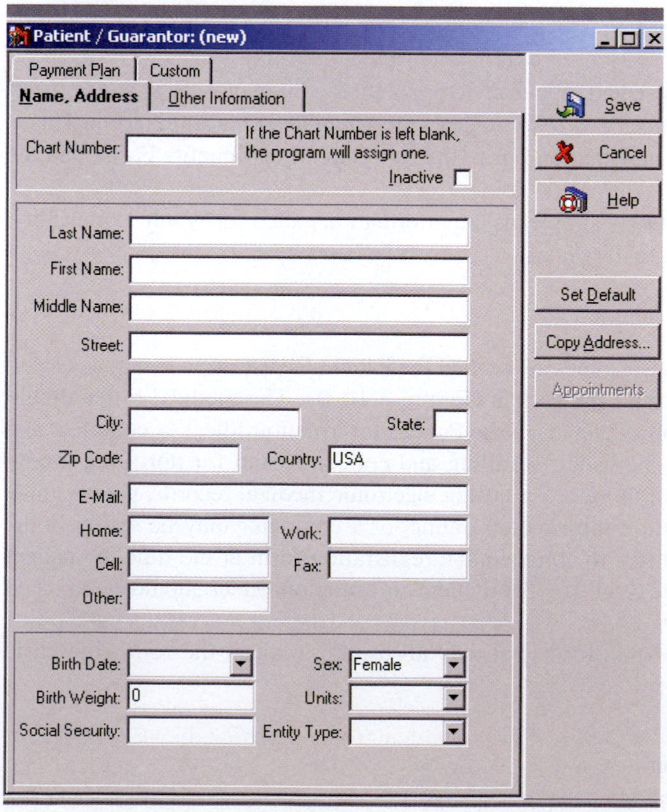

FIGURE 3-11

Electronic Patient Registration Form

- Date of birth
- Social Security number, or the ID number from the patient's insurance, or the driver's license number if the patient does not have insurance
- Person responsible for payment, or insured's name
- Spouse's name and occupation
- Information about patient referral
- Driver's license number
- Emergency contact
- Insurance billing information

Obtain the names, addresses, and policy and group numbers of all carriers insuring the patient. This is important because of coordination of benefits clauses included in most health insurance policies. If the patient has an insurance card, make a copy of the card to keep in the patient's file. Insurance coverage should be verified before rendering services. The insurance information should be rechecked every time the patient comes in for an appointment, as this information may change. For Medicaid patients, the insurance card should be checked at each visit to ensure that coverage still exists.

ACTIVITY #3

Completing Patient Information Sheets

Directions: Complete a Patient Information Sheet and create patient charts for Dr. Paul Provider's office for the following five patients. Individual folders may be used to keep information for each patient. Refer to the Patient Information Table and Provider Information Table in Appendix A for information. (These five patients will be used throughout this guide for illustrative purposes. Other patients may be used as well.)

1. Abby Addison
2. Bobby Brumble
3. Cathy Crenshaw
4. Daisy Doolittle
5. Edward Edmunds

PRACTICE **PITFALLS**

Patients should be asked to present their insurance card and a valid form of identification. This is done to ensure that the person seeking treatment is actually the person to whom the insurance card has been issued. A copy of both the insurance card and identification should be made and placed in the patient's chart.

GUARANTOR. A **guarantor** is a person who undertakes the responsibility for payment of a debt. This situation is most commonly presented in a medical practice when services are rendered for care of a child. The parent or guardian of that child is legally obligated for payment of the child's medical services. A form should be signed indicating that the guarantor will be responsible for the payment fees for medical services rendered. This signature requirement is usually located on the Patient Information Sheet. An anticipated insurance payment does not replace the guarantor's obligation to pay any outstanding balance.

EMANCIPATED MINOR. **Emancipation** is a legal process whereby a child assumes responsibility for himself or herself, and the child's parent or legal guardian is no longer legally responsible for the child. A child can become an **emancipated minor** in several ways. In some states, a minor can become emancipated just by claiming so; in other states, court approval is required. However,

FIGURE 3-12

Sample Encounter Form

Pearson Physicians Group   312-123-1234

Patient Number	Ticket Number	Service Date	Prior Balance
			Pat
Patient Name		Gender	Ins
Address		Phone	Other
SSN	Referring Dr.		Total
Primary Insurance Co.	Policy/Group ID		Paymt
Secondary Insurance Co.	Policy/Group ID		Bal Due

Location

Cardiologist

☐ Other:

X	Code	Service
		New Patient
	99203	Limited/Simple (30m)
	99204	Comprehensive (45m)
	99205	Complex (60m)
		New Patient Consult (Need Referring MD)
	99243	Brief (40m)
	99244	Full Consult (60m)
	99245	Very Complex (80m)
		Established Patient
	99211	Nurse Visit
	99212	Very Brief FU (10m)
	99213	Limited/Simple FU (15m)
	99214	Comprehensive FU (25m)
	99215	Complex FU (40m)
		New Cons. 2nd Opin.
	99274	Moderate 2nd Opinion
	99275	Complex 2nd Opinion
		Home Health
	99375	Home Health 30 days
		Drugs:
	J3420	B-12 Injection
	J1940	Lasix
	90724	Flu (Dx V-04.8)
	G0008	MC Flu Admin Fee
		Misc Rx
	90782	IM Injections
	90784	IV Injections
	A4615	O2 Cannula

X	Code	Service
		Office Procedures
	93000	EKG w/ Interp
	93015	Stress Tread w/ Interp
	93040	Rhythm strip w/ Interp
	93307	2D Echo Compl.
	93320	Doppler Compl.
	93325	Color Flow Compl.
	93308	2D Echo F/U
	93321	Doppler F/U
	ES	Stress Echo
	BUB	Echo/Bubble/Doppler
		Event Monitor
	93268	Loop- Non MC
	G0005	Loop - Hookup - MC
	G0007	Loop - Interp - MC
	93012	Chest Plate Tech - Non MC
	93014	Chest PI - Interp Non MC
	G0016	Chest PI - Interp MC
		Holter Monitor
	93224	Holter w/ Interp Global
		Other
	92960	Cardioversion
	93734	Pacer Eval - Single
	93735	Pacer Eval - Sngl w/ Prg
	93731	Pacer Eval - Dual
	93732	Pacer Eval - Dual w/ Prg
	99499	Review outside records
	99080	Special Reports

X	Code	Service
		Diagnostic w/o Interp (Technical only)
	93005	EKG
	93017	Stress Tread
	93225	Holter Hookup
	93226	Holter Scan
	93307-TC	2D Echo
	93320-TC	Doppler Compl.
	93325-TC	Color Flow
	93308-TC	2D Echo F/U
	93321-TC	Doppler F/U
	93880-TC	Carotid Doppler
	Phys	**Interpretation**-Supervision, Interpretation & Report Only
	93010	EKG Interp & Reortt only
	TR	Regular Stress Test–S, I & R
	NU	Nuclear Stress Test–S, I & R
	ES-26	Stress Echocardiogram–S, I & R
	307	Echocardiogram 2-D
	320-26	Doppler Echocardiogram
	325-26	Color Flow
	308	Echocardiogram 2-D F/U
	321-26	Doppler F/U
	227	Holter Monitor - I & R only
	71250-26	UltraFast CT
	XXXXX	**LAB ORDERED** (see attached sheet)
	36415	VeniPuncture (non MC)
	99000	Specimen Collection (Lab)

Next Appointment:
Return in: ___ (Wks) (Mo) (Yr)

Before next appointment:
☐ Ekg ☐ Echo ☐ Doppler ☐ CXR ☐ Event Monitor
☐ TM ☐ Stress Echo ☐ CFD ☐ Holter ☐ Lab

BI:

Hospital Admission:
☐ Admit Cath
☐ Admit to _____ unit at:

☐ BAP ☐ WMC ☐ CMC ☐ SHMC
☐ Other:

Notes:

Cardiac Diagnoses

regardless of the process used to attain emancipation, once a minor is considered emancipated, the child is entitled to make his or her own medical decisions and also is responsible for payment for any medical services received.

Encounter Form

Encounter Forms are used to record both clinical and financial information about the patient's visit and are used as billing and routing documents. These forms also are referred to as charge tickets, fee slips, and superbills in the provider's office, and as a chargemaster in the hospital. The Encounter Form should be filled out and attached to the front of the patient's medical chart when a patient comes for a visit. These forms should be sequentially numbered so that they may all be accounted for.

To fully capture revenue, the Encounter Form is submitted to the billing department and the biller transfers the information onto a CMS-1500 Form. When this form is completed, it should contain all the patient's insurance information, demographic information, diagnosis and procedure codes, pricing, and physician information. An example of an Encounter Form is shown in Figure 3-12 ●.

Release of Information Form

The **Release of Information Form** is used to allow the provider to request additional information from other providers of service or to share information with an insurance carrier (Figure 3-13 ●).

PAUL PROVIDER, M.D.
5858 PEPPERMINT PLACE
ANYTOWN, USA 12345
(765) 555-6768

RELEASE OF INFORMATION FORM

I AUTHORIZE any provider, medical practitioner, hospital, clinic, or other medical or medically related facility, insurance or reinsurance company, the Medical Information Bureau, Inc., consumer reporting agency, or employer having information available as to diagnosis, treatment, and prognosis with respect to any physical or mental condition, and/or treatment of me or my minor children and any other non-medical information about me and my minor children to give to the group policyholder, my employer, or its legal representative any and all such information.

I UNDERSTAND the information obtained by the use of this Authorization will be used to determine eligibility for insurance, and eligibility for benefits under any existing policy. Any information obtained will not be released by/to any person or organization EXCEPT to the group policyholder, my employer, reinsuring companies, or other persons or organizations performing business or legal services in connection with my application, claim, or as may be otherwise lawfully required or as I may further authorize.

I KNOW that I may request to receive a copy of this Authorization.

I AGREE that a photographic copy of this Authorization shall be as valid as the original.

I AGREE this Authorization shall be valid for one year from the date shown below.

Signature of Insured and/or Spouse _____ Date _____

Name(s) of minor child(ren) _____

FIGURE 3-13

Release of Information Form

If the provider submits an insurance claim for the patient, the patient must sign a Release of Information Form before information may be given to an insurance company, attorney, or other third party. According to the HIPAA Privacy Rule, it is illegal to release any information regarding a patient without the patient's knowledge and written consent.

The patient's signature is good for the length of time indicated on the form, allowing the provider to release the information requested for one year maximum. If the patient is a child, the parent or guardian must sign the release. Often a release-of-information statement is included on the actual claim form describing treatment. This brief statement does not take the place of having a completed and signed Release of Information Form in the patient's file.

Request for Additional Information Form

The **Request for Additional Information Form** is designed for gathering information or records from various sources. The medical biller will usually use a Request for Additional Information Form to request additional information needed to bill for services rendered. All information needed from a particular source should be requested at the same time.

Assignment of Benefits Form

The **Assignment of Benefits Form** is a request for all insurance payments to be directed to the provider holding the assignment (Figure 3-14 ●). Most providers consider this a necessity for those patients who have insurance, because the assignment ensures that monies paid for services provided are issued directly to the provider and not to the patient or subscriber. Assignment of benefits indicates that the payer is authorized to send payment directly to the provider of services. The Assignment of Benefits Form should be signed, dated (preferably date stamped), and

---

PAUL PROVIDER, M.D.
5858 PEPPERMINT PLACE
ANYTOWN, USA 12345
(765) 555-6768

ASSIGNMENT OF BENEFITS

I authorize payment directly to the above named provider of medical expense benefits otherwise payable to me but not to exceed my indebtedness to said provider for any services furnished to me by that provider.

The signature on this form or a photocopy is valid for one year from the date indicated.

Signature _____ Date _____

FIGURE 3-14

Assignment of Benefits Form

attached to the insurance verification form. If the patient has signed an Assignment of Benefits, you would type "Signature on File" (or "SOF") in the signature field on the claims form or other document to indicate that payment is to be made to the provider. The information contained on an Assignment of Benefits Form may be contained at the bottom of a Patient Information Sheet. If this is the case, there is no need for the patient to sign an additional form to authorize assignment of benefits.

Patient History Form

The **Patient History Form** is important to the provider (Figure 3-15 ●). It helps identify previous medical history that may be important in treating the patient's present condition. This is usually a detailed form with basic health questions requiring only yes or no answers. (Patient History Forms are more extensive than shown in Figure 3-15, which is for sample purposes only.) The provider gives the patient a complete physical in the exam room and includes the findings on the Patient History Form. Some providers may dictate a medical history report (see Chapter 14: The CMS-1500 Form and Medical Billing Procedures).

The Patient Information Sheet, Release of Information Form, Assignment of Benefits Form, and Patient History Form should all be completed by the patient at the time of the first visit. In an effort to simplify patient registration, some physician offices will mail the Patient History Form to the patient's home so it can be filled out and brought to the initial visit. Physician offices with electronic records may put these forms on their Web site. However, it is the job of the person receiving the forms from the patient to ensure that these forms are complete. If the answer to a question is "no," the patient should write the word "no" in the field. If the information is not applicable, the patient should write "N/A" in the field. This ensures that the patient has looked at and responded to all of the fields. This can prevent problems when a patient mistakenly skips over a question, particularly when the answer could be important for proper care.

Insurance Verification

An **Insurance Coverage Form** is used to verify and document insurance coverage information. The patient's portion of the charges is usually collected at the time service is rendered. Each office has a standard form for verification of coverage. Figure 3-16 ● shows a sample Insurance Coverage Form that can be used if information is being manually tracked.

This form covers much of the pertinent information needed to determine the patient's portion of the claim, and it assists in gaining the maximum reimbursement for the patient. Maximum reimbursement may be obtained by following any requirements set forth in the insurance contract, such as obtaining preauthorization for certain services or taking advantage of benefits that

Paul Provider, M.D.
5858 Peppermint Place
Anytown, USA 12345
(765) 555-6768

Patient History

Date: _____

Patient Name _____ Age _____

Any allergies to food or medicine?   No   Yes
If yes: Allergic to _____

Have you ever been hospitalized?   No   Yes
If yes: Indicate date and reason_____

Have you ever been diagnosed or experienced:

Bladder Infections	_____	Underweight	_____	Anemia	_____
Ear Infections	_____	Epilepsy	_____	Overweight	_____
Sinus Infections	_____	Seizures	_____	Hay Fever	_____
Vision Problems	_____	Mumps	_____	Chickenpox	_____
Frequent Headaches	_____	Sickle Cell Anemia	_____	Heart Murmur	_____

Other _____

Are you currently taking any medication(s)?
If yes: Name of medication(s) _____

Date of last Tuberculosis and/or Tetanus shot: _____

Check any of the following that any blood relative has or has had:

Anemia	_____	Heart Disease	_____	Thyroid Problems	_____
Sickle Cell Anemia	_____	Heart Attack	_____	Diabetes	_____
Stroke	_____	Birth Defects	_____	Asthma	_____
Cancer	_____	Mental Retardation	_____	Kidney Disease	_____
Tuberculosis	_____	Alcoholism	_____	High Blood Pressure	_____

Patient Signature: _____ Date: _____

FIGURE 3-15

Patient History Form

Paul Provider, M.D.
5858 Peppermint Place
Anytown, USA 12345
(765) 555-6768

Insurance Coverage Form

INSURED: _____ BIRTH DATE: _____

SSN: _____ EFFECTIVE DATE: _____

INSURANCE POLICY: _____

ADDRESS: _____

ID/MEMBER #: _____ GROUP #: _____

DEPENDENT AGE LIMIT: _____

_____

INDIV. DEDUCTIBLE AMOUNT: _____ 3 MO CARRYOVER: _____

FAMILY DEDUCTIBLE: _____ AGGREGATE/NONAGGREGATE

STANDARD COINSURANCE: _____ LIFETIME MAXIMUM: _____

COINSURANCE LIMIT _____

_____

BENEFITS PAID AT OTHER THAN THE STANDARD COINSURANCE % [Including benefit, coinsurance amount and special circumstances (i.e., SSO allowed at 100%, required for hysterectomy, coronary bypass, etc.)]:

_____

_____

PREAUTHORIZATION REQUIRED FOR: _____

_____

_____

ACCIDENT BENEFIT AMOUNT: _____ TREATMENT TO BE RECEIVED WITHIN _____ DAYS

OTHER NOTES/COMMENTS: _____

_____

TOTAL PAYMENTS (CCYY)

Indicate below the names of the insured and his or her dependents. When any of the following information is received, write it in pencil followed by the date. This will help you to realize when a patient's deductible has been met and if the patient is nearing any maximum benefit.

	INSURED	DEPENDENT	DEPENDENT	DEPENDENT	DEPENDENT
NAME:	_____	_____	_____	_____	_____
DEDUCTIBLE:	_____	_____	_____	_____	_____
COINS PD:	_____	_____	_____	_____	_____
LIFETIME:	_____	_____	_____	_____	_____

FIGURE 3-16

Insurance Coverage Form

might be paid at a higher percentage (e.g., preadmission testing, outpatient instead of inpatient surgeries, etc.).

Some forms will contain room for information on family members so that family deductible and coinsurance maximum amounts can be tracked.

> ### PRACTICE **PITFALLS**
>
> Make sure you get preauthorization or preapproval of benefits for services specifically indicated in the contract that require such. Otherwise, a payment penalty may be imposed, which will significantly reduce the benefits paid, or benefits may be completely denied.

The insurance carrier must be contacted in order to complete this form accurately. During the call, provide the insurance carrier with the name of the patient, the name of the insured, and the policy name/number. The carrier can then provide the information needed to complete each field.

Some carriers may prefer to have the Insurance Coverage Sheet faxed to them rather than spend time on the phone. If this is the case, also fax the Release of Information Form with the patient's signature on it.

ACTIVITY #4

Completing Insurance Coverage Forms

Directions: Using the Patient Information Table and the Insurance Carrier Contracts found in Appendix A, complete an Insurance Coverage Form for Abby Addison, Bobby Brumble, Cathy Crenshaw, Daisy Doolittle, and Edward Edmunds.

Additional Suggestions

There are a number of things to keep in mind when dealing with patients. Of course, client service should always be your first and foremost concern, but at the same time you need to have regard for the medical office. It is important to obtain all necessary information from the patient. Remember that one of the primary objectives of the medical biller is to minimize the amount of time between the provider's service and the complete reimbursement of the bill. Getting the bill paid quickly is also a service to patients, so they are assured that their insurance will pay the bill and they do not have worry about large medical bills. The information that can facilitate this process may include the following:

1. Ask the patient to fill out all necessary forms for setting up the patient file. Give the patient sufficient time to fill out the forms and check that they are complete before accepting them. Many offices mail the forms to the patient before their first visit to ensure their completeness.
2. Be sure you understand the policies of the office for which you work regarding the completion of forms and payment for bills. This way you can explain them accurately to the patient at the time of the first visit.
3. Use the office forms consistently and accurately so tracking information runs smoothly, regardless of who enters the information.
4. Secure all the details of the insurance information. If the patient or insured has a card, make a copy of it for your files. Make sure the information contains the subscriber's name, the policy number, the effective date, the company that holds the policy or the name of the policy, and the insurance carrier's address.
5. Make sure the patient understands the provider's policy regarding any amounts that the insurance carrier does not pay or does not cover.

Summary

- Maintaining patient files in a proper manner is one of a medical biller's most important jobs.
- The medical biller/receptionist, medical assistant, and the provider are the individuals most likely responsible for maintenance of the patient chart.
- It is important that everyone who makes notations in a patient chart follows the rules of proper medical charting.
- It is important for the medical biller to know how to properly store charts and how to retrieve stored charts.
- SOAP notes may be useful in abstracting information for billing purposes.
- Several forms must be included in all medical charts. These forms include the Patient Information Sheet, the Assignment of Benefits Form, the Authorization to Release Information Form, and the Patient History Form. Many of these forms will need to be completed by the patient at the time of the first visit.

Review Questions

Directions: Answer the following questions without looking back into the material just covered. Write your answers in the space provided.

1. What are ten of the fifteen medical documentation rules?

   a. _____

   b. _____

   c. _____

   d. _____

   e. _____

   f. _____

   g. _____

   h. _____

   i. _____

   j. _____

2. What information do you need on a master list when storing patient records?

   _____

   _____

3. What is alphabetical filing?

   _____

   _____

4. How long should you keep medical records, and why?

   _____

   _____

5. What three people often will be involved in documenting in a patient chart?

   _____

_____

_____

6. List five of the items that should be included on the Patient Information Sheet.

_____

_____

_____

_____

7. What is the purpose of the Patient Information Sheet? _____

_____

_____

8. Define the term *provider.* _____

_____

_____

9. What is the purpose of the Insurance Coverage Sheet? _____

_____

_____

10. What is an Assignment of Benefits Form? _____

_____

_____

If you are unable to answer any of these questions, refer back to that section in the chapter, and then fill in the answers.

Activity #5: Matching Key Terms

Directions: Match the following terms with the proper definition by writing the letter of the correct definition in the space next to the term.

1. _____ Assignment of Benefits Form

   a. A form used to allow the provider to request additional information from other providers of service or to share information with an insurance carrier

2. _____ Electronic prescriptions

   b. A form used to collect general information regarding the patient

3. _____ Insurance Coverage Form

   c. A form designed to ask for information or records from various sources

4. _____ Patient Information Sheet

   d. A form used by many practices to verify insurance coverage and document this information

5. _____ Release of Information Form

   e. A form requesting all insurance payments to be directed to the provider holding the assignment

6. _____ Request for Additional Information Form

   f. Prescriptions that are entered into the provider's computer, then electronically sent to the computer at the patient's pharmacy

SECTION
HEALTH INSURANCE PROGRAMS

2

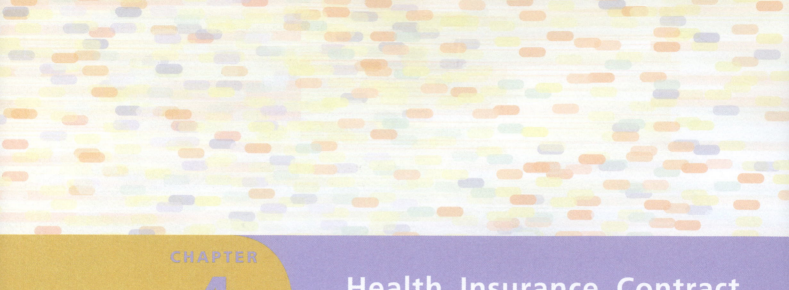

Health Insurance Contract Interpretation

Key Words and Concepts you will learn in this chapter:

Accident

Actively-at-work provision

Aggregate deductible

Allowed amount

Authorized Treatment Record Form

Basic benefits

Carryover provision

Coinsurance

Concurrent review

Conversion factor

Coordination of benefits (COB)

Copayment

Deductible

Eligibility

Exclusions

Family deductible

Fee-for-service

Fee schedule

Geographical Cost Practice Index (GPCI)

Health Savings Account (HSA)

Indemnity insurance plans

Insurance premium

Mandatory program

After completion of this chapter you should be able to:

Describe indemnity plans.

Define the basic terms used in an insurance contract.

Explain how the various elements of a contract can affect billing.

Properly complete a Treatment Authorization Request Form.

Describe the common basic benefits that are included in a contract.

Accurately calculate deductible amounts given a contract and scenario.

Describe how major medical limits can affect the insurance carrier's payment on a claim.

Explain what COBRA is and how it affects coverage for preexisting conditions.

Explain how exclusions and allowed amounts can affect payment on a claim.

Describe the precertification process.

Mental health expenses
Nonaggregate deductible
Order of Benefit Determination (OBD)
Preadmission testing
Preauthorization
Precertify
Preexisting condition
Prospective review
Relative value unit
Relative value scale
Retrospective review
Second surgical opinion (SSO)
consultation
Unnecessary surgery
Usual, Customary, and Reasonable (UCR)
Utilization review
Voluntary program

Describe what utilization review is and how it can affect benefit payments.

List situations in which a surgery may be considered unnecessary.

State the purposes of second surgical opinions and how they can affect claim payments.

Describe the two types of second surgical opinion programs.

List the thirteen Order of Benefit Determination rules.

Interpreting and understanding contracts is one of the most important aspects of being a medical biller. The health care contract is the one document that is used to determine the benefits that the insurance carrier will pay for services rendered.

The wording and terminology of health insurance contracts can often be confusing to someone who is not well versed in the insurance field. For this reason, medical billers often will be called on to interpret the provisions of a contract for billing purposes or to explain benefits to a patient.

Also, many medical practices prefer to collect the patient's portion of the bill (that portion not covered by insurance) at the time services are rendered (Figure 4-1 ●). To properly calculate the amount due from the patient, it is important that medical billers be able to interpret the benefits covered in the contract.

FIGURE 4-1

A medical biller collecting payment from a patient
© Michal Heron/Pearson Education

In addition, an astute medical biller should be able to explain the policy options to the patient or provider. For example, a contract may provide 100 percent coverage for certain services that are performed on an outpatient basis. If a patient has inpatient surgery scheduled for a listed procedure, it can be beneficial for the medical biller to inform the provider of the increased payment for outpatient surgery. It is then up to the provider and the patient to determine if the increased coverage is beneficial to the patient in the particular circumstance or situation.

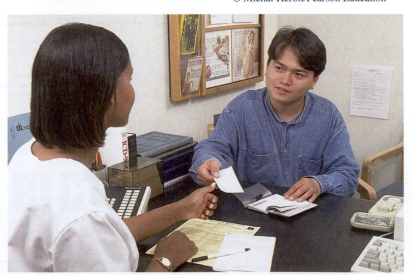

Indemnity Insurance Plans

Indemnity insurance plans, also called **fee-for-service**, have been the traditional form of commercial health insurance. Indemnity insurance is a principle of insurance that provides medical coverage when a loss occurs and restores the insured party to the approximate financial condition he or she was in had before the loss occurred. Under an indemnity plan, the covered person chooses his or her own physician, specialist, hospital, or other provider. Indemnity plans require the insured person to pay an **insurance premium** (the actual amount of money charged by insurance companies for active coverage). Once the plan has become active, the insured person has a deductible that must be paid. The **deductible** is a predetermined portion of annual out-of-pocket medical expenses. These plans also require the covered person to pay a predetermined percentage of additional annual expenses up to a preset maximum; that share is called the coinsurance requirement.

These plans often pay benefits at a set amount, such as 80 percent of the covered services. The patient is responsible for the remaining 20 percent, as well as any amounts not covered by the insurance carrier (Figure 4-2 ●).

The concepts discussed in this chapter apply to all types of contracts, including Blue Cross/Blue Shield (BC/BS), managed care contracts (discussed more fully in Chapter 10) and preferred provider plans. Although many people consider BC/BS to be different from other insurance carriers, in truth BC/BS contracts cover many of the same procedures and have many of the same benefits as other indemnity plans.

▶ **CRITICAL THINKING QUESTION:** Why is it important for the medical biller to be able to interpret insurance contracts?

FIGURE 4-2

A sample of a Blue Cross Blue Shield card that indicates the patient responsibilities, such as deductible and co-pay

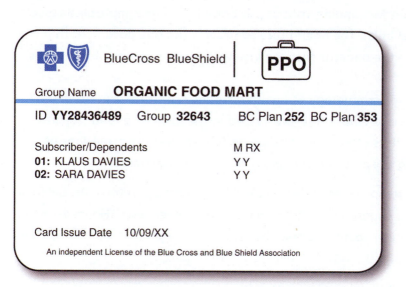

Contract Provisions

Billers who are familiar with the provisions of a specific contract may be able to provide added benefits related to the scheduling of a patient or the manner in which a claim is filed.

Appendix A contains the information for three company contracts. You are familiar with the information in these contracts from when you completed the patient Insurance Coverage Forms in Chapter 3. In this chapter, we once again refer to these contracts but for the purpose of enhancing an understanding of the types of provisions that can be seen in contracts.

Eligibility

The first item that is considered in the contract is **eligibility**, or the qualifications that make the person eligible for coverage. To be eligible for benefits under most group insurance policies, the member must be a full-time employee at the company. For example, in the Creative Creations Corporation/White Corporation contract, an employee must work a minimum of thirty hours per week to be covered by this contract. The contract also covers anyone who is considered a dependent of the employee. Keep in mind that companies sometimes offer benefits to part-time employees but at a higher cost.

Of course, if a person has purchased individual coverage and is not associated with the employer, no minimum work requirement would apply. However, there would still be qualifications for coverage of a dependent under this plan (Figure 4-3 ●).

Coverage for children has changed with federal legislation introduced in 2010. This legislation states that health plans that offer dependent coverage must offer health insurance to enrollees' adult children age twenty-six and younger, even if the adult children no longer live with their parents, are not dependents on their parents' tax return, or are no longer students. This new rule applies to both married and unmarried children, although their spouses and children do not qualify for coverage.

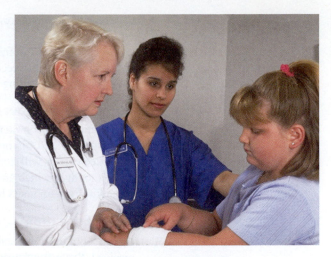

FIGURE 4-3

A child being treated by a provider

© Michal Heron/Pearson Education

ACTIVITY #1

Determining Eligibility Requirements

Directions: Review the company contracts in Appendix A and answer the following questions.

What are the eligibility requirements for:

Creative Creations Corporation/White Corporation _____

_____

_____

Rover Insurers, Inc./Red Corporation _____

_____

_____

Ball Insurance Carrier/Blue Corporation _____

_____

_____

Effective Date

The next item to be considered is whether or not the contract was in force at the time the services were rendered. This often is defined as the minimum length of time that an employee has worked for a company.

There also is an **actively-at-work provision** that is included in many contracts. The actively-at-work provision states that a person must be at work (or actively engaged in his or her normal activities) on the date coverage becomes effective. If the enrollee is not at work or actively engaged in his or her normal activities, the contract does not become effective until the employee returns to work.

As a medical biller, it is important to verify that a patient is covered under an insurance policy and eligible to receive benefits. Medical offices will typically contact the insurance company prior to performing a procedure to ensure that the patient is covered.

Termination of Coverage

This section of a contract provides information regarding when coverage will terminate for both the employee and his or her dependents. It is important to note when coverage ceases as the insurance carrier will not pay benefits after this date. Coverage will often continue until the end of the month in which an employee terminates. If this is the case, it would be important to schedule any follow-up visits before the end of that month.

Preauthorization

A number of insurance carriers require that certain benefits be preauthorized before the services are received. **Preauthorization** is the means of clarifying what charges the insurance carrier will cover for services that are to be performed, as well as obtaining approval to perform those services.

Many insurance carriers have a standard Preauthorization Request Form (Figure 4-4 ●). This form is used to give the insurance carrier information regarding the patient, the diagnosis, and the procedures to be performed.

To complete a Preauthorization Request Form, you must enter the following information:

Name of Patient: Enter the name of the patient who will receive the services.

Address: Enter the patient's address.

City, State, Zip: Enter the city, state, and zip code of the patient.

Sex: Enter M for male or F for female.

Marital Status: Enter the patient's marital status. This is especially important when the patient is a dependent of the insured.

Date of Birth: Enter the patient's date of birth.

Insurance Policy Name/Group Number: Enter the insurance policy name or number under which the patient is insured.

Name of Insured: Enter the name of the insured. This may be a spouse or parent of the patient. In rare instances it may be a different relation to the insured (e.g., the patient is a grandchild of the insured and the insured has custody). The relationship should be indicated.

Treatment Authorized By/Treatment Authorization Number: If treatment is to be authorized, all individuals who have provided authorization should be noted along with any authorization number that may have been received.

Diagnosis Description: Enter the English-language description of the patient's illness, injury, or condition.

ICD-9-CM or ICD-10-CM Code: Enter the ICD-9-CM or ICD-10-CM code(s) associated with the patient's condition. These codes indicate the patient's diagnosis.

Reason for Services: Describe the reason or the medical justification for the services that will be rendered. If necessary, include any laboratory reports, x-rays, pictures, or other documentation to justify the need for services.

Specific Services: Enter the specific services for which the provider is seeking authorization. These should be identified by specific CPT or HCPCS procedure codes (which identify service or item). Each service or item should be listed on a separate line.

Units: Enter the number of units or the number of times the provider estimates this service should be performed (e.g., 10 for requesting 10 psychiatric visits).

Charges: Enter the charges for each service or item. This should be the charge for a single unit of service, not the total amount for all the units being requested.

Signature: The provider must sign the Preauthorization Request.

In addition to preauthorization, precertification and/or predetermination are sometimes needed. *Precertification*, as discussed in Chapter 3, is sometimes required by insurance companies. To **precertify** means to get preapproval from the insurance company for admission for elective, non-emergency hospitalization or other procedures deemed by the insurance company as

Paul Provider, M.D.
5858 Peppermint Place
Anytown, USA 12345

PREAUTHORIZATION REQUEST

Name of Patient: _____

Address: _____

City, State, Zip: _____

Sex: _____   Marital Status: _____   Date of Birth: _____

Insurance Policy Name/Group Number: _____

Name of Insured: _____

Treatment authorized by: _____

Treatment authorization number: _____

Diagnosis Description: _____

_____

ICD-9-CM or ICD-10-CM Code(s): _____

Reason for Services: _____

_____

_____

_____

_____

Specific services you are requesting authorization for: _____

___CPT Code: _____   Units: _____   Charges: _____

_____

_____

_____

_____

_____

I hereby certify that the above information is true and correct to the best of my knowledge.

Signature: _____   Date: _____

FIGURE 4-4

Preauthorization Request Form

needing precertification. *Predetermination* involves the provider sending the patient's insurance carrier a statement listing proposed treatments and/or tests. The insurance company will typically respond with a statement of the amount of reimbursement the company will pay for the test or treatment. Some insurance companies do not require predetermination, whereas most require precertification. The difference between predetermination and preauthorization is that with predetermination the medical office is providing the insurance company information to determine if the insurance carrier agrees with the provider that the proposed treatment is required. When obtaining preauthorization, the treatment necessity is not in question; rather, authorization for the treatment is being obtained.

PAUL PROVIDER, M.D.
5858 Peppermint Place
Anytown, USA 12345
(765) 555-6768

Authorized Treatment Record Form

Patient Name: _____

Policy Name: _____

Above patient has been authorized for the following treatment(s):

    Diagnosis: _____

    Authorized Procedure(s): _____

    Allowed Number of Treatments: _____

    Treatment Authorized by: _____

    Treatment Authorization Number: _____

TREATMENT RECORD

Visit	Date	Procedure(s)	Provider
1			
2			
3			
4			
5			
6			
7			
8			
9			
10			
11			
12			
13			
14			
15			
16			
17			
18			
19			
20			

FIGURE 4-5

Authorized Treatment Record Form

Authorized Treatment Record Form

An **Authorized Treatment Record Form** (Figure 4-5 ●) is used to track the performance of predetermined services rendered by a provider's office. Once the medical office receives the preauthorization request back from the insurance carrier, the treatments provided for those particular services should be tracked using the Authorized Treatment Record Form.

Contract Benefits

The next section of the contract usually details the benefits that the contract covers. These can include basic benefits and major medical benefits. Premiums are based on the number and amount of benefits that a contract covers; the greater the coverage, the higher the cost of the premiums. For example, a contract that covers charges at 90 percent of the allowed amount (allowed amounts are discussed later) and has a $100 deductible usually will cost more than a comparable contract that covers charges at 70 percent of the allowed amount and has a $250 deductible.

Basic Benefits

Basic benefits are those benefits usually paid at 100 percent and before major medical benefits are paid. The Affordable Care Act mandates that certain preventative services are covered at 100 percent, although these services will change, the listing of this coverage is in the basic benefits section. Therefore, it is possible for the insurance plan to pay basic benefits even when the patient has not yet met the deductible. Most basic benefit plans have been replaced with managed care plans.

Some contracts have a basic benefit that is based on the unit value (a number based on the difficulty of a procedure and the overhead needed; see "Allowed Amount") being multiplied by a basic **conversion factor** (see Ball Insurance Carrier contract in Appendix A). This allows a small portion of most services to be paid at 100 percent with the remaining portion paid at the normal coinsurance percentage. These types of basic benefits do not apply to all procedures.

Accident Benefits

One of the most common basic benefits is an accident benefit. An **accident** is defined as an unintentional injury that has a specific time, date, and place. Under the Creative Creations Corporation/White Corporation contract, the first $300 of services that are a result of an accident occurrence are paid at 100 percent. After that, the remaining charges are paid at 90 percent. This benefit is for the first $300 of charges that are incurred within 120 days of the date of the accident, so follow-up care should be scheduled within that 120-day period to get the higher rate. Also, be aware that if other providers charge for the same accident, it is the first $300 of *all* charges that are paid at the 100 percent benefit. Remember, if Tommy Tucker gets hit by a car, there may be ambulance charges, hospital charges, provider's charges, X-ray technician charges, and other charges. Thus, it is important to get your claim in as quickly as possible to ensure the provider you work for is reimbursed at 100 percent and not at 90 percent.

ACTIVITY #2

Determining Accident Benefits

Directions: Study the contracts in Appendix A and answer the following questions.

What are the terms of the accident benefit for:

Creative Creations Corporation/White Corporation _____

_____

_____

Rover Insurers, Inc./Red Corporation _____

_____

_____

Ball Insurance Carrier/Blue Corporation _____

_____

_____

In addition, services provided due to an accident should be indicated as such on the bill. On the CMS-1500 claim form, the place is boxes 10b and 10c, and the date of the accident is indicated in box 14. (The CMS-1500 claim form will be explained in detail in Chapter 14.) If the office does not use the CMS-1500, there may be another place to indicate that this was an accident, or that information should be typed on the bottom of the bill. Such data also should be noted in the patient's chart so that when the Explanation of Benefits (EOB) is received from the insurance carrier, it can be determined if the correct benefits were applied (e.g., the bill was paid at 100 percent).

Preadmission Testing

In the past, a patient would enter the hospital the day before surgery for routine tests such as a chest x-ray and a blood test. The hospital would then admit the patient and watch to ensure that he or she had nothing to eat or drink during the twenty-four hours before the surgery. Insurance carriers realized there would be a great savings if the patient were to visit the hospital for the tests, return home, and then return the next day for the surgery, which would eliminate their payment for an overnight stay in the hospital.

To encourage this practice, some insurance companies began offering an extra incentive for **preadmission testing**, or testing done before the patient enters the hospital for surgery. Some insurance carriers now cover these charges at 100 percent rather than at their normal coinsurance percentage.

Tests performed at the facility where the patient will be admitted, and performed within twenty-four hours of admittance, are usually allowed under this benefit. If it is appropriate for the patient's condition, this option should be considered and the patient made aware of it.

Second Surgical Opinions

Some insurance carriers cover a second surgical opinion at 100 percent. This originally started out as a cost-cutting measure. The hope was that only those surgeries that were considered necessary would be approved, with some patients receiving alternative (and less expensive) treatments, or that treatment would be considered completely unnecessary.

Second surgical opinions have become less popular among insurance carriers because the cost savings seems to be minimal, if any. Many providers are reluctant to go against the word or prescribed treatments of another provider. They do not want to contradict their peers or open themselves up to a lawsuit by suggesting a less radical treatment that may eventually prove less effective. Therefore, they often will simply confirm the diagnosis and the prescribed treatment of the original provider.

Outpatient Facility Charges

Some surgeries are simple or routine enough to be performed on an outpatient basis. This means that the patient enters the facility in the morning, has surgery, and, after a brief recovery period, returns home the same day. There are no overnight or room and board charges. To encourage outpatient surgery when and where possible, some insurance carriers will cover such charges at 100 percent.

ACTIVITY #3

Reading Insurance Contracts to Understand Basic Benefits

Directions: Study the contracts in Appendix A and answer the following questions.

What basic benefits does each contract have?

Creative Creations Corporation/White Corporation _____

_____

_____

Rover Insurers, Inc./Red Corporation _____

_____

_____

Ball Insurance Carrier/Blue Corporation _____

_____

_____

Major Medical Benefits

This section of the contract lists the particular benefits and stipulations that a contract provides.

DEDUCTIBLE. The first item usually listed is the amount of the deductible. The deductible is the amount that the individual patient must pay before benefits are paid by the insurance carrier. Deductibles are usually accumulated according to a calendar year. Thus, each January 1, the amount the patient has paid toward the designated deductible returns to zero and the patient must start paying again.

The exception to this is in contracts that have a **carryover provision**. A deductible carryover provision means that any amounts that the patient pays toward the deductible in the last three months of the year will carry over and will be applied toward the next year's deductible. Remember, the patient pays the deductible before the insurance is required to pay any benefits; therefore, if the patient is still paying a deductible in the last three months of the year, the insurance carrier has not had to pay any major medical benefits on this patient up to that time.

For example, if the month is September, and it is appropriate for the patient's condition, ask the patient if he or she would like to schedule services for after October 1. If the plan has a carryover provision, the deductible payments will then apply not only for this year but also for the following year.

Family Deductible   Family deductibles work the same way that individual deductibles do in that once a certain limit is reached, no more deductible is taken. For a **family deductible**, once the specified number of family members meets their individual deductible, the family deductible is considered met for the remaining family members. There are two types of family deductibles:

ACTIVITY #4

Determining Deductibles

Part 1. Directions: Indicate the individual and family deductible amounts for the following contracts (based on the information provided in Appendix A.

Creative Creations Corporation/White Corporation _____

_____

_____

Rover Insurers, Inc./Red Corporation _____

_____

_____

Ball Insurance Carrier/Blue Corporation _____

_____

_____

Part 2. Directions: Fill in the deductible amount that should be paid on this claim.

The Barton family is covered under the Creative Creations Corporation/White Corporation insurance contract. The following is an accumulation of their deductible amounts:

Family Member	Deductible Met
Billy	$25
Barry	$45
Bobby	$85
Betty	$0
Total Family Deductible Met to date	$155

Betty now submits a claim for $500 in services. She need only pay $_____ toward her deductible as, when added to the family total, the $200 family deductible limit is met. Even though none of the family members have met their individual limit, the family limit has been satisfied. Therefore, no more deductible will be taken on any member of this family.

In nonaggregate family deductible limits, the added sum of what each family member has paid is not important. Rather, a specified number of individuals in the family must meet their individual deductible limit in order for the family limit to be met. Nonaggregate family limits often require that the family pay more money toward the deductible.

ACTIVITY #5

Determining Deductibles

Directions: Fill in the deductible amount that should be paid on this claim.

The Barton family is now covered under the Ball Insurance Carrier contract. The following is an accumulation of their deductible amounts:

Family Member	Deductible Met
Billy	$25
Barry	$45
Bobby	$85
Betty	$0
Total Family Deductible Met to date	$155

Betty now submits a claim for $500 in services. She must pay the $_____ toward her deductible. Even then, the family deductible has still not been satisfied.

If the next claim is for Billy for $75, the full $75 amount would be considered part of the deductible, thus bringing the amount Billy has paid toward his deductible to $100. However, the family deductible still has not been met because only one family member (Betty), not two, has reached the individual family limit.

Only when Billy, Barry, or Bobby has paid $125 toward their deductible will the family deductible be considered met. At that time, no more deductible would be taken on any member of the family.

aggregate and nonaggregate. An **aggregate deductible** requires all major medical deductibles applied for all family members to be added together to attain the family limit. A **nonaggregate deductible** requires a specified number of individual deductibles to be satisfied before the family limit is met.

PRACTICE **PITFALLS**

As a biller, try to be aware of where each member of a family stands in relation to deductible payments. This can be done fairly simply by looking at the patient ledger for each family member and also asking the patient if other services received and paid for have resulted in meeting the patient's deductible. The patient with the most charges during the year has probably gone the farthest toward meeting his or her deductible. Also, if the insurance carrier has previously made several payments, the deductible has usually (although not always) been satisfied.

If more than one member of a family is being treated, consider submitting the bill for the member(s) with the highest payments on his or her deductible. Then submit the claims for the other family members at a later date.

For example, let's assume that the entire Barton family came down with an illness and had to come in for office visits. The whole family comes in and is treated on the same day. You check their charts and discover that they are covered by the Ball contract and:

Family Member	Deductible Met
Billy	$25
Barry	$45
Bobby	$85
Betty	$0
Total Family Deductible Met to date	$155

As a biller, it would be best to submit the claims for Bobby and Barry first, and then submit the claims for the remaining family members about a week later. This would ensure that only an additional $120 in deductible ($40 on Bobby and $80 on Barry) would have to be covered by the family. If all the bills were submitted at once, the claims examiner may choose to process the claims for Betty and Billy first, thus taking a deductible of $225 ($125 on Betty and $100 on Billy).

Health Savings Account (HSA)   A **health savings account** is a medical savings account that is available to individuals who are enrolled in high-deductible health insurance plans. At the time of depositing funds into the account, the funds are not subject to federal income tax. Any funds not spent roll over each year. Funds can be used to pay for various types of medical expenses without incurring any federal tax liability.

COINSURANCE AND COPAYMENTS. Coinsurance is an agreement between the member and the insurance carrier to share expenses. This is usually expressed in percentages (e.g., the insurance covers 80 percent of the approved amount of a bill, and the patient covers 20 percent). A **copayment** is a fixed amount a member must pay for a covered service regardless of whether or not a deductible has been met.

It is important for the biller to know the coinsurance percentage on a patient's insurance in order to collect the proper payment from the patient at the time services are rendered. Let's say you are visited by a patient who is covered under the Ball Insurance Carrier contract and has not yet met his or her deductible. If the services totaled $500, you should collect $200 from the patient. First collect the $125 deductible for which the patient will be responsible and then collect 20 percent of the remaining $375 ($75).

Collecting the patient's portion of the payment before the patient leaves the office is one way to ensure that most of the bill will be paid.

COINSURANCE LIMIT OR OUT-OF-POCKET LIMIT. Many insurance companies are aware that the costs of a catastrophic illness can ruin a family financially. Because insurance carriers want to keep people enrolled, they must leave them with enough resources to consistently pay premiums. For this reason, many insurance carriers have a coinsurance limit, also called an out-of-pocket limit. This limit stipulates that if the coinsurance portion of a patient's bills reaches a certain amount, all subsequent claims will be paid at 100 percent of the allowed amount. For example, the Ball contract has a coinsurance limit of $400. Because the coinsurance amount is based on 20 percent of the allowed amount (with insurance covering 80 percent of the allowed amount), the patient must have bills with approved amounts totaling over $2,125 in a calendar year ($125 is applied toward the deductible, $2,000 multiplied by 20 percent equals the $400 limit).

In the past, insurance companies were able to place annual and lifetime maximums on what the plan would pay, but that changed with the Affordable Care Act.

As a medical biller, if your patient has an illness that generates numerous claims totaling large amounts, you should attempt to schedule as many of the visits in the same year as possible. This will allow bills that are over the coinsurance limit to be paid at a higher percentage than those under it, thus decreasing the burden on the family and increasing the likelihood of the provider collecting the full amount.

ACTIVITY #6

Determining the Coinsurance Limit

Directions: Study the contracts in Appendix A and answer the following questions. Write your answers in the space provided.

What is the coinsurance limit for each of the following?

Creative Creations Corporation/White Corporation _____

_____

Rover Insurers, Inc./Red Corporation _____

_____

Ball Insurance Carrier/Blue Corporation _____

_____

MENTAL HEALTH EXPENSES. Mental health expenses include claims submitted for psychiatric services, marriage and family counseling services, and drug and alcohol treatment. Often there

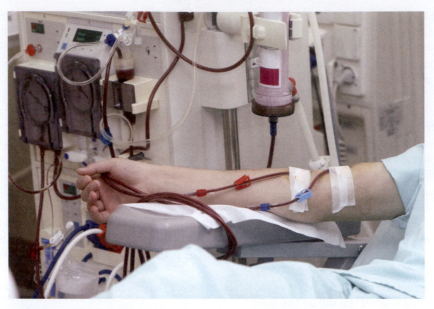

FIGURE 4-6

A patient with a preexisting condition that requires the patient to undergo hemodialysis
© Picsfive/Shutterstock.com

are different limits, copayments, and/or coinsurance percentages for mental health expenses. Many contracts have a calendar year maximum or a maximum number of visits for these types of services.

It is important for the biller to understand any limits on the number of treatments or amounts covered by insurance. Make the provider aware of these limits so that the provider can suggest or schedule treatments accordingly.

PREEXISTING CONDITIONS. Many contracts will not cover conditions that existed before a patient was covered under a contract (called **preexisting conditions**).

The term *preexisting* has a different meaning for each contract. Most often, it is defined as a condition for which the patient has sought treatment within a given time period before insurance coverage has begun. If the patient has sought treatment for such a condition, before coverage, benefits for treatment may not be covered or may be limited to a certain dollar amount. Prior to HIPAA, discussed below, insurance companies could disallow preexisting condition coverage for as long as two years.

Some contracts also have a "treatment-free" period. With this provision, if the patient can go without treatment for a specified period of time (often ninety days), then the insurance carrier will no longer consider the condition to be preexisting and will cover the illness or condition under the normal terms of the contract.

Treatment includes any kind of contact in regard to the illness, including any office visit or testing that was used to diagnose the illness. It also includes treatment of the condition, tests or office visits to monitor the condition, and filling of prescriptions related to the condition.

HIPAA/Health Insurance Portability and Accountability Act   On August 26, 1996, new laws regarding health insurance were signed into law by President William Clinton. This group of laws was called the Health Insurance Portability and Accountability Act of 1996 (HIPAA). The most important changes address preexisting condition limitations and prior coverage certification.

Under 1996 HIPAA law, preexisting condition exclusions were limited to six months, and credit was required for prior coverage.

Preexisting condition limitations were disallowed for pregnancy or newborns. Therefore, if a woman transfers coverage while she is pregnant, then the new insurance carrier must cover the costs associated with the pregnancy.

Companies also are now required to provide written certification of all prior coverage. They must provide this information to the patient upon termination of coverage.

Patient Protection and Affordable Care Act In 2010, President Obama implemented the Patient Protection and Affordable Care Act (PPACA), which drastically changes the provisions allowed in an insurance contract. The main changes include elimination of preexisting conditions limitations, elimination of annual and lifetime maximum benefits, mandated coverage of preventative care services, and extension of dependent care coverage. These changes took effect over a four year time period.

● **ONLINE INFORMATION:** For further information on the protections provided under HIPAA and the Patient Protection and Affordable Care Act (PPACA), visit www.cms.gov and search for the topic of information desired.

Consolidated Omnibus Budget Reconciliation Act (COBRA) Congress passed the landmark COBRA health benefit provisions in 1986. The law amends the Employee Retirement Income Security Act (ERISA), the Internal Revenue Code, and the Public Health Services Act to provide continuation of group health coverage that otherwise would be terminated.

COBRA contains provisions giving certain former employees, retirees, spouses, and dependent children the right to temporary continuation of health coverage at group rates. This coverage, however, is only available in specific instances. Group health coverage for COBRA participants is usually more expensive than health coverage for active employees, as usually the employer formerly paid a part of the premium. It is ordinarily less expensive, however, than individual health coverage.

Employees are no longer allowed to continue COBRA coverage on a policy if they are covered under a new policy. In the past, many employees would continue coverage on an old policy until the preexisting condition limitation had been satisfied on the new insurance. Because the new insurance is no longer allowed to apply preexisting condition limitations, the need for this duplicate coverage has been eliminated. Many people may still elect to continue coverage on the old policy until they have satisfied any length of employment requirements (e.g., must be employed for ninety days). However, the waiting period is not considered a break in coverage for purposes of the 63-day break in coverage. Therefore, if an employee terminates at one company (and ceases coverage) and is hired at a second company within 63 days, the person is considered continuously covered even if a 90-day waiting period must be satisfied before coverage begins with the new employer. To understand this concept further visit the U.S. Department of Labor website, www.dol.gov, and search "COBRA" for the latest updates on this law.

When hiring, employers are not allowed to discriminate against those with higher medical costs. This is true even though the higher costs will eventually show an increase in the company's insurance premiums.

Until the PPACA is fully implemented, those who do not satisfy the continuous coverage requirements for preexisting condition exclusions are limited to conditions for which treatment was received within six months before coverage. Exclusions are only allowed to remain in effect for twelve months. Therefore, after twelve months the carrier must cover the condition, whether it was preexisting or not. If a person did not enroll upon becoming eligible, then preexisting condition exclusions are allowed to continue for up to eighteen months. One of the PPACA benefits is a federal insurance policy available to anyone denied coverage due to preexisting conditions. Many states also offer such plans.

PRACTICE **PITFALLS**

When a patient transfers insurance, changes employers, or loses insurance eligibility (e.g., a child reaches maximum dependent age), a certificate that details the previous coverage should be issued. Because this is a new situation, many patients may not be aware of the significance of having this certificate.

Ask patients to provide a copy of this certificate and file this copy in the patient's chart. If the patient then receives treatment for a condition that would be considered preexisting, include a copy of the certificate with the patient's claim. This will help to prevent denial of the claim.

ACTIVITY #7

Working with Coverage Certification

Directions: Read each of the following scenarios and determine whether or not the certificate of prior insurance should be included with the claim, and why or why not. (PY = prior year; CY = current year)

1. Jennifer received treatment for a chronic ulcer on 7/1/PY and again on 8/1/PY. On 10/1/PY she quit her old job and began working for a new employer on 10/15/PY. She immediately signed up for insurance and her coverage became effective after a thirty-day waiting period, on 11/15/PY. On 1/15/CY she was seen by a provider for additional ulcer treatment. Should you send in a copy of her coverage certificate with the 1/15/CY claim? _____
   _____
   _____

2. Mary received treatment for diabetes on 7/1/PY and again on 8/1/PY. On 10/1/PY she quit her old job and began working for a new employer two weeks later on 10/15/PY. She immediately signed up for insurance, and her coverage became effective after a ninety-day waiting period on 1/15/PY. On 10/15/CY she was seen by a provider for additional diabetes treatment. Should you send in a copy of her coverage certificate with the 10/15/CY claim? _____
   _____
   _____

3. Tom received treatment for kidney disease 2/1/CY and again on 3/1/CY. On 10/1/CY he quit his old job and began working for a new employer two weeks later, on 10/15/CY. He immediately signed up for insurance and his coverage became effective after a thirty-day waiting period on 11/15/CY. On 12/15/CY he was seen by a provider for additional kidney disease treatment. Should you send in a copy of his coverage certificate with the 12/15/CY claim? _____
   _____
   _____

4. Betty received a routine visit for pregnancy on 7/1/PY and again on 8/1/PY. On 10/1/PY she began working for a new employer. She immediately signed up for insurance, and her coverage became effective after a thirty-day waiting period, on 12/15/PY. She did not have prior coverage. On 1/15/CY she was seen by a provider for an additional routine visit. Should you send in a copy of her coverage certificate with the 1/15/CY claim? _____
   _____
   _____

5. Jessie received treatment for anorexia on 7/1/PY and again on 8/1/PY. On 10/1/PY she quit her old job and chose not to continue coverage under COBRA rules. On 12/15/PY she began working for a new employer. She immediately signed up for insurance and her coverage became effective after a thirty-day waiting period on 1/15/CY. On 10/25/PY she was seen by a provider for additional anorexia treatment. Should you send in a copy of her coverage certificate with the 10/25/PY claim? _____
   _____
   _____

Exclusions

Every contract will have a list of **exclusions**. These are items that the insurance carrier does not cover. It is important to check the list of exclusions before scheduling surgery or other expensive treatments for a patient. If the procedures or treatments are not covered, the patient will be responsible for the entire amount of the bill. Many providers who routinely perform procedures that are not covered (e.g., cosmetic surgeons) often will require payment in full before scheduling the surgery.

Allowed Amounts

Insurance carriers limit payment to a specified amount. The **allowed amount** is what the insurance company considers to be a reasonable charge for the procedure performed, and it is often less than the amount that the provider bills. For instance, let's say the allowed amount is $100 but within that allowed amount the patient is responsible for 20 percent and the payer is responsible for 80 percent, equaling 100 percent of the allowed amount.

A nationwide listing of allowable amounts is not really equitable because it costs a lot more to do business in Los Angeles (e.g., higher nurse and secretary salaries, rents, costs of supplies, etc.) than it does in a rural medical clinic in Louisiana. Because of this, a system called **Usual, Customary, and Reasonable (UCR)** was established. The UCR is mostly used in reference to fee-for-service reimbursement. The usual fee is the fee that a provider typically charges for a specific procedure. The customary fee is the range of usual fees that providers in the same geographic area charge for the same procedure. To determine if a fee is reasonable, both the usual and customary are taken into account and the payment is the lesser of the two.

Another method used to calculate fees is the **relative value scale**. When using this method the procedure that is performed has been given a numeric value (called a **relative value unit**) based on how difficult the procedure is to perform, the overhead involved, and the chance of incurring a malpractice lawsuit. For example, it takes a lot more skill, time, and medical supplies to perform brain surgery than it does to clean a skinned knee and put a bandage on it. Therefore, brain surgery is given a much higher unit value than cleaning and bandaging a skinned knee. Because each procedure has a different unit value, there are often several codes for the same type of procedure. For example, there are five different codes for an office visit of a new patient. The code used depends on how difficult the patient's condition is to treat and the skill level involved in this treatment. Because different unit values are assigned to each code, it is important that the biller code the procedures correctly.

This unit value is multiplied by a Geographical Cost Practice Index (GPCI). A **Geographical Cost Practice Index** is a numerical factor used to multiply to arrive at a sum. Geographical Cost Practice Index is determined by the first three digits of the zip code in which the services were performed and the type of services provided.

Although the unit value for a procedure would remain the same no matter where in the nation it was performed, the Geographical Cost Practice Index would change depending on the cost of doing business in a given area. Thus, the factors for Louisiana would be far less than those for Los Angeles. The base relative value unit is multiplied by the Geographical Cost Practice Index to get the adjusted relative value.

The adjusted relative value is multiplied by the conversion factor (a standard dollar value) to calculate the allowed amount. Usually insurance companies establish different conversion factors for different types of services.

The types of services are divided into four groups:

- Medical Services (office visits)
- Surgical Services (procedures that invade the body)
- X-ray and Laboratory Procedures (x-rays taken and lab tests performed)
- Anesthesia Services

Applicable deductible and coinsurance amounts are subtracted from the allowed amount before the insurance carrier makes payment.

● **ONLINE INFORMATION:** To learn more about the relative value unit, visit the Centers for Medicare and Medicaid Services at www.cms.gov. Once at the site, type "RVU" in the search box.

Some insurance plans do not use allowed amounts or usual and customary charges in determining claim payments but instead base payment on a fee schedule. A **fee schedule** is a list of predetermined charges for medical services and supplies. Reimbursement for services rendered to patients under a fee schedule–based plan is limited to the maximum charge allowed by the fee schedule at the time of the service or the provider's fee, whichever is lower. Depending on the specialty of the provider the fee schedule will reflect the charges for the types of procedures performed in that specialty. For instance, a fee schedule for a pediatrician would include a fee for well-baby checks. On a gynecologist fee schedule, the fee for performing a pap smear would be included.

PRACTICE **PITFALLS**

If the claim is for $125 but the allowed amount of the procedure(s) is $75, the insurance carrier will only apply that $75 toward the deductible. Thus, even though the patient is paying $125 for the services, only $75 of the deductible limit has been met. The patient would still need another $50 (under the Ball Insurance Carrier contract) of allowed charges to meet their deductible.

Likewise, if the claim is for $500 and the allowed amount is $350, the patient could be responsible for quite a large a bill. Under the Ball contract, the $125 deductible would be subtracted from the allowed amount, leaving $225. This would then be multiplied by the 80 percent coinsurance rate and the insurance carrier would send a check for $180. The patient would be responsible for the remaining $320.

Not all insurance carriers use the same list of relative value units. Therefore, the allowed amount for one insurance carrier will be different from the allowed amount of a different insurance carrier.

In addition, the insurance carrier will never pay more than the billed amount. Therefore, if the allowed amount for a bill is $200, but the provider only charged $150, the insurance carrier will consider the billed amount to be the allowed amount of $150. The carrier will then subtract any remaining deductible to be paid, and multiply the remainder by the coinsurance percent.

As a biller, if you notice that the provider's charges for a particular procedure are always the same as the allowed amount, it may mean that the provider is charging less than what the insurance carriers consider to be reasonable for that procedure. Discuss this with the provider and consider raising the billed amount for this procedure.

Likewise, if the allowed amount is always significantly lower than the billed amount, you may wish to discuss lowering the fee with the provider. Be aware that allowed amounts are nearly always lower than billed amounts, so lowering of fees should not be done without serious consideration.

Precertification of Inpatient Admissions

To precertify means to get preapproval for admission on elective, nonemergency hospitalization. Contact is made with either the plan administrator or another entity sanctioned to determine the necessity of the admission. Most often, these entities are composed of a specialized group of nurses working under the direction of a provider. The nurses deal directly with the provider's office and the facility to determine whether the admission is necessary and whether the number of days of care is medically necessary. If the patient stays longer than the approved number of days, the additional days of care may not be paid for or the usual payment may be reduced by a percentage specified by the plan. The objective in this program is to prevent unnecessary admissions and to get the patient out of the hospital as soon as is medically appropriate.

For these reasons, it is important that all medical billers check the terms of the contract whenever possible. Often information on precertification is included on the patient's insurance card. This information will say something like the following:

All voluntary inpatient admissions must be precertified 48 hours prior to admission. In case of emergency admission, please contact the carrier within 24 hours of admission or benefits may be reduced or services not covered.

Some programs provide for precertification only before or on the day of hospitalization. Other programs provide for a complete approach to managing the care, which entails a utilization review program.

As part of HIPAA, the federal government has mandated that no precertification can be required on maternity confinements. The law stipulates that a confinement for a normal delivery cannot be limited to less than forty-eight hours (two days) or in the case of a Cesarean section ninety-six hours (four days). The law, however, does not state that a concurrent review cannot be done. Therefore, if the patient stays hospital confined beyond the two days for a normal delivery or four days for a C-section and the plan has concurrent review and extended-stay provisions, applicable penalties can be imposed on those extra days.

Utilization Review

As previously indicated, precertification or a **prospective review** determines the need and appropriateness of the recommended care. **Utilization review** is the process of monitoring the use and delivery of medical services. Utilization review (UR) programs contain the following three components:

1. Precertification (before) or prospective review
2. Concurrent review (during the confinement)
3. Retrospective review (after termination of confinement)

Concurrent review determines whether the estimated length of time and scope of the inpatient stay are justified by the diagnosis and symptoms. This review is conducted periodically during the projected length of time the patient is in the hospital. If the length of stay exceeds the criteria or if there is a change in treatment, the matter is referred to the medical consultant for review.

At no time does the consultant dictate the method of treatment or the length of stay. These decisions are left entirely to the patient and the attending provider. However, the consultant is entitled to inform the patient, provider, and facility that the continued stay exceeds the approved number of days and may not be covered by the plan as medically necessary. It is then the patient's responsibility to decide which course to take.

Retrospective review is used to determine after discharge whether the hospitalization and treatment were medically necessary and covered by the terms of the benefit program. This type of review may be used as a substitute for admission and concurrent reviews when the failure to notify the UR program of an admission prevents the regular review procedures. However, the main drawback to the retrospective review is that the patient and providers are not notified about the services that will not be covered until after they have been provided. The best programs always work most effectively when the patient is notified beforehand that he or she will be primarily responsible for payment of services. This approach deters the member from incurring unnecessary expenses.

Second Surgical Opinion Consultations

Surgical claims represent the second-highest categorical cost to carriers (hospitalization ranks first). The United States has the world's highest rate of surgical treatment because neither the provider nor the patient has much financial incentive to consider less expensive alternatives.

About 80 percent of all surgeries can be considered "elective"—that is, they are not required because of a life-threatening situation. The objective of a **second surgical opinion (SSO) consultation** is to eliminate elective surgical procedures that are classified as unnecessary.

Unnecessary surgery is surgery that is recommended as an elective procedure when an alternative method of treatment may be preferable for a number of reasons, including the following:

- The surgery itself may be premature, taking into consideration all pathologic indications.
- The risk to the patient may not justify the benefits of surgery.
- An alternative medical treatment may be superior for both medical and cost-effective reasons.
- A less severe surgical procedure may be preferable under the circumstances, or no medical or surgical procedure may be necessary at all.

In the SSO consultation, the patient consults an independent specialist to determine whether the recommended elective surgical procedure is advisable. This process is not intended to interfere with the patient–provider relationship or to prevent the patient from receiving necessary elective operations.

This program may be administered in one of two ways:

1. A **mandatory program** requires the patient to obtain an SSO for special procedures, or there is an automatic reduction or denial of benefits. For an example of this type of program, see the Rover Insurers, Inc. contract in Appendix A.
2. A **voluntary program** encourages participants to have an SSO, but there is no automatic reduction of benefits if the patient does not comply.

In both approaches, the SSO and related tests are usually paid at 100 percent so that the patient will not have any out-of-pocket expenses for conforming to the program.

The SSO program has met with much criticism because it has not effectively reduced the number of elective surgeries. One of the main reasons for this ineffectiveness is that providers may be reluctant to tell a patient that a surgery is unnecessary. This attitude stems from the growing number of malpractice lawsuits. For example, if a provider states that a patient does not need surgery and a sudden emergency situation arises that is related to the original need for surgery, the provider may be held liable under a malpractice suit. Consequently, many plans are abandoning the SSO plan provision.

ACTIVITY #8

Determining Second Surgical Benefits

Directions: Review the contracts at in Appendix A and indicate which contracts have a second surgical benefit provision.

_____

_____

Coordination of Benefits

Coordination of benefits (COB) is a process that occurs when two or more plans provide coverage on the same person. Coordination between the two plans is necessary to allow for payment of 100 percent of the allowable expense.

Before standardized coordination rules were adopted by the benefits industry, a person covered under two policies could collect full benefits from both. Thus, the member could actually make a profit by being sick or injured. Because each plan would prefer to pay as the secondary payer, it became necessary to develop rules to determine when a plan should pay as primary, secondary, or tertiary.

The thirteen rules determining the order of payment are referred to as the **Order of Benefit Determination (OBD)**:

1. The plan without a COB provision will be primary to a plan with a COB provision.
2. When a plan does not have OBD rules, and as a result the plans do not agree on the OBD, the plan without these OBD rules will determine the order of payment.
3. The plan that covers an individual as an employee will be primary to a plan that covers that individual as a dependent.
4. If an individual is an employee under two plans, the primary plan is the one under which the employee has been covered longer.
5. If an employee is an active employee under one plan and a retiree (or laid off) under another, the active plan will pay as primary.

The parent birthday rule, explained in 6 and 7, affects the OBD for dependent children of parents who are living together and married (not divorced or legally separated).

6. The plan of the parent whose birthday (based on month and day only) occurs first during the calendar year is the primary plan.
7. When both parents' birthdays are the same (based on month and day), the benefits of the plan that covered one parent longer is the primary plan.

For dependents of legally separated or divorced parents and those whose parents have remarried, the Order of Benefit Determination is based on the following rules.

8. The plan of the parent specified as having legal responsibility for the health care expense of the child is the primary plan.

For dependents of separated parents with no court decree, the following applies.

9. The plan of the parent with custody is the primary plan.
10. The plan of the stepparent (if any) with whom the child resides is secondary.
11. The plan of the natural parent without custody is tertiary.
12. The stepparent (if any) who does not reside with the child has no legal right to declare dependency. Therefore, no coordination should be performed because the child is probably not an eligible dependent under the plan.
13. For joint custody, with no additional responsibility designation, the plan of the parent whose coverage has been in effect longer would be the primary payer. However, this rule

may vary by administrator. Some parents pay costs on a 50/50 basis, thereby sharing equally in the health care risk.

ACTIVITY #9

Determining Primary, Secondary, and Tertiary Coverage

Directions: Assume that all of the adults in the following questions have active coverage. For each scenario, indicate which party would be primary, secondary, tertiary, and so on, by writing 1, 2, 3, or 4 in the blank space next to the person. If the person is not responsible for the dependent(s) at all, write N/A.

1. A remarried mother has custody of her children six months of the year. Her coverage was effective 6/1/1999, and her date of birth (DOB) is 10/15/CCYY-35. The natural father's coverage was effective 5/1/2000, and his date of birth is 8/10/CCYY-41. The mother's husband's coverage was effective 5/1/1998, and his date of birth is 9/1/CCYY-32. The father's wife's coverage was effective 6/15/1999, and her date of birth is 7/4/CCYY-44.

   _____ Mother _____ Father _____ Stepfather _____ Stepmother

2. A remarried mother has custody of her children. However, by court decree, the father has financial responsibility for their health care costs. The mother's DOB is 4/1/CCYY-34, and her coverage was effective 2/15/2000. The father's DOB is 3/15/CCYY-37, and his coverage was effective 3/1/1997. The stepfather's DOB is 12/15/CCYY-37, and his coverage was effective 3/1/1996. The stepmother's DOB is 8/17/CCYY-35, and her coverage was effective 6/1/1999.

   _____ Mother _____ Father _____ Stepfather _____ Stepmother

3. Two natural parents are married. The mother's DOB is 7/1/CCYY-28. The father's DOB is 7/1/CCYY-29. The mother's effective date of coverage is 6/1/1998. The father's effective date of coverage is 6/1/1999.

   _____ Mother _____ Father _____ Stepfather _____ Stepmother

4. Two natural parents are married. The mother's DOB is 7/1/CCYY-28. The father's DOB is 7/1/CCYY-29. The mother's effective date of coverage is 6/1/1998. The father's effective date of coverage is 6/1/1999. The mother's plan does not have a COB provision.

   _____ Mother _____ Father _____ Stepfather _____ Stepmother

5. Two natural parents are divorced and neither has remarried. By court decree, the grandparents have legal custody of the children. Also by court decree, the father has financial responsibility for the children's medical care. The mother's DOB is 4/1/CCYY-34, and her coverage was effective 2/15/2000. The father's DOB is 3/15/CCYY-37, and his coverage was effective 3/1/1997. The grandmother's DOB is 12/15/CCYY-60, and her coverage was effective 3/15/1986. The grandfather's DOB is 8/17/CCYY-65, and his coverage was effective 6/1/1989.

   _____ Mother _____ Father _____ Grandfather _____ Grandmother

CHAPTER REVIEW

Summary

- It is vital that medical billers understand how to properly interpret the basic and major medical benefits of a contract.
- It will take research to keep updated on insurance coverage legislation that impacts patient benefits.
- Medical billers must understand provisions in a contract, such as preauthorization and pre-certification, that can impact payment on a patient's claim.

Review Questions

Directions: Answer the following questions without looking back into the material just covered. Write your answers in the space provided.

1. What is eligibility? _____

   _____

2. Basic benefits are usually paid at 100 percent and are _____

   _____

3. Define *accident*. _____

   _____

4. What is preadmission testing? _____

   _____

5. What is outpatient surgery? _____

   _____

6. What is a deductible? _____

   _____

7. Define *aggregate family deductible*. _____

   _____

8. What is coinsurance? _____

   _____

9. What happens when a patient reaches his or her coinsurance limit? _____

   _____

10. What are mental health expenses? _____

    _____

11. What is a preexisting condition? _____

    _____

12. What is an exclusion? _____

    _____

13. What is an allowed amount? _____

    _____

14. How do you calculate the allowed amount?

    _____

If you are unable to answer any of these questions, refer back to that section in the chapter, and then fill in the answers.

Activity #10: Calculating the Amount of Deductible

Directions: Calculate the amount of deductible that will be taken and answer the following questions.

The Apple family is covered under the Creative Creations Corporation/White Corporation contract. Their previous deductible payments are as follows:

	Annie	Adam	April	August	Ashley
Carryover paid	0.00	5.00	10.00	55.00	0.00
Deductible paid	10.00	0.00	5.00	5.00	0.00

1. What is the individual deductible limit on this contract?   1. _____

2. What is the family deductible limit on this contract?   2. _____

3. Is the family limit aggregate or nonaggregate?   3. _____

4. How much has been paid toward the family deductible?   4. _____

5. Annie incurs allowed charges of $35. How much will be applied to the deductible?   5. _____

6. How much has Annie now met on her deductible?   6. _____

7. How much has now been paid toward the family deductible?   7. _____

8. August incurs allowed charges of $55. How much will be applied to the deductible?   8. _____

9. How much has August now met on his deductible?   9. _____

10. How much has now been paid toward the family deductible?   10. _____

11. April incurs allowed charges of $55. How much will be applied to the deductible?   11. _____

12. How much has April now met on her deductible?   12. _____

13. How much has now been paid toward the family deductible?   13. _____

14. Adam incurs allowed charges of $60. How much will be applied to the deductible?   14. _____

15. How much has Adam now met on his deductible?   15. _____

16. How much has now been paid toward the family deductible?   16. _____

17. Annie incurs allowed charges of $35. How much will be applied to the deductible?   17. _____

18. How much has Annie now met on her deductible?   18. _____

19. How much has now been paid toward the family deductible?   19. _____

Activity #11: Calculating the Amount of Deductible

Directions: Calculate the amount of deductible that will be taken and answer the following questions.

The Bear family is covered under the Rover Insurers, Inc./Red Corporation contract. Their previous deductible payments are as follows:

	Brad	Bonnie	Barbra	Brian
Carryover paid	0.00	5.00	10.00	55.00
Deductible paid	10.00	0.00	5.00	5.00

1. What is the individual deductible limit on this contract?   1. _____

2. What is the family deductible limit on this contract?   2. _____

3. Is the family limit aggregate or nonaggregate?   3. _____

4. How many people are needed to meet the family deductible for this year?   4. _____

5. Bonnie incurs allowed charges of $55. How much will be applied to the deductible?   5. _____

6. How much has Bonnie now met on her deductible?   6. _____

7. How many people are now needed to meet the family deductible?   7. _____

8. Brian incurs allowed charges of $85. How much will be applied to the deductible?   8. _____

9. How much has Brian now met on his deductible?   9. _____

10. How many people are now needed to meet the family deductible?   10. _____

11. Barbra incurs allowed charges of $105. How much will be applied
    to the deductible?   11. _____

12. How much has Barbra now met on her deductible?   12. _____

13. How many people are now needed to meet the family deductible?   13. _____

14. Brad incurs allowed charges of $60. How much will be applied to the
    deductible?   14. _____

15. How much has Brad now met on his deductible?   15. _____

16. How many people are now needed to meet the family deductible?   16. _____

17. Bonnie incurs allowed charges of $35. How much will be applied to the
    deductible?   17. _____

18. How much has Bonnie now met on her deductible?   18. _____

19. How many people are now needed to meet the family deductible?   19. _____

20. Brian incurs allowed charges of $35. How much will be applied to the
    deductible?   20. _____

21. How much has Brian now met on his deductible?   21. _____

22. How many people are now needed to meet the family deductible?   22. _____

23. Barbra incurs allowed charges of $55. How much will be applied to the
    deductible?   23. _____

24. How much has Barbra now met on her deductible?   24. _____

25. How many people are now needed to meet the family deductible?   25. _____

26. Brad incurs allowed charges of $60. How much will be applied to the
    deductible?   26. _____

27. How much has Brad now met on his deductible?   27. _____

28. How many people are now needed to meet the family deductible?   28. _____

29. Bonnie incurs allowed charges of $35. How much will be applied
    to the deductible?   29. _____

30. How much has Bonnie now met on her deductible?   30. _____

31. How many people are now needed to meet the family deductible?   31. _____

Activity #12: Calculating the Amount of Deductible

Directions: Calculate the amount of deductible that will be taken and answer the following
questions.

The Carpenter family is covered under the Ball Insurance Carrier/Blue Corporation contract
Their previous deductible payments are as follows:

	Carry	Connie	Cathy	Chris
Carryover paid	0.00	5.00	10.00	55.00
Deductible paid	10.00	0.00	5.00	5.00

1. What is the individual deductible limit on this contract?   1. _____

2. What is the family deductible limit on this contract?   2. _____

3. Is the family limit aggregate or nonaggregate?   3. _____

4. How many people are needed to meet the family deductible?   4. _____

5. Connie incurs allowed charges of $35. How much will be applied to the
   deductible?   5. _____

6. How much has Connie now met on her deductible?   6. _____

7. How many people are now needed to meet the family deductible?   7. _____

8. Carry incurs allowed charges of $55. How much will be applied to the deductible?

8. _____

9. How much has Carry now met on her deductible?

9. _____

10. How many people are now needed to meet the family deductible?

10. _____

11. Chris incurs allowed charges of $60. How much will be applied to the deductible?

11. _____

12. How much has Chris now met on his deductible?

12. _____

13. How many people are now needed to meet the family deductible?

13. _____

14. Chris incurs allowed charges of $35. How much will be applied to the deductible?

14. _____

15. How much has Chris now met on his deductible?

15. _____

16. How many people are now needed to meet the family deductible?

16. _____

17. Connie incurs allowed charges of $95. How much will be applied to the deductible?

17. _____

18. How much has Connie now met on her deductible?

18. _____

19. How many people are now needed to meet the family deductible?

19. _____

20. Carry incurs allowed charges of $45. How much will be applied to the deductible?

20. _____

21. How much has Carry now met on her deductible?

21. _____

22. How many people are now needed to meet the family deductible?

22. _____

23. Cathy incurs allowed charges of $105. How much will be applied to the deductible?

23. _____

24. How much has Cathy now met on her deductible?

24. _____

25. How many people are now needed to meet the family deductible?

25. _____

26. Carry incurs allowed charges of $85. How much will be applied to the deductible?

26. _____

27. How much has Carry now met on her deductible?

27. _____

28. How many people are now needed to meet the family deductible?

28. _____

29. Chris incurs allowed charges of $85. How much will be applied to the deductible?

29. _____

30. How much has Chris now met on his deductible?

30. _____

31. How many people are now needed to meet the family deductible?

31. _____

32. Cathy incurs allowed charges of $90. How much will be applied to the deductible?

32. _____

33. How much has Cathy now met on her deductible?

33. _____

34. How many people are now needed to meet the family deductible?

34. _____

Activity #13: Matching Key Terms

Directions: Match the following terms with the proper definition by writing the letter of the correct definition in the space next to the term.

1. _____ Authorized Treatment Record Form

a. Claims submitted for psychiatric services, marriage and family counseling, and drug and alcohol treatment

2. _____ Carryover provisions

b. Used to eliminate elective surgical procedures that are classified as unnecessary

3. _____ Coordination of benefits

c. A deductible that requires a specified number of individual deductibles be satisfied before the family limit is met

4. _____ Indemnity insurance plans

d. Under this system, each procedure that is performed has been given a number value (called a relative unit value) based on how difficult the procedure is to perform, the overhead involved, and the chance of incurring a malpractice lawsuit.

5. _____ Mental health expenses

e. The thirteen rules determining the order of insurance benefit payment

6. _____ Nonaggregate deductible

f. A form used to track the usage of preauthorized services rendered by a provider's office

7. _____ Order of Benefit Determination

g. Conditions that existed before a patient was covered under a contract

8. _____ Preexisting conditions

h. Any amounts that the patient pays toward his or her deductible in the last three months of the year will carry over and will be applied toward the next year's deductible.

9. _____ Second surgical opinion consultation

i. A principle of insurance that provides medical coverage when a loss occurs and restores the insured party to the approximate financial condition that he or she was in before the loss occurred

10. _____ Usual, Customary, and Reasonable (UCR)

j. A process that occurs when two or more plans provide coverage on the same person. Coordination between the two plans is necessary to allow for payment of 100 percent of the allowable expense.

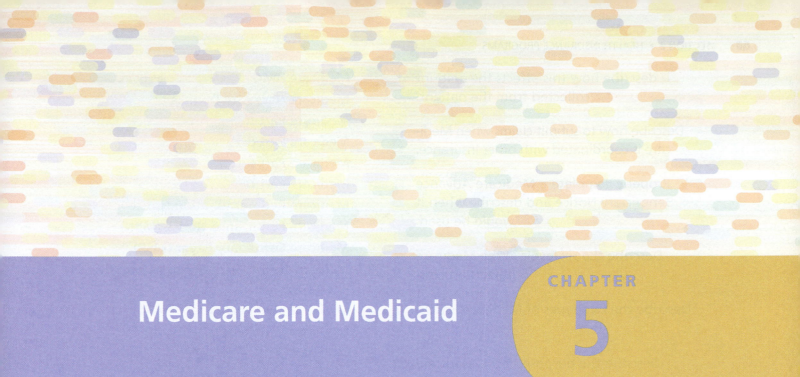

Medicare and Medicaid

After completion of this chapter you should be able to:

State the eligibility requirements for Medicare.

Describe the types of Medicare coverage and the benefits for each.

Differentiate between Medigap and Medicare supplements.

State the exceptions when patients may submit a Medicare bill themselves.

State the guidelines for collecting the patient portion of a Medicare claim.

List the claims that require acceptance of assignment.

Describe how to post Medicare payments.

Describe Assignment of Benefits and how it can affect the amount collected on a Medicare claim.

Properly "balance bill" a Medicare claim.

State the most common reasons for a "not medically necessary" denial and

Key Words and Concepts you will learn in this chapter:

Advance Beneficiary Notice (ABN)

Benefit period

Categorically needy

Centers for Medicare and Medicaid Services (CMS)

Clean claim

CMS-1500

Diagnosis-related group (DRG)

Downcoding

Durable medical equipment (DME)

Durable Medical Equipment Regional Carriers (DMERCs)

Early and Periodic Screening, Diagnosis, and Treatment (EPSDT) Program

Eligibility card Fiscal intermediaries

End-stage renal disease (ESRD)

Limiting charge

Medicaid

Medicaid Remittance Advice (MRA)

Medically needy

Medicare

Medicare Health Insurance Claim Number (HICN)

describe how this affects the amount collected from the patient.

Describe how to submit claims when Medicare is coordinated with other insurance.

Properly complete a Medicare Advance Beneficiary Notice and describe when it would be used.

Describe the six levels in the Medicare appeals process.

Describe the two types of Medicare HMOs.

Describe the purpose of the Medicaid program.

Explain how to verify a patient's eligibility for Medicaid coverage.

List the benefits covered under the Medicaid program.

Define and describe the EPSDT program.

State the rule for time limits for Medicaid claims and the exceptions to this rule.

List the services that require a Treatment Authorization Request.

Properly complete a Treatment Authorization Request.

State the guidelines for submitting Medicaid claims.

Medicare HMO

Medicare Necessity Denials

Medicare Part A

Medicare Part B

Medicare Part C

Medicare Part D

Medicare Redetermination Notice

Medicare Remittance Notice (MRN)

Medicare Secondary Payer (MSP)

Medicare Severity-Diagnosis Related Group (MS-DRG)

Medicare Summary Notice (MSN)

Medicare Supplemental Insurance

Medigap

National Provider Identifiers (NPIs)

Nonparticipating providers

Notice of Noncoverage

Participating providers

Payer of last resort

Resource-based relative value scale (RBRVS)

Share of cost

Medicare

Medicare is the Federal Health Insurance Benefit Plan for the Aged and Disabled, enacted under Title XVIII of the Social Security Act. This program is for people sixty-five years of age or older, people under sixty-five years of age with certain disabilities, and people of any age with end-stage renal disease. The **Centers for Medicare and Medicaid Services (CMS)** is the organization that oversees the Medicare program. CMS was formerly known as the Health Care Financing Administration (HCFA).

Social Security Administration offices throughout the United States take applications for Medicare, determine eligibility, and provide general information about the program. Many different insurance companies, usually one or two within each state, administer the actual processing of the claims.

Medicare Eligibility

Following are some of the guidelines governing Medicare eligibility.

Based on Age

An individual is eligible for Medicare coverage on the first day of the month in which he or she reaches age sixty-five. People born on the first day of the month are eligible on the first day of the month preceding their birth date.

EXAMPLE:

Birthday: June 25, eligible for Medicare June 1

Birthday: June 1, eligible for Medicare May 1

Based on Disability

Medicare coverage for totally disabled persons begins on the first day of the twenty-fifth month from the date approved for Social Security Disability or Railroad Retirement benefits (Figure 5-2 ●). Those covered include disabled workers of any age, disabled widows between the ages of fifty and sixty-five, disabled beneficiaries age eighteen and over who receive Social Security benefits because of disability before age twenty-two, the blind, and Railroad Retirement annuitants.

Based on End-Stage Renal Disease

End-stage renal disease (ESRD) occurs when a person's kidneys fail to function. As a result, the patient usually begins dialysis treatments or has a kidney transplant operation (Figure 5-3 ●). Because of the multiple problems associated with this disease, patients are considered to be totally disabled, even though some individuals with this disease continue to work. Eligibility for Medicare ESRD is dependent on the type of treatment the patient is receiving. As a result, the following special rules apply to ESRD patients.

The employer's group health plan is the primary payer for the first thirty months after a patient (under age sixty-five) with ESRD becomes eligible for Medicare. This thirty-month period begins based on the earlier of (1) the month in which a regular course of renal dialysis is initiated or (2) the month the patient is hospitalized for a kidney transplant.

Medicare is the secondary payer during this thirty-month period but will revert to the primary status beginning with the thirty-first month. As a general rule, all services under a dialysis program are Medicare assigned (defined later in this section).

FIGURE 5-1

Effective communication skills are vital in the medical office.

© Michal Heron/Pearson Education

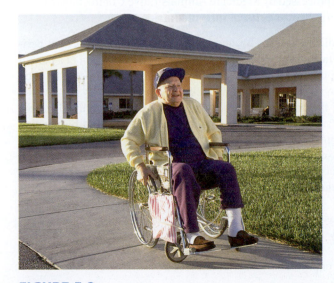

FIGURE 5-2

Medicare provides coverage for totally disabled persons.

© Michal Heron/Pearson Education

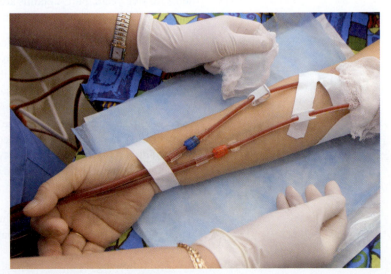

FIGURE 5-3

Patient on dialysis with dialysis shunt

© Bork/Shutterstock.com

Medicare coverage is also available for ESRD beginning the fourth month if the patient does not have insurance coverage and is receiving hemodialysis. Medicare effective dates for home/self dialysis and transplants vary depending on the type of treatment and where the treatment is performed.

The Parts of Medicare

The Medicare program has four parts: Parts A, B, C, and D. The services covered under each part are as follows:

1. **Medicare Part A** is considered the basic plan or hospital insurance. This part covers facility charges for acute inpatient hospital care, skilled nursing, home health care, and hospice care.
2. **Medicare Part B** is the medical (supplementary, voluntary) insurance that covers provider services, outpatient hospital services, home health care, outpatient speech and physical therapy, and durable medical equipment.
3. **Medicare Part C** is the Medicare Advantage portion and includes coverage in an HMO, PPO, and so on.
4. **Medicare Part D** is the prescription drug component (effective 2006).

Medicare Part A

Part A, the hospital coverage portion of Medicare, is automatic upon enrollment for the following individuals:

- All people age sixty-five and over, if entitled to (a) monthly Social Security benefits or (b) a pension under the Railroad Retirement Act
- All people who reached the age of sixty-five before 1968, whether or not under the Social Security or Railroad Retirement programs
- Workers who reached the age of sixty-five in 1975 or after need twenty quarters of Social Security work credits if female, or twenty-four quarters of Social Security work credits if male, to be fully insured.
- Some spouses may receive Medicare benefits derived strictly from their eligible spouse's work credits. Using the eligible spouse's Social Security number with the appropriate letter behind it designates that benefits are based on the eligible spouse.

Effective July 1, 1973, all people age sixty-five years and older who are not otherwise eligible for Part A may enroll by paying the full cost of such coverage, provided they also enroll in Part B. Aliens may be eligible for coverage in the Medicare program if they have been U.S. residents for five years. Part A claims are processed by Medicare Administrative Contractors (MAC), insurance companies that were formerly known as **fiscal intermediaries**.

BENEFITS OF PART A. The use of Medicare benefits for an inpatient is measured by benefit periods. The Part A deductible amount is taken from the first inpatient hospital admission in a benefit period. A **benefit period** begins with the first day of admission to the hospital. A benefit period ends after the patient has been discharged from the hospital or skilled nursing facility for a period of sixty consecutive days (including the day of discharge). If the patient is readmitted for the same or different reason within the sixty-day period, the patient remains covered by the first deductible. A new benefit period begins and another inpatient deductible is taken the next time the patient is admitted after the sixty-day period. The benefit period deductible is not based on the calendar year as many insurance companies' deductibles are. The deductible is adjusted each calendar year and can be found on the Medicare Web site. For 2011, the Part A deductible is $1,132 per benefit period.

If a member remains in the hospital for an extended time, additional copayments are required. Medicare deducts the copay amount from the billed amount and then pays the amount in excess of the copay.

The following inpatient hospital copayments were in effect for 2011:

- 1st day–60th day = a total of $1,132
- 61st day–90th day = $283 copayment per day
- 91st day–150th day = $566 copayment per day

Days 91 to 150 are known as the 60-day Lifetime Reserve. These copayments are not renewable with a new benefit period or a new calendar year. After the 60 Lifetime Reserve days are used, the patient owes the entire cost of care.

A separate copayment schedule and requirement apply to skilled nursing facilities (SNFs). To be eligible for this benefit, a doctor must certify the necessity of skilled nursing and rehabilitative care on a daily basis. Custodial care is not covered, nor is it available for occasional rehabilitative care. In addition, the Medicare intermediary must approve the stay.

The following SNF copayments were in effect for 2011:

- 1st day–20th day = No copayment. Because admission is usually from an acute care facility, during which time the deductible was met, 100 percent of the allowable amount is generally paid by Medicare.
- 21st day–100th day = $141.50 copayment per day

Multiple admissions can occur during a calendar year. However, the maximum number of allowable days is 100 per benefit period.

Medicare Part B

Part B is the supplementary medical insurance, which covers provider and outpatient hospital services. It is considered a supplemental plan because each participant must pay a stipulated amount each month for the benefits. MACs also process Part B claims. Part B MACs were formerly known as carriers.

The rules, limits, and maximums under this coverage are subject to change annually.

BENEFITS. A $162.00 deductible was in place for 2011. After the deductible has been satisfied, generally 80 percent of the approved charge would be paid.

Since January 1, 2006, the Medicare Part B deductible has been indexed to the increase in the average cost of Part B services for Medicare beneficiaries. In other words, the amount charged for the Part B deductible depends on the amount spent by Medicare for payments for services.

Medicare Part C

Medicare beneficiaries may choose to have covered items and services furnished to them through a Medicare Health Maintenance Organization (Medicare HMO; see "Medicare and Managed Care" later in this chapter). If a Medicare beneficiary selects this coverage, he or she is no longer covered by Parts A and B and must receive services according to the selected carrier's arrangements. When patients are enrolled in a Medicare HMO, claims for these patients must be submitted to the HMO.

> ### PRACTICE **PITFALLS**
>
> Beneficiaries may enroll, disenroll, or change their Medicare HMO. For this reason, frequent verification of patient eligibility is important. To determine if the patient is enrolled in a Medicare HMO, ask the patient at the initial interview, or see if a sticker is attached to the Medicare identification card indicating that the beneficiary has coverage through a Medicare HMO.

Medicare Part D

In an effort to provide better health coverage for Medicare beneficiaries, in 2006 Medicare Part D was enacted as part of the Medicare Prescription Drug, Improvement, and Modernization Act of 2003. With this program Medicare beneficiaries receive limited coverage for prescription drug benefits.

▶ **CRITICAL THINKING QUESTION:** Why would a patient choose to select one part of Medicare but not another?

Allowable Charges

In 1992 the federal government established a standardized provider payment schedule based on a **resource-based relative value scale (RBRVS).** The RBRVS was designed to address the soaring cost of provider health care in the United States, the imbalance between practicing in high-cost or low-cost geographic areas, and provider specialties.

Payments for services in the RBRVS system are determined by the resource costs required to provide the particular service. The RBRVS basically contains three components: the provider's total work, relative specialty practice cost, and professional liability insurance. Payments are calculated by multiplying the combined relative values of a service by a conversion factor (a monetary amount that is determined by the CMS). Payments also are adjusted for geographical differences in resource costs.

An RBRVS for a particular procedure is comprised of a provider's total work (50 percent), practice costs (45 percent), and malpractice costs (5 percent). Total work is defined by six factors: time, technical skill, mental effort, physical effort, judgment, and stress. These factors are measured before, during, and after the specific service or procedure. Practice costs are defined as overhead costs including office rent, staff salaries, equipment, and supplies.

● **ONLINE INFORMATION:** For a copy of the RBRVS scale and for examples of its use, visit www.aap.org/visit/RBRVSbrochure.pdf.

ACTIVITY #1

Demonstrating Your Understanding of Medicare

Directions: Name the four parts of Medicare and list the benefits provided under each part.

1. _____
   _____

2. _____
   _____

3. _____
   _____

4. _____
   _____

Medicare Health Insurance Card

A Medicare health insurance card (HIC) may be identified by its red, white, and blue coloring and is issued to every person who is entitled to Medicare benefits. When billing for a patient who is a Medicare recipient, always request the patient's Medicare HIC. This card indicates whether the patient has Part A (hospital), Part B (medical, provider services), Part C (HMO, PPO), or Part D (prescription drug) coverage, and when each became effective. A copy of this card should be made and placed in the patient's chart (Figure 5-4 ●).

FIGURE 5-4

Sample Medicare card

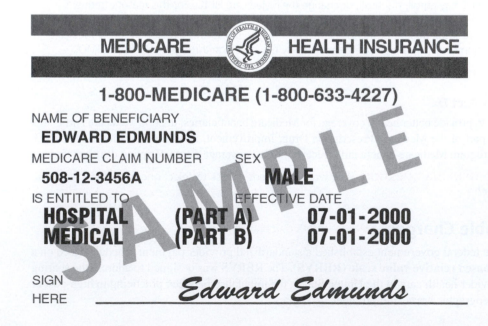

MEDICARE · HEALTH INSURANCE

1-800-MEDICARE (1-800-633-4227)

NAME OF BENEFICIARY
EDWARD EDMUNDS

MEDICARE CLAIM NUMBER   SEX
508-12-3456A   **MALE**

IS ENTITLED TO   EFFECTIVE DATE
HOSPITAL (PART A)   07-01-2000
MEDICAL   (PART B)   07-01-2000

SIGN
HERE   _Edward Edmunds_

The card identifies the Medicare beneficiary and includes the following information:

- Name as it appears on the Social Security records
- Medicare Health Insurance Claim Number (HICN)
- Beginning date of Medicare entitlement for particular services
- Sex
- Place for beneficiary signature

The patient's **Medicare health insurance claim number (HICN)** is a unique identification number assigned to Medicare beneficiaries, which normally consists of a Social Security number followed by a letter of the alphabet and possibly another letter or number (e.g., 123-45-6789A). The alpha character at the end of the number indicates how the beneficiary became entitled but does not indicate the type of coverage that the patient has. The beneficiary or provider must include the HICN on all claims submitted to Medicare for payment, as well as on all related bills or documents.

The Medicare card also contains a letter code indicating the recipient's status. The letter codes are as follows:

Code	Identification
A	Primary claimant (wage earner)
B	Aged wife, age 62 or over
B1	Aged husband, age 62 or over
B3	Aged wife, age 62 or over, second claimant
B5	Young wife, with a child in her care, second claimant
B6	Divorced wife, age 62 or over
BY	Young husband, with a child in his care
C1-C9	Child (includes minor, student, or disabled child)
D	Aged widow, age 60 or over
D1	Aged widower, age 60 or over
D2	Aged widow (2nd claimant)
D3	Aged widower (2nd claimant)
D6	Surviving divorced wife
E	Widowed mother
E1	Surviving divorced mother
E4	Widowed father
E5	Surviving divorced father
F1	Father
F2	Mother
F3	Stepfather
F4	Stepmother
F5	Adopting father
F6	Adopting mother
HA	Disabled claimant (wage earner)
HB	Aged wife of disabled claimant, age 62 or over
M	Uninsured—Premium Health Insurance Benefits (Part A)
M1	Uninsured—Qualified for but refused Health Insurance Benefits (Part A)
T	Uninsured—Entitled to Health Insurance Benefits (Part A) under deemed or renal provisions; or Fully Insured who have elected entitlement only to Health Insurance Benefits
TA	Medicare Qualified Government Employment (MQGE)
TB	MQGE aged spouse

W	Disabled widow
W1	Disabled widower
W6	Disabled surviving divorced wife

Medicare entitlement extends to Railroad Retirement beneficiaries. The HICN assigned to these individuals usually begins with an alphabetical prefix and is followed by six or nine digits (e.g., A 123-45-6789).

PRACTICE **PITFALLS**

The Medicare card should be checked at least once every year, as Medicare HICN can change according to the beneficiary's record of entitlement. This is especially true in the case of female beneficiaries, as their name, HICN, and suffix can change according to marital status. Also, a copy of the Medicare card should be made and placed in the patient's chart.

National Provider Identifier Number

As mandated by the Health Insurance Portability and Accountability Act of 1996 (HIPAA), the CMS has established a provider identification system called **National Provider Identifiers (NPIs)**. The objective of the National Provider Identifier system is to assign a unique national identifier number to every provider of Medicare health care services.

The NPI is a standard unique health identifier for providers and consists of nine numbers plus a check-digit in the tenth position. Since May 23, 2007, all covered entities must use the NPI for all claims or payers. NPIs replaced the use of previous identification numbers such as Unique Provider Identification Numbers (UPINs) and Provider Identification Numbers (PINs). The NPI is a lifetime number regardless of where a provider works.

● **ONLINE INFORMATION:** To learn more about the NPI visit the Web site for Centers for Medicare and Medicaid Services at www.cms.hhs.gov/NationalProvIdentStand

Medicare Billing Notices

The **Medicare Remittance Notice (MRN)** is used to convey payments to providers who accept assignment for Medicare claims. This document is sent to a provider by the Medicare carrier or intermediary and lists all the claims submitted by the provider that were paid for a specified time period (Figure 5-5 ●). MRNs provide a report of claim determination, check for the payable amount, and an explanation of how or why a claim was processed as it was. Each carrier/intermediary uses its own variation of this format.

The MRN lists the patient's name, the date services were rendered, the services that were rendered, the billed amount, and the Medicare approved amount. It also shows the part of the approved amount that was applied toward the patient's deductible, the patient's coinsurance amount, and the amount Medicare is paying.

The **Medicare Summary Notice (MSN)** is an explanation of benefits sent to the Medicare beneficiary, detailing the processing of claims submitted for payment (Figure 5-6 ●).

Following is an explanation of the MSN:

1. *Date:* Date MSN was sent.
2. *Customer Service Information:* Who to contact with questions about the MSN. Provide the date of the MSN (1), your Medicare number (3), and the date of the service (7).
3. *Medicare Number:* The number on the Medicare Card.
4. *Name and Address:* Lists the Medicare beneficiary's address.
5. *Be Informed:* Message regarding Medicare fraud and abuse.
6. *(Part A) Hospital Insurance—Inpatient Claims;* or *(Part B) Medical Insurance—Outpatient Facility Claims;* or *(Part B) Medical Insurance—Assigned Claims;* or *(Part B) Medical Insurance—Unassigned Claims:* Indicates type of service provided.

```
CARRIER NAME                                          MEDICARE
ADDRESS 1                                          REMITTANCE
ADDRESS 2                                              NOTICE
CITY, STATE ZIP
(909) 111-2222

        PROVIDER NAME              PROVIDER #:          1111111111
        ADDRESS 1                  PAGE #:              1   OF   1
        ADDRESS 2                  CHECK/EFT #:         00001111111
        CITY, STATE ZIP            STATEMENT #:         F21103AA0101SYS
```

IMPORTANT INFORMATION FOR SUPPLIERS

PERF PROV SERV DATE	POS NOS PROC MODS	BILLED	ALLOWED	DEDUCT	COINS	GRP/RC-AMT	PROV PD
NAME EDMUNDS, EDWARD	HIC 508123456A ACNT 34567890 ICN 02105104002000					ASG Y MOA MA01	
1111111111 0315 031502 12	1 L0310 GZ	500.00	0.00	0.00	0.00	OA-50 250.00	0.00
REM: M25						CO-50 250.00	
1111111111 0315 031502 12	1 L0317 GAGK	250.00	250.00	0.00	50.00	OA-100 0.00	200.00
PT RESP 50.00	CLAIM TOTALS	750.00	250.00	0.00	50.00	500.00	200.00
ADJ TO TOTALS: PREV PD	0.00 INTEREST .19 LATE FILING CHARGE					0.00 NET	200.19
NAME EDMUNDS, EDWARD	HIC 508123456A ACNT 123456789 ICN 02105104012200					ASG Y MOA MA130 MA13	
1111111111 0301 030102 12	1 K0010	50.00	0.00	0.00	0.00	CO-16 50.00	0.00
PT RESP 0.00	CLAIM TOTALS	50.00	0.00	0.00	0.00	50.00	0.00
ADJ TO TOTALS: PREV PD	0.00 INTEREST 0.00 LATE FILING CHARGE					0.00 NET	0.00

SUMMARY OF NON-ASSIGNED CLAIMS

PERF PROV SERV DATE	POS NOS PROC MODS	BILLED	ALLOWED	DEDUCT	COINS	GRP/RC-AMT	PROV PD
NAME EDMUNDS, EDWARD	HIC 508123456A ACNT 123456789 ICN 02102104012100					ASG Y MOA MA15 MA18 MA01	
1111111111 0303 030302 12	1 E0143 NU	150.00	111.97	0.00	22.39	OA-100 89.58	0.00
REM: M3 M25						PR-42 38.03	
PT RESP 150.00	CLAIM TOTALS	150.00	111.97	0.00	22.39 127.61	0.00	
ADJ TO TOTALS: PREV PD	0.00 INTEREST 0.00 LATE FILING CHARGE					0.00 NET	0.00
CLAIM INFORMATION FORWRDED TO: ACE INS							

TOTALS:	# OF CLAIMS	BILLED AMT	ALLOWED AMT	DEDUCT AMT	COINS AMT	TOTAL RC-AMT	PROV PD AMT	PROV ADJ AMT	CHECK AMT
	3	950.00	361.97	0.00	72.39	677.61	200.00	0.19-	200.19

PROVIDER ADJ DETAILS:	PLB REASON CODE	FCN	HIC	AMOUNT
	L6			0.19-

GLOSSARY: GROUP, REASON, MOA, REMARK AND REASON CODES

CO   Contractual obligation. The patient may not be billed for this amount.

OA   Other adjustment

PR   Patient responsibility

16   Claim/service lacks information which is needed for adjudication. Additional information is supplied using remittance advice remark codes whenever appropriate.

42   Charges exceed our fee schedule or maximum allowable amount.

50   These are non-covered services because this is not deemed a "medical necessity" by the payer.

100   Payment made to patient/insured/responsible party.

M3   Equipment is the same or similar to equipment already being used.

M25   Payment has been (denied for the/made only for a less extensive) service because the information furnished does not substantiate the need for the (more extensive) service. If you believe the service should have been fully covered as billed, or if you did not know and could not reasonably have been expected to know that we would not pay for this (more extensive) service, or if you notified the patient in writing in advance that we would not pay for this (more extensive) service and he/she agreed in writing to pay, ask us to review your claim within 120 days of the date of this notice. If you do not request review, we will, upon application from the patient, reimburse him/her for the amount you have collected from him/her (for the/in excess of any deductible and coinsurance amounts applicable to the less extensive) service. We will recover the reimbursement from you as an overpayment.

MA01 If you do not agree with what we approved for these services, you may appeal our decision. To make sure that we are fair to you, we require another individual that did not process our initial claim to conduct the review. However, in order to be eligible for a review, you must write to us within 120 days of the date of this notice, unless you have a good reason for being late.

An institutional provider, e.g., hospital, Skilled Nursing Facility (SNF), Home Health Agency (HHA) or hospice may appeal only if the claim involves a reasonable and necessary denial, a SNF recertified bed denial, or a home health denial because the patient was not homebound or was not in need of intermittent skilled nursing services, or a hospice care denial because the patient was not terminally ill, and either the patient or the provider is liable under Section 1879 of the Social Security Act, and the patient chooses not to appeal.

If your carrier issues telephone review decisions, a professional provider should phone the carrier's office for a telephone review if the criteria for a telephone review are met.

MA13 You may be subject to penalties if you bill the beneficiary for amounts not reported with the PR (patient responsibility) group code.

MA15 Your claim has been separated to expedite handling. You will receive a separate notice for the other services reported.

MA18 The claim information is also being forwarded to the patient's supplemental insurer. Send any questions regarding supplemental benefits to them.

MA130 Your claim contains incomplete and/or invalid information, and no appeal rights are afforded because the claim is unprocessable. Please submit a new claim with the correct/complete information.

L6   Interest.

FIGURE 5-5

Sample Medicare Remittance Notice

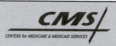

Medicare Summary Notice

Page 1 of 2

July 1, 2011

BENEFICIARY NAME
STREET ADDRESS
CITY, STATE   ZIP CODE

CUSTOMER SERVICE INFORMATION

Your Medicare Number: 111-11-1111A

If you have questions, write or call:
Medicare (#12345)
555 Medicare Blvd., Suite 200
Medicare Building
Medicare, US XXXXX-XXXX

Call: 1-800-MEDICARE (1-800-633-4227)
Ask for Doctor Services
TTY for Hearing Impaired: 1-877-486-2048

BE INFORMED: Beware of telemarketers offering free or discounted medicare items or services.

This is a summary of claims processed from 05/10/2011 through 08/10/2011.

PART B MEDICAL INSURANCE – ASSIGNED CLAIMS

Dates of Service	Services Provided	Amount Charged	Medicare Approved	Medicare Paid Provider	You May Be Billed	See Notes Section
Claim Number: 12435-84956-84556						
Paul Jones, M.D., 123 West Street, Jacksonville, FL 33231-0024						a
Referred by: Scott Wilson, M.D.						
04/19/11	1 Influenza immunization (90724)	$5.00	$3.88	$3.88	$0.00	b
04/19/11	1 Admin. flu vac (G0008)	5.00	3.43	3.43	0.00	b
	Claim Total	**$10.00**	**$7.31**	**$7.31**	**$0.00**	
Claim Number: 12435-84956-84557						
ABC Ambulance, P.O. Box 2149, Jacksonville, FL 33231						a
04/25/11	1 Ambulance, base rate (A0020)	$289.00	$249.78	$199.82	$49.96	
04/25/11	1 Ambulance, per mile (A0021)	21.00	16.96	13.57	3.39	
	Claim Total	**$310.00**	**$266.74**	**$213.39**	**$53.35**	

PART B MEDICAL INSURANCE – UNASSIGNED CLAIMS

Dates of Service	Services Provided	Amount Charged	Medicare Approved	Medicare Paid You	You May Be Billed	See Notes Section
Claim Number: 12435-84956-84558						
William Newman, M.D., 362 North Street, Jacksonville, FL 33231-0024						a
03/10/11	1 Office/Outpatient Visit, ES (99213)	$47.00	$33.93	$27.15	$39.02	c

THIS IS NOT A BILL – Keep this notice for your records.

FIGURE 5-6

Sample Medicare Summary Notice

Your Medicare Number: 111-11-1111A

Notes Section:

a This information is being sent to your private insurer. They will review it to see if additional benefits can be paid. Send any questions regarding your supplemental benefits to them.

b This service is paid at 100% of the Medicare approved amount.

c Your doctor did not accept assignment for this service. Under Federal law, your doctor cannot charge more than $39.02. If you have already paid more than this amount, you are entitled to a refund from the provider.

Deductible Information:

You have met the Part B deductible for 2011.

General Information:

You have the right to make a request in writing for an itemized statement which details each Medicare item or service which you have received from your physician, hospital, or any other health supplier or health professional. Please contact them directly, in writing, if you would like an itemized statement.

Compare the services you receive with those that appear on your Medicare Summary Notice. If you have questions, call your doctor or provider. If you feel further investigation is needed due to possible fraud and abuse, call the phone number in the Customer Service Information Box.

Appeals Information – Part B

If you disagree with any claims decisions on this notice, your appeal must be recieved by **November 1, 2011.** Follow the instructions below:

1) Circle the item(s) you disagree with and explain why you disagree.

2) Send this notice, or a copy, to the address in the "Customer Service Information" box on Page 1. (You may also send any additional information you may have about your appeal.)

3) Sign here _____   Phone number _____

Revised 08/11

FIGURE 5-6

(Continued)

7. *Dates of Service:* Dates service was provided.
8. *Claim Number:* Number that identifies this specific claim.
9. *Benefit Days Used (Part A):* Shows the number of days used in the benefit period. *Amount Charged (Part B):* Amount the provider billed Medicare.
10. *Non-Covered Charges (Part A):* Shows the charges for services denied or excluded by the Medicare program for which the patient may be billed. *Medicare Approved (Part B):* Amount Medicare approved for this service or supply.
11. *Deductible and Coinsurance (Part A):* The amount applied to the patient's deductible and coinsurance. *Medicare Paid Provider (Part B):* Amount Medicare paid the provider. For unassigned claims this section is called "Medicare Paid You."
12. *You May Be Billed:* The amount the provider may bill the patient.
13. *See Notes Section:* If letter appears, refer to (16) for explanation.
14. *Provider's Name and Address:* Provider's name and billing address.
15. *Services Provided (Part B):* Brief description of the service or supply received.
16. *Notes Section:* Explains letters in (13) for more detailed information about this claim.
17. *Deductible Information:* How much of the deductible the patient has met.
18. *General Information:* Important Medicare news and information.
19. *Appeals Information:* How and when to request an appeal.

ACTIVITY #2

Testing Your Understanding of the MRN and MSN

Directions: Answer the following questions. Refer to the text if necessary.

1. What is an MRN and to whom is it sent?

   _____

   _____

   _____

2. What is an MSN and to whom is it sent?

   _____

   _____

   _____

Advanced Beneficiary Notice (ABN)

Providers are responsible for knowing the Medicare policies for their state and for informing patients in writing when Medicare is likely to deny payment for a planned procedure. If a provider fails to provide a proper **Advance Beneficiary Notice (ABN)** in situations that require one, the provider can be held liable under the provisions of Limitation of Liability (LOL) laws (Title XVIII, section 1879). An ABN is a written notice a provider gives a Medicare beneficiary before rendering services, which informs a patient that a particular procedure may not be considered medically necessary by Medicare, and that if payment is denied by Medicare the patient will be responsible for paying for the procedure. LOL provisions require only that the beneficiary be notified, and the beneficiary's signature indicating receipt can, and very likely will, result in the beneficiary's financial liability.

The provider must have reasonable cause to believe the procedure will be denied as not medically necessary. Reasonable cause can include a procedure that is listed as not covered under Medicare guidelines (e.g., cosmetic surgery) or a procedure that has been previously denied under similar circumstances.

Medicare has set forth strict guidelines as to the content of this form. To be acceptable, an ABN must be on the approved Form CMS-R-131-G, or on CMS-R-131-L for laboratory tests. When an ABN has been obtained, use the –GA modifier to alert Medicare that the ABN has been obtained. Failure to obtain the ABN could result in denial of payment. The forms in Figures 5-7 ● and 5-8 ●, when completed, meet all ABN requirements.

Patient's Name: Edmunds, Edward

Medicare # (HICN): 508-12-3456A

Paul Provider, M.D.

5858 Peppermint Place, Anytown, USA 12345

ADVANCE BENEFICIARY NOTICE (ABN)

NOTE: You need to make a choice about receiving these health care items or services.

We expect that Medicare will not pay for the laboratory test(s) that are described below. Medicare does not pay for all of your health care costs. Medicare only pays for covered items and services when Medicare rules are met. The fact that Medicare may not pay for a particular item or service does not mean that you should not receive it. There may be a good reason your doctor recommended it. Right now, in your case, **Medicare probably will not pay for -**

Items or Services:
Insurance Physical

Because:
Routine service; not covered under Medicare benefits.

The purpose of this form is to help you make an informed choice about whether or not you want to receive these items or services, knowing that you might have to pay for them yourself. Before you make a decision about your options, you should **read this entire notice carefully.**

> Ask us to explain if you don't understand why Medicare probably won't pay.
> Ask us how much these items or services will cost you (Estimated Cost: $ 90.00),
> in case you have to pay for them yourself or through other insurance.

PLEASE CHOOSE **ONE** OPTION. CHECK **ONE** BOX. **SIGN & DATE** YOUR CHOICE.

☐ **Option 1. YES**   I want to receive these items or services.

I understand that Medicare will not decide whether to pay unless I receive these items or services. Please submit my claim to Medicare. I understand that you may bill me for items or services and that I may have to pay while Medicare is making its decision. If Medicare does pay, you will refund me any payments I made to you that are due to me. If Medicare denies payment, I agree to be personally and fully responsible for payment. That is, I will pay personally, either out of my pocket or through any other insurance that I have. I understand I can appeal Medicare's decision.

☐ **Option 2. NO.**   I have decided not to receive these items or services.

I will not receive these items or services. I understand that you will not be able to submit a claim to Medicare and that I will not be able to appeal your opinion that Medicare won't pay.

_____

Date

_____

Signature of patient or person acting on patient's behalf

Note: Your health information will be kept confidential. Any information that we collect about you on this form will be kept confidential in our offices. If a claim is submitted to Medicare, your health information on this form may be shared with Medicare. Your health information, which Medicare sees, will be kept confidential by Medicare.

OMB Approval No. 0938-0566   Form No. CMS-R-131-L (June 2002)

FIGURE 5-7

Advance Beneficiary Notice (ABN) for general use

Patient's Name: Edmunds, Edward
Medicare # (HICN): 508-12-3456A

Laboratory Provider
5859 Peppermint Place, Anytown, USA 12345

ADVANCE BENEFICIARY NOTICE (ABN)

NOTE: You need to make a choice about receiving these laboratory tests.

We expect that Medicare will not pay for the laboratory test(s) that are described below. Medicare does not pay for all of your health care costs. Medicare only pays for covered items and services when Medicare rules are met. The fact that Medicare may not pay for a particular item or service does not mean that you should not receive it. There may be a good reason your doctor recommended it. Right now, in your case, Medicare probably will not pay for the laboratory test(s) indicated below for the following reasons:

Medicare does not pay for these tests for your condition	Medicare does not pay for these test as often as this (denied as too frequent)	Medicare does not pay for experimental or research use tests
1. Complete Blood Cell Count (CBC)		

The purpose of this form is to help you make an informed choice about whether or not you want to receive these laboratory tests, knowing that you might have to pay for them yourself. Before you make a decision about your options, you should read this entire notice carefully.

    Ask us to explain, if you don't understand why Medicare probably won't pay.

    Ask us how much these laboratory tests will cost you (**Estimated Cost: $25.00**),

    in case you have to pay for them yourself or through other insurance.

PLEASE CHOOSE **ONE** OPTION. CHECK **ONE** BOX. **SIGN & DATE** YOUR CHOICE.

☐ **Option 1. YES.** I want to receive these laboratory tests.

I understand that Medicare will not decide whether to pay unless I receive these laboratory tests. Please submit my claim to Medicare. I understand that you may bill me for laboratory tests and that I may have to pay while Medicare is making its decision. If Medicare does pay, you will refund me any payments I made to you that are due to me. If Medicare denies payment, I agree to be personally and fully responsible for payment. That is, I will pay personally, either out of my pocket or through any other insurance that I have. I understand I can appeal Medicare's decision.

☐ **Option 2. NO.** I have decided not to receive these laboratory tests.

I will not receive these laboratory tests. I understand that you will not be able to submit a claim to Medicare and that I will not be able to appeal your opinion that Medicare won't pay. I will notify my doctor who ordered these laboratory tests that I did not receive them.

_____
Date

_____
Signature of patient or person acting on patient's behalf

Note: Your health information will be kept confidential. Any information that we collect about you on this form will be kept confidential in our offices. If a claim is submitted to Medicare, your health information on this form may be shared with Medicare. Your health information, which Medicare sees, will be kept confidential by Medicare.

OMB Approval No. 0938-0566   Form No. CMS-R-131-L (June 2002)

FIGURE 5-8

Advance Beneficiary Notice (ABN) for laboratory tests

Collecting Amounts Due from the Patient

You must bill the patient for any amounts that Medicare lists as the patient's responsibility (after any other coverage has been billed) and honestly attempt to collect these amounts. This means billing the patient at least three times before writing off any portion of the patient's amount. In addition, you must use the same collection attempts for Medicare patients as you do for non-Medicare patients.

If the patient's portion of the bill is written off, why this was done should be documented. Hardship conditions should be fully noted, as should bankruptcies or other conditions. The patient should be asked to sign a statement verifying this information.

Two cases may be allowed for noncollection attempts: hardship of the patient and amounts that are too minimal to be cost-effective for established collection procedures. Hardship will usually only be accepted if the medical office can show that patients' portions were waived in only a limited number of cases. In cases of cost-effectiveness, the provider should have a cost analysis performed that determines all the costs involved in collecting on an account. Amounts below this level can be considered not cost-effective. The cost analysis should be updated periodically and kept on file. Failure to bill Medicare patients for their part of the fee can result in fines and penalties, exclusion from the Medicare program, and possible criminal charges.

▶ **CRITICAL THINKING QUESTION:** When trying to collect the patient's portion of the bill, how can you demonstrate sensitivity to issues that the patient may have about his or her ability to pay the bill?

Billing Deceased Patients

Because Medicare pays for health care for an aged population, it is inevitable that some of the patients will die while enrolled. Before you process any claims, be sure to obtain a signed Assignment of Benefits form from the patient and place it in the patient file.

There are two ways to handle unpaid bills for deceased patients. If assignment is accepted, Medicare will process. If assignment is not accepted, Medicare may wait until the patient's estate is settled before making payment.

If the family of the deceased pays the bill, it should complete form CMS-1660 showing that the bill has been paid and attach the receipt. Medicare will then send payment to the person who paid the bill.

Posting Medicare Payments

Payments received from Medicare may be lower than the provider's billed charge. If the provider accepts Medicare's assignment, it is important that the medical biller knows how to post payments to the patient's ledger and make adjustments.

On receipt of the MRN, the patients' charts indicated on the MRN should be pulled. Post each payment individually to each patient ledger card (in today's world, most patient account programs are computerized; however, the premise of the program in this book is manually based) and to the daily journal. Separate entries should be made for each patient on the daily journal (not in a lump sum).

If the Medicare allowed amount is less than the billed charge, an adjustment or write-off will need to be made on the ledger card. After the payment has been posted, the next entry on the ledger card should be the adjustment to the charges. Enter the difference between the billed amount and the Medicare approved amount. This amount will be entered on the ledger card in the adjustment column and will be subtracted from the remaining balance. This entry will ensure that Medicare recipients are not being billed for charges that exceed the Medicare approved amount.

Assignment of Benefits

To be a participating provider, the provider must agree to accept assignment on all Medicare claims. By doing this, the provider receives payment directly from Medicare rather than the payment going to the beneficiary. In addition, the provider has agreed to accept the amount approved by the Medicare carrier for the covered services. The patient is not responsible for any amount in excess of the approved amount.

Providers Who Accept Assignment

When a provider agrees to accept Medicare assignment for a bill, Medicare will pay the provider directly for that bill. The provider may bill the patient only for any deductibles or coinsurance that Medicare has deducted from the assigned bill. As a result, the total fee that providers may receive from Medicare and from beneficiaries for an assigned bill is limited to what Medicare deems to be an appropriate fee for the particular service or procedure (the Medicare "allowance").

To encourage providers to accept assignment, the Medicare allowance is higher for providers who agree to accept assignment for all bills for Medicare-eligible persons. These providers are called **participating providers**. Thus, participating providers agree not to practice "balance billing," which would entail charging patients for more than the Medicare allowed amount.

Providers who treat Medicare patients but who decide whether to accept assignment on a case-by-case basis are called **nonparticipating providers**. If assignment is accepted on a claim, the rules for participating providers apply. If assignment is not accepted, the Medicare payment is made directly to the beneficiary.

PRACTICE **PITFALLS**

Providers may collect reimbursement for excluded services, unmet deductibles, and coinsurance from the beneficiary.

To accept or not accept assignment of Medicare benefits for a claim, the provider must enter an X in the square for either Yes or No in block 27 of the CMS-1500 form.

Mandatory Assignment

Providers have the option to accept or not accept Medicare assignment. However, some services require providers to accept assignment. These include the following:

- Clinical diagnostic laboratory services
- Medicare patients who also are eligible for Medicaid
- Ambulatory surgery centers
- Method II home dialysis supplies and equipment
- Provider's assistant, nurse midwives, nurse specialists, nonprovider anesthetists, clinical psychologists, and clinical social workers services
- Effective February 1, 2001, all providers, nonprovider practitioners, and suppliers must take assignment on all claims for drugs and biologicals furnished to any patient enrolled in Medicare Part B.

Limiting Charges

Federal law prohibits a doctor who does not accept assignment from charging more than 15 percent above Medicare's approved amount. This is called the **limiting charge.** Balance billing by nonparticipating providers is strictly limited to this amount. Participating providers are not affected because they are not allowed to balance bill Medicare patients for any services. The limiting charge applies only to providers' services. Ambulance companies and other nonprovider providers are not subject to limiting charge regulations.

Some providers routinely write off any amounts not covered by Medicare. This practice is prohibited by law, as it means that Medicare covers 100 percent of the bill. Thus, there is no monetary incentive to the patient not to overuse services.

SURGERY DISCLOSURE NOTICE. Specific requirements must be followed for nonparticipating providers who perform elective surgeries priced at over $500. For surgeries that are elective (i.e., surgery scheduled in advance, not an emergency, when delay would not result in impairment or death), are not assigned, and for which a charge greater than $500 is expected, the provider must notify the patient of certain information in writing. This information includes the following:

- Name and description of the procedure
- Fact that the surgery is elective
- Expected charge for the surgery
- Approximate Medicare allowable

- Amount by which the provider's charge exceeds the allowable
- The amount of the patient's responsibility

Failure to provide this information could result in penalties being assessed. Medicare carriers may contact providers and request a signed copy of the notification.

ACTIVITY #3

Calculating Collectible Amounts and Adjustments

Directions: Calculate the adjustment and the amount that you may bill the patient in the following examples. Assume in all cases that the patient has fully met the deductible for the year and that the provider is a nonparticipating provider.

	Billed Amount	Medicare Approved	Medicare Paid	Collectible Amount	Adjustment	Balance Due from Patient
1.	175.00	115.40	92.32	_____	_____	_____
2.	35.00	3.00	2.40	_____	_____	_____
3.	375.00	323.60	258.88	_____	_____	_____
4.	45.00	40.00	32.00	_____	_____	_____
5.	1,500.00	1225.60	980.48	_____	_____	_____
6.	950.00	138.05	110.44	_____	_____	_____
7.	20.00	4.72	3.78	_____	_____	_____
8.	95.00	86.86	69.49	_____	_____	_____
9.	175.00	135.70	108.56	_____	_____	_____
10.	75.00	50.30	40.24	_____	_____	_____
11.	260.00	250.00	200.00	_____	_____	_____
12.	545.00	295.95	236.76	_____	_____	_____
13.	1,200.00	968.53	774.82	_____	_____	_____
14.	450.00	445.00	356.00	_____	_____	_____
15.	750.00	560.15	$448.12	_____	_____	_____

Medicare Necessity Denials

The most common reason for denial of claims by Medicare, which are known as **Medicare necessity denials,** is for services that are considered not medically necessary. In Medicare claim processing, this phrase has a wide variety of meanings. The three most common situations that generate a "not medically necessary" denial are the following:

1. The diagnosis does not match the service. If no clear connection can be made between the diagnosis and the related services, additional information should be provided to justify the medical necessity of services.
2. Frequency of services is greater than allowed. Medicare has specific limits for the number of times a specific service can be performed. For example, a patient age sixty-five and over is allowed one mammography screening every two years. If the second mammogram is done before the two-year limit is up, it will be denied as not medically necessary.
3. Level of service does not match diagnosis. This denial is most often used with office visit codes. For example, if the diagnosis for a patient were a simple fracture of the arm, a Level V office visit would be denied. Some Medicare agencies will down-code the level to the appropriate Level II code, but others will simply deny the visit as not medically necessary. **Downcoding** occurs when an insurance carrier changes a code to a similar code that has a lower level of service.

If a claim is denied as not medically necessary, any amounts paid by the patient must be refunded within thirty days of the notification of denial. If you wish to appeal the denial, send in the claim and any related documentation to the Medicare carrier and request a formal review. Be sure to detail exactly which services you are appealing (instead of asking the carrier to review the entire claim), and include documentation to support the medical necessity of services. The information will be reviewed to make a new determination regarding medical necessity.

PRACTICE **PITFALLS**

Claims with incidental services may list certain procedures that are not medically necessary. In such cases, Medicare is not stating that the service is not medically necessary but, rather, that the second procedure is incidental to or an integral part of the first procedure. For example, a laparoscopy is an integral part of removal of a liver lesion. The removal procedure would be allowed and paid; however, the laparoscopy procedure would be denied as not medically necessary if billed as a second procedure since it is an integral part of the first procedure (the removal). In essence, this is a form of downcoding, but the use of the "not medically necessary" denial can lead to confusion and concerns among your patients. It is important to check the Current Procedural Terminology (CPT) and Healthcare Common Procedure Coding System (HCPCS) codes carefully to be sure that a single code does not cover both procedures.

If the claim is denied, you may request that the Medicare carrier provide you with all the information it used to make the denial determination. The request must be made in writing and should list the patient's name, the date of services, the services that were denied, and the reasons Medicare indicated on the forms for the denial. It should also be stated that you are requesting the information under the Freedom of Information Act. Any information sent by the carrier should be studied and retained for future reference.

Medicare Secondary Payer

Some individuals covered by Medicare also have other insurance to pay their medical bills. Medicare pays secondary (**Medicare Secondary Payer [MSP]**) to employer-sponsored group insurance, individual policies carried by the employee, workers' compensation insurance, beneficiary entitled to Black Lung benefits, automobile or no-fault insurance, and third-party liability. Medicare pays primary to Medicare supplemental plans (Medigap insurance), Medicaid, and after thirty months of end-stage renal disease. The patient should be questioned during the first visit to determine all insurance coverage(s) that could affect payment of a claim.

Certain diagnoses have been identified as being covered by workers' compensation. If the patient is diagnosed with one of these conditions, the Medicare carrier will probably request additional information or deny the claim as covered by workers' compensation. This list of diagnoses can be obtained from the U.S. Department of Labor.

When submitting a claim for secondary payments to Medicare, a copy of the claim as originally submitted to the primary carrier should be submitted. The primary insurance's explanation of benefits (EOB) should be attached, along with any necessary evidence to support services. No changes should be made on the claim, including altering the "amount paid" and "amount now due" boxes to reflect the payment made by the primary carrier.

If a Medicare patient is covered by primary insurance and receives a payment from the primary insurance that is greater than the Medicare allowed amount, the provider cannot charge the patient for any amounts (including the 20 percent coinsurance normally collected). The full allowed amount has been collected from the primary insurance carrier. The provider is allowed to keep any amounts paid by the primary insurance that are over the Medicare-allowed amount without violating the agreement with Medicare. If the patient's insurance pays less than the amount Medicare determines to be the patient's responsibility (deductible and coinsurance amounts), the provider is allowed to bill the patient for the difference between the amount collected from the primary insurance and the patient's responsibility as determined by Medicare.

If a third party is determined to be liable for expenses (e.g., from an auto or other accident), that carrier should be billed first. If the carrier denies payment, a copy of the EOB should be filed with the Medicare claim. If the patient later sues and is granted monetary compensation, Medicare will demand a repayment of the benefits paid. The patient may be asked to sign a form that states that he or she will inform Medicare of the court's decision or a settlement. If the patient receives payment without informing Medicare, the patient is responsible for repaying Medicare. See the Medicare Secondary Payer Table shown in Figure 5-9 ●.

Medicare Secondary Payer Table

If the patient. . .	And this condition exists. . .	Then this program pays first. . .	And this program pays second. . .
Is age 65 or older, and is covered by a Group Health Plan through a current employer or spouse's current employer	The employer has less than 20 employees	**Medicare**	Group Health Plan
	The employer has 20 or more employees, or at least one employer is a multi-employer group that employs 20 or more individuals	Group Health Plan	**Medicare**
Has an employer retirement plan and is age 65 or older or is disabled and age 65 or older	The patient is entitled to Medicare	**Medicare**	Retiree coverage
Is disabled and covered by a Large Group Health Plan from work, or is covered by a family member who is working	The employer has less than 100 employees	**Medicare**	Large Group Health Plan
	The employer has 100 or more employees, or at least one employer is a multi-employer group that employs 100 or more individuals	Large Group Health Plan	**Medicare**
Has end-stage renal disease and Group Health Plan coverage	Is in the first 30 months of eligibility or entitlement to Medicare	Group Health Plan	**Medicare**
	After 30 months	**Medicare**	Group Health Plan
Has end-stage renal disease and COBRA coverage	Is in the first 30 months of eligibility or entitlement to Medicare	COBRA	Medicare
	After 30 months	**Medicare**	COBRA
Is covered under Workers' Compensation because of job-related illness or injury	The patient is entitled to Medicare	Workers' Compensation (for health care items or services related to job-related illness or injury)	**Medicare**
Has black lung disease and is covered under the Federal Black Lung Program	The patient is eligible for the Federal Black Lung Program	Federal Black Lung Program (for health care services related to black lung disease)	**Medicare**
Has been in an auto accident where no-fault or liability insurance is involved	The patient is entitled to Medicare	No-fault or liability insurance (for accident-related health care services)	**Medicare**
Is age 65 or older OR is disabled and covered by Medicare and COBRA	The patient is entitled to Medicare	**Medicare**	COBRA
Has Veterans Health Administration (VHA) benefits	Receives VHA authorized health care services at a non-VHA facility	VHA	Medicare may pay when the services provided are Medicare-covered services and are not covered by the VHA

FIGURE 5-9

Medicare Secondary Payer Table

Medicare and Veterans

Veterans may be eligible for benefits with the Veterans Health Administration (VHA) and at the same time be eligible for Medicare coverage. In these cases, when the patient is eligible for both, Medicare pays first and VHA is the secondary insurance. Coverage scenarios also change depending on whether there is a Veterans Affairs (VA) hospital and/or military base within a reasonable driving distance.

Durable Medical Equipment

Durable medical equipment (DME) is equipment that meets all of the following requirements:

- Can withstand repeated use
- Is primarily and customarily used to serve a medical purpose
- Is generally not useful to a person in the absence of an illness or injury
- Is appropriate for use in the home

Often a provider will prescribe special equipment for use by a beneficiary in the home. The equipment may provide therapeutic benefits or enable the beneficiary to perform certain tasks that could not otherwise be undertaken because of certain medical conditions or illnesses. DME includes, but is not limited to the following:

- Diabetic supplies
- Canes, crutches, walkers
- Commode chairs
- Home oxygen equipment
- Hospital beds
- Wheelchairs

The CMS has four carriers that process durable medical equipment, prosthetics, orthotics, and supplies (DMEPOS) claims. These carriers are referred to as **Durable Medical Equipment Regional Carriers (DMERCs).** Each DMERC covers a specific geographic region of the country.

Medicare Denials

Medicare may deny claims for numerous reasons. If a claim is denied, the reason for the denial will appear on the MRN. This will often be a code, which refers to an in-depth explanation.

One of the most common denials is "incorrect patient information." The information actually may not be incorrect; it may just be different from what Medicare's computer system can process. For example, if a patient is listed on the Medicare records as Sam S. Smith, and you list him as Samuel S. Smith, or Sam Simpson Smith, or Sam Smith, the Medicare computer software may reject the claim. To prevent this from happening, copy the patient's data exactly as it appears on the Medicare card. This is the information you should have in your records and computer data banks, even if Mr. Smith completes his Patient Information Sheet differently.

Another message commonly found on Medicare claims is the following:

We understand that you may not have known that Medicare would not pay for this service. If you believe this service should have been covered, or if you did not know or could not have been expected to know that Medicare would not pay for this service, or if you notified the beneficiary in writing in advance that Medicare would not pay for this service and he/she agreed to pay, ask us to review your claim.

This indicates that the provider has provided a service that Medicare considers "medically unnecessary." If the provider could not be expected to know that this service would be considered medically unnecessary (e.g., Medicare never informed the provider either on a previous MRN or through a newsletter or personal letter), then Medicare is obligated to pay the provider if the claim is submitted for review. For this reason, you should submit all denied Medicare claims for review.

Medicare Appeals Process

Before requesting a Medicare appeal, first determine if the denial was a result of an error or an omission on your part. If so, resubmit the claim with the errors corrected. If you need further clarification regarding the reason a claim was denied, telephone your Medicare carrier or intermediary. If an appeal goes beyond the initial request for review, the provider of the services should be involved in most cases.

There are five levels to the Medicare appeals process:

1. Redetermination
2. Reconsideration
3. Hearing by an administrative law judge
4. Review by the Medicare Appeals Council
5. Judicial review

You should go through each level of appeal before moving on to the next level. The goal is to improve your reimbursement at the lowest level possible.

Redetermination

You have the right to a review if you are dissatisfied with the settlement of a claim. You must request a review within 120 days from the date of the original claim determination, and there is no minimum amount in controversy for this level of review. This request may be made on Form CMS-20027. If you are not using this form, simply submit a statement that explains why you are dissatisfied with the reimbursement on the claim. A written request not made on form CMS-20027 must include the following:

• Beneficiary name
• Medicare Health Insurance Claim (HIC) number
• Specific service and/or item(s) for which a redetermination is being requested
• Specific date(s) of service
• Name and signature of the party or the representative of the party

Attach any supporting documentation to the redetermination request. End the request with a thank you. Have the provider sign it. The redetermination request should be sent to the contractor that issued the initial determination.

Medicare should respond within sixty days. If you do not hear from the claims reviewer within that time, call and ask about the status of the review. If the claim was assigned, the claims reviewer can inform the provider of the results of the review. If the claim was unassigned, the claims reviewer will inform the patient rather than the provider.

When requesting a redetermination, do not use previous payments as justification for why a payment should be made. Medicare may decide that all payments were in error and that you owe a refund.

The redetermination letter issued by the Medicare Appeals Department is called the **Medicare Redetermination Notice**. It will contain all the information necessary to request the next level of appeal.

PRACTICE PITFALLS

It is very helpful to submit an explanation as to why the service(s) should be paid. It is especially helpful to include any documentation that would support this explanation. Supporting documentation may include but is not limited to any or all of the following:

- Operative reports
- X-ray reports
- Test results
- Consultation reports
- Progress notes
- Office notes
- A letter from the provider of service(s)

Reconsideration

If you are not satisfied with the results of the redetermination, you can request a hearing. To proceed to this level, the hearing must be requested within 180 days of the review determination. There is no minimum appeal amount required in order to appeal at this level.

The hearing request form (Figure 5-10 ●) is usually sent to a different office from where the review was done, and the people who process these requests are typically more experienced than those at the lower levels. There are three types of hearings:

1. *On the record.* Based on the written material and data, which you have already submitted to Medicare, and any additional data you provide.
2. *Telephone hearing.* Allows you to introduce new information over the telephone and speak directly with the reviewer. You may be required to substantiate your phone information with additional written records. The provider should always be available for the telephone hearing so that he or she may answer any questions regarding treatment.
3. *In person.* The patient, the provider, and other parties meet in person. The proceedings are typed or recorded, and the tape or transcript is usually available on request.

A decision is generally made within 120 days, unless there are extenuating circumstances. You should receive a written explanation of the findings from the hearing. You may receive further reimbursement, or you may again be denied.

Hearing by an Administrative Law Judge

A request for a hearing by an administrative law judge (ALJ) must be made within sixty days of the fair hearing decision and involve at least $130 in controversy. A decision will generally be issued by the ALJ within ninety days of receipt of the request To succeed at this level, you must prove that yours is an unusual case and that it deserves special consideration. Disagreement with Medicare policies will not be addressed at this level.

Your file will be looked at again. It may be immediately reversed (and payment made), or it may be forwarded to a non-Medicare employee. At this point, you will be contacted regarding details for proceeding with the ALJ hearing.

The Medicare carrier will usually not have a representative present at the ALJ hearing. An authorized representative from the provider's office will need to be present to answer questions. You may submit additional information showing special complications or situations that made your case unusual.

Medicare Appeals Council Review

An Appeals Council Review request must be made within sixty days of the ALJ decision. There are no requirements for the amount of money in controversy. The Appeals Council may, on its own, review the ALJ decision if there is a question that the ALJ decision was not made in accordance with the law. The Appeals Council will generally issue a decision within ninety days of receipt of a request for review.

DEPARTMENT OF HEALTH AND HUMAN SERVICES
CENTERS FOR MEDICARE & MEDICAID SERVICES

REQUEST FOR HEARING
PART B MEDICARE CLAIM
Medical Insurance Benefits - Social Security Act
NOTICE—Anyone who misrepresents or falsifies essential information requested by this form may upon conviction be subject to fine and imprisonment under Federal Law.

CARRIER'S NAME AND ADDRESS

1 NAME OF PATIENT

2 HEALTH INSURANCE CLAIM NUMBER

3 I disagree with the review determination on my claim, and request a hearing before a hearing officer of the insurance carrier named above.

MY REASONS ARE: (Attach a copy of the Review Notice. NOTE: If the review decision was made more than 6 months ago, include your reason for not making this request earlier.)

4 CHECK ONE OF THE FOLLOWING

☐ I have additional evidence to submit.
(Attach such evidence to this form or forward it to the carrier within 10 days.)

☐ I do not have additional evidence.

CHECK **ONLY ONE** OF THE STATEMENTS BELOW:

☐ I wish to appear in person before the Hearing Officer.

☐ I do not wish to appear and hereby request a decision on the evidence before the Hearing Officer.

5 EITHER THE CLAIMANT OR REPRESENTATIVE SHOULD SIGN IN THE APPROPRIATE SPACE BELOW

SIGNATURE OR NAME OF CLAIMANT'S REPRESENTATIVE	CLAIMANT'S SIGNATURE
ADDRESS	ADDRESS
CITY, STATE, AND ZIP CODE	CITY, STATE, AND ZIP CODE
TELEPHONE NUMBER / DATE	TELEPHONE NUMBER / DATE

(Claimant should not write below this line)

- -

ACKNOWLEDGMENT OF REQUEST FOR HEARING

Your request for a hearing was received on _____ . You will be notified of the time and place of the hearing at least 10 days before the date of the hearing.

SIGNED

DATE

Form CMS-1965 (05/03)

FIGURE 5-10

Request for Medicare Hearing Form

Federal District Court Hearing

If a provider is still dissatisfied following consideration by the Medicare Appeals Council, and the amount in controversy is at least $1,300, the provider may file an appeal in the federal district court where the provider is located or in the District of Columbia.

At least $1,300 must be in controversy at this level, and an attorney must represent your case. You must appeal within sixty days of the Appeals Council decision. The provider's attorney will handle the case. The provider may want to contact his or her medical society for attorneys experienced at this level of the appeals process.

Reviews or Hearings After the Deadline

A review or hearing request must be filed within six months. You may file after the six-month deadline if you can show good cause for not doing so sooner. Attach a letter to the request for review or hearing that explains the good cause. Medicare defines good cause as any of the following:

- There were circumstances beyond your control or significant communication difficulties.
- The delay resulted from your efforts to obtain documentation, which you did not realize could have been provided after filing for the review or hearing.
- Your records were destroyed or damaged, delaying the filing of the request.

It may be difficult to convince your carrier to provide an extension of time to request a review or hearing. You may need to consider if the benefits are worth the time and effort.

ACTIVITY #4

Check Your Understanding of the Medicare Appeals Process

Directions: List the five levels of the Medicare appeals process.

1. _____
2. _____
3. _____
4. _____
5. _____

Medicare Supplemental Insurance

Medicare Supplemental Insurance (also known as **Medigap** policies) are separate plans written exclusively for Medicare participants that pay for charges that Medicare does not cover. Be careful not to confuse these policies with Medicare Part B, also called supplementary medical insurance (as discussed earlier). Medigap policies are specifically designed to supplement Medicare's benefits and are regulated by federal and state law. Supplemental programs offered by most insurance companies have many variations between them. Also, the benefit structures of these programs are formulated by a Medicare-approved contract the patient may choose to buy to supplement Medicare. A supplemental plan may be written with a variety of optional benefits that the policyholder may choose from, such as the following common options:

1. *Providers' services.* Covers Part B deductible and 20 percent coinsurance for reasonable charges.
2. *Hospital services.* Covers Part A deductible and may or may not cover the various copays not covered by Medicare.
3. *Nursing care, prescriptions, and the nonreplaced fees on the first three pints of blood.*

With the changes in Medicare, supplemental plans have become much more flexible. Therefore, the benefits can be very complex and comprehensive or very basic.

Medicare and Managed Care

In the mid-1980s, Medicare began looking at the managed care market as a way to save costs.

A **Medicare HMO** is an HMO that has contracted with the federal government under the Medicare Advantage program (formerly called Medicare+Choice) to provide health benefits to persons eligible for Medicare who choose to enroll in the HMO, instead of receiving their benefits and care through the traditional fee-for-service Medicare program.

ACTIVITY #5

Researching Medicare HMOs

To learn more about Medicare HMOs, go to the Web site www.medicarehmo.com. Review the information available at this Web site and then write a short synopsis of what you learned.

_____

_____

_____

_____

_____

_____

_____

_____

_____

Medicare Notice of Noncoverage

A **Notice of Noncoverage** must be provided to all Medicare HMO members at the time of discharge from an inpatient facility. This is a letter that advises enrollees of their right to an immediate professional review on a proposed discharge. This allows patients who feel they are being discharged too early to appeal the decision.

In addition, all providers and groups must provide Medicare members with a copy of "An Important Message from Medicare" at the time of admission to any inpatient facility. This letter informs patients of their rights with regard to treatment. Inpatient facilities include hospitals, skilled nursing facilities, convalescent hospitals, psychiatric hospitals, and any other facility where the patient will be staying overnight or receiving twenty-four-hour care.

When filling in the variable fields on the letter, make sure the entries are easily understood. The notice should be hand-delivered to the member, and the member's signature should be obtained, acknowledging receipt of the notice. A copy of the notice, signed by the member, must be placed in the patient chart.

If a Medicare member disagrees with a plan for discharge from an inpatient medical facility, he or she has the right to request an immediate review of the proposed discharge. If the review is requested by noon of the day following receipt of the notice, the member is not financially liable for the inpatient services until receipt of notification that the review board has agreed with the discharge. If the patient does not file the request for review within the specified time period, he or she may still request a review. However, the patient will be financially responsible for treatment after the proposed discharge date if the request is denied.

Medicare Billing Guidelines

When billing Medicare, the provider must complete the appropriate billing forms. The **CMS-1500** (Figure 5-11 ●) form should be used to bill for Medicare services performed outside a hospital setting, thus the CMS-1500 is the uniform claim form for billing provider services. Detailed instructions for completing the CMS-1500 are covered Chapter 14.

Special requirements on the CMS-1500 for Medicare claims include the following:

- *Block 1a.* Enter the Medicare HICN, complete with any prefixes and suffixes.
- *Blocks 4 and 7.* Enter the primary insurance policyholder's name and address (if different from the patient's name and address).

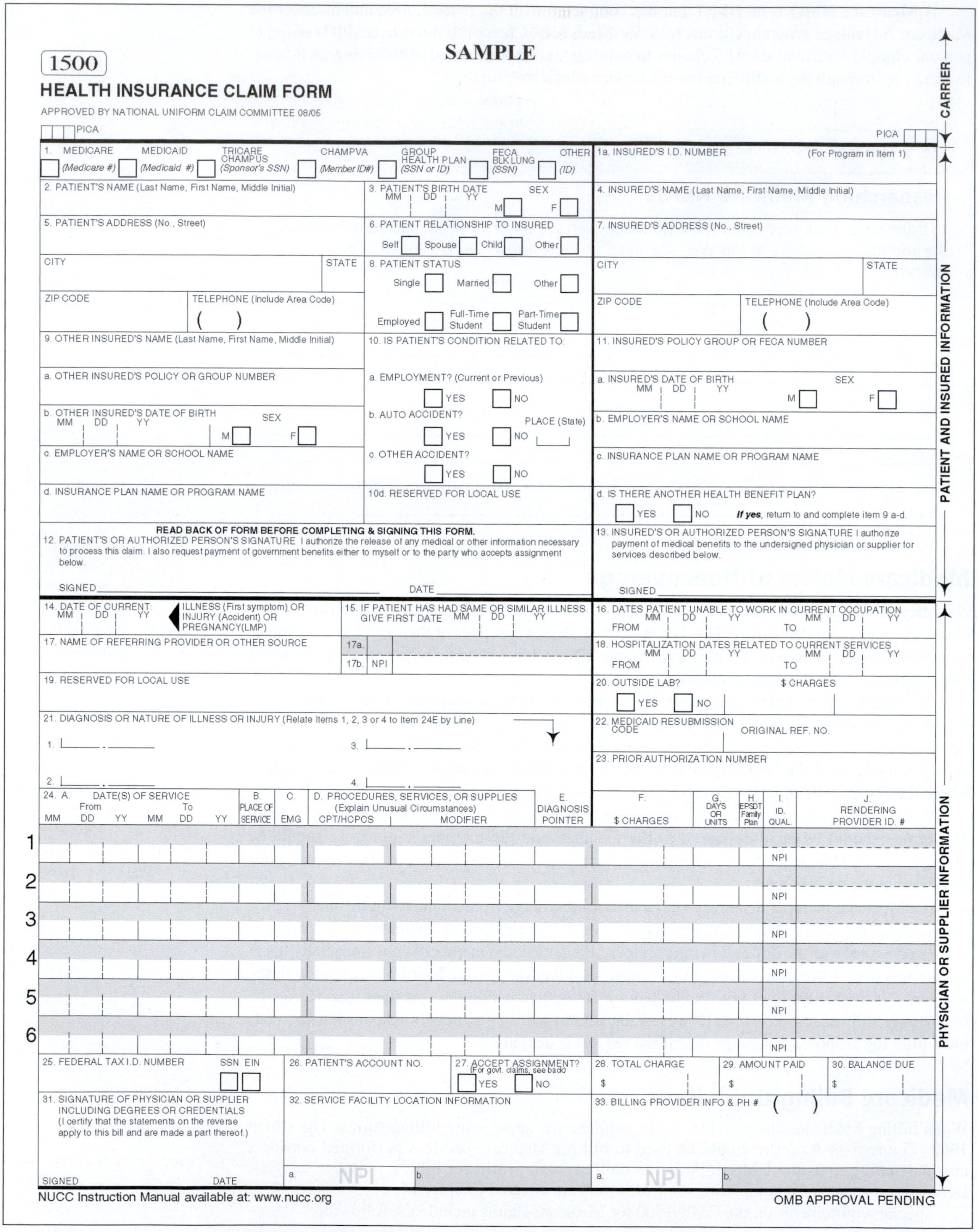

SAMPLE

1500

HEALTH INSURANCE CLAIM FORM

APPROVED BY NATIONAL UNIFORM CLAIM COMMITTEE 08/05

PICA | PICA

CARRIER

1. MEDICARE (Medicare #) | MEDICAID (Medicaid #) | TRICARE CHAMPUS (Sponsor's SSN) | CHAMPVA (Member ID#) | GROUP HEALTH PLAN (SSN or ID) | FECA BLK LUNG (SSN) | OTHER (ID)

1a. INSURED'S I.D. NUMBER (For Program in Item 1)

2. PATIENT'S NAME (Last Name, First Name, Middle Initial)

3. PATIENT'S BIRTH DATE MM DD YY SEX M F

4. INSURED'S NAME (Last Name, First Name, Middle Initial)

5. PATIENT'S ADDRESS (No., Street)

6. PATIENT RELATIONSHIP TO INSURED Self Spouse Child Other

7. INSURED'S ADDRESS (No., Street)

CITY STATE

8. PATIENT STATUS Single Married Other

CITY STATE

ZIP CODE TELEPHONE (Include Area Code) ( )

Employed Full-Time Student Part-Time Student

ZIP CODE TELEPHONE (Include Area Code) ( )

9. OTHER INSURED'S NAME (Last Name, First Name, Middle Initial)

10. IS PATIENT'S CONDITION RELATED TO:

11. INSURED'S POLICY GROUP OR FECA NUMBER

a. OTHER INSURED'S POLICY OR GROUP NUMBER

a. EMPLOYMENT? (Current or Previous) YES NO

a. INSURED'S DATE OF BIRTH MM DD YY SEX M F

b. OTHER INSURED'S DATE OF BIRTH MM DD YY SEX M F

b. AUTO ACCIDENT? YES NO PLACE (State)

b. EMPLOYER'S NAME OR SCHOOL NAME

c. EMPLOYER'S NAME OR SCHOOL NAME

c. OTHER ACCIDENT? YES NO

c. INSURANCE PLAN NAME OR PROGRAM NAME

d. INSURANCE PLAN NAME OR PROGRAM NAME

10d. RESERVED FOR LOCAL USE

d. IS THERE ANOTHER HEALTH BENEFIT PLAN? YES NO ***If yes***, return to and complete item 9 a-d.

READ BACK OF FORM BEFORE COMPLETING & SIGNING THIS FORM.

12. PATIENT'S OR AUTHORIZED PERSON'S SIGNATURE I authorize the release of any medical or other information necessary to process this claim. I also request payment of government benefits either to myself or to the party who accepts assignment below.

SIGNED DATE

13. INSURED'S OR AUTHORIZED PERSON'S SIGNATURE I authorize payment of medical benefits to the undersigned physician or supplier for services described below.

SIGNED

PATIENT AND INSURED INFORMATION

14. DATE OF CURRENT: MM DD YY ILLNESS (First symptom) OR INJURY (Accident) OR PREGNANCY(LMP)

15. IF PATIENT HAS HAD SAME OR SIMILAR ILLNESS. GIVE FIRST DATE MM DD YY

16. DATES PATIENT UNABLE TO WORK IN CURRENT OCCUPATION MM DD YY FROM TO MM DD YY

17. NAME OF REFERRING PROVIDER OR OTHER SOURCE

17a.

17b. NPI

18. HOSPITALIZATION DATES RELATED TO CURRENT SERVICES MM DD YY FROM TO MM DD YY

19. RESERVED FOR LOCAL USE

20. OUTSIDE LAB? YES NO $ CHARGES

21. DIAGNOSIS OR NATURE OF ILLNESS OR INJURY (Relate Items 1, 2, 3 or 4 to Item 24E by Line)

1. ___ . ___ 3. ___ . ___

2. ___ . ___ 4. ___ . ___

22. MEDICAID RESUBMISSION CODE ORIGINAL REF. NO.

23. PRIOR AUTHORIZATION NUMBER

24. A. DATE(S) OF SERVICE From MM DD YY	To MM DD YY	B. PLACE OF SERVICE	C. EMG	D. PROCEDURES, SERVICES, OR SUPPLIES (Explain Unusual Circumstances) CPT/HCPCS MODIFIER	E. DIAGNOSIS POINTER	F. $ CHARGES	G. DAYS OR UNITS	H. EPSDT Family Plan	I. ID. QUAL.	J. RENDERING PROVIDER ID. #
1									NPI	
2									NPI	
3									NPI	
4									NPI	
5									NPI	
6									NPI	

25. FEDERAL TAX I.D. NUMBER SSN EIN

26. PATIENT'S ACCOUNT NO.

27. ACCEPT ASSIGNMENT? (For govt. claims, see back) YES NO

28. TOTAL CHARGE $

29. AMOUNT PAID $

30. BALANCE DUE $

31. SIGNATURE OF PHYSICIAN OR SUPPLIER INCLUDING DEGREES OR CREDENTIALS (I certify that the statements on the reverse apply to this bill and are made a part thereof.)

SIGNED DATE

32. SERVICE FACILITY LOCATION INFORMATION

a. NPI b.

33. BILLING PROVIDER INFO & PH # ( )

a. NPI b.

PHYSICIAN OR SUPPLIER INFORMATION

NUCC Instruction Manual available at: www.nucc.org

OMB APPROVAL PENDING

FIGURE 5-11

Sample of CMS-1500 Claim Form

- *Blocks 9–9d.* Enter the Medigap or other policy information. If the patient and insured are the same, enter "SAME" in block 9. If Medicare is the primary insurer, leave 9–9d empty.
- *Block 11.* Enter "NONE" unless the claim is for Medicare as the secondary payer. If so, then list the requested information in blocks 11–11c.
- *Block 13.* Enter "SOF" or "Signature on File" if the provider is a participating provider.
- *Block 17 and 17a.* Enter the full name and credentials of the referring, ordering, or other source in 17, and enter the UPIN or NPI number in 17a.
- *Block 24K.* Enter the UPIN or PIN number of the performing provider of service or supplier if a group name is entered in block 33.
- *Block 30.* Enter amount.

Mandatory Claims Submission

Federal law makes it mandatory for providers to submit claims for Medicare patients. It is also mandatory that providers submit claims to Medicare electronically. The laws and regulations permit a number of exceptions to the electronic billing requirement under special circumstances. Providers are not allowed to charge for the service of billing Medicare. Providers who do not submit a claim or who impose a charge for completing the claim are subject to

PRACTICE **PITFALLS**

The following suggestions help with properly completing the billing forms and complying with Medicare guidelines.

1. It is important that the proper ICD-9-CM or ICD-10-CM code be used to denote the diagnosis. All diagnoses must be coded to the highest digit possible. If a five-digit code exists, it should be used rather than a four-digit code. In addition, an appropriate ICD-9-CM or ICD-10-CM code should be cross-referenced from block 21 to block 24E for each service indicated in block 24D of the CMS-1500.

2. Keep for reference a fee schedule, list of unbundled services, list of denied services, list of procedures with limits on the number of services, and list of those procedures that require preauthorization from the carrier. Having these items readily available will assist the provider in making informed decisions regarding the care and treatment of the patient, while still receiving the maximum possible reimbursement for services rendered.

3. If modifiers are not self-explanatory, be sure to include any necessary documentation that substantiates the services rendered.

4. If you have a claim that contains numerous procedures or potentially confusing information, send a cover letter that clarifies the services performed and the documentation for the necessity of services.

5. Document everything. If you have received information over the phone, document the full name, title, and department of the person who gave you the information, as well as the date and time of the contact. Sending a follow-up letter that thanks the person for helping and puts in writing your understanding of the important points of the conversation is also a wise practice. At the bottom of the letter include a note as follows: "If I misunderstood the information, please contact me at the above number or address to clarify." This letter provides proof of the contact should you need it in an audit. If a contact is received stating that you misunderstood the information, be sure to document it, then notate it on the original letter.

6. Read and retain your Medicare bulletins. They are considered legal notification that you have been made aware of Medicare rules and regulations.

7. Providers may collect any deductible and coinsurance from the patient at the time of service. However, it may be best to wait until after receiving the Medicare Remittance Notice. This prevents the medical office from having to return any amounts that were for services that Medicare deemed not medically necessary, and it allows a more accurate calculation of the amount the patient owes.

8. Medicare rules state that the carrier must pay claims within thirty days for "clean claims." A **clean claim** is one that can be paid as soon as it is received because the claim is complete in all aspects and does not need additional investigation. Claims for non-participating providers are not processed as quickly as those for participating providers. Also, claims submitted electronically are processed faster than those submitted on paper and often contain fewer errors, as reentry of the data is not required.

9. Be courteous and kind when dealing with Medicare representatives.

10. If the amounts listed on the Medicare Remittance Notice (MRN) do not match your data regarding allowed amounts or benefits, contact the carrier for clarification.

11. If a check is received from Medicare that contains an overpayment, first check the records to be sure the payment is incorrect. If an overpayment has occurred, deposit the check and write to Medicare regarding the overpayment. Include in the letter copies of the MRN, the check, and the claim, along with an explanation of the amount that has been overpaid. If an overpayment has occurred, Medicare will deduct the overpayment from the provider's next check.

sanctions. The patient may not submit the claim for payment themselves, except in the following situations:

1. If the patient has other insurance, which should pay as primary, the patient may submit the claim and attach a copy of the other carrier's EOB.
2. If the services are not covered by Medicare, but the patient wishes a formal coverage determination for their records, the patient may submit the claim.
3. If the provider refuses to submit the claim (which is a violation of law and the provider may be penalized for such actions), the patient may submit it.
4. If services are provided outside the United States, the patient may submit the claim.
5. When the patient has purchased durable medical equipment from a private source, the patient may submit the claim.

Claim Filing Time Limit

Medicare regulations require that claims be filed no later than twelve months, or one calendar year, after the date of service. Medicare will deny a claim if the service was provided more than twelve months ago. When a claim is denied for filing after the deadline, that determination cannot be appealed. However, if documentation is submitted that shows that the delay was a result of an administrative error on the part of the Social Security Administration or the Medicare carrier or intermediary, the time limit may be waived. However, claim payment for assigned claims will be reduced by 10 percent if the claim is not filed within one year of the date of service. Providers may not bill the patient for this reduction.

Medicare Severity-Diagnosis Related Group

Although we have focused on Medicare as it applies to office settings rather than hospital settings, it is important to have some understanding of diagnosis-related group billing. Effective October 1, 1983, Medicare instituted the **Medicare Severity-Diagnosis Related Group (MS-DRG)** payments for inpatient hospital claims. In August 2007, a major restructuring of the DRG system occurred, resulting in the program now known as MS-DRG rather than DRG.

Under MS-DRG, instead of the hospital itemized billing system, a flat-rate payment is made based on complications or comorbidities (CCs) or major CCs (MCCs) that the patient may be experiencing along with the principal diagnosis. By billing using the MS-DRG system, if the hospital can treat the patient for less, it retains the savings. If treatment costs more, the hospital must absorb the loss. Neither Medicare nor the patient is responsible for the excess amount for hospital claims only, and this does not involve billing from provider offices. It is very important to code diagnoses accurately (to the fifth digit, if warranted and using ICD-9-CM codes), as payments are based on principal diagnosis.

Provisions have been made for cases atypically expensive (based on the diagnosis) because of complications or an abnormally long confinement. Known as outliers, these cases are reimbursed on an itemized or cost percentage basis instead of MS-DRG. The bill from the hospital must indicate that it is an outlier.

Excluded from MS-DRG are long-term care, children's care, and care in psychiatric or rehabilitative hospitals. In addition, several states have obtained waivers from MS-DRG.

MS-DRG Benefit Payment Calculations

As shown in the following examples, the maximum liability under a plan includes only the expenses that are covered by the plan and that the insured is legally obligated to pay.

EXAMPLE 1 Itemized hospital bill exceeds Medicare MS-DRG allowance.

Hospital bill	$8,700
DRG allowance	$7,000
Medicare payment	$5,868
(Medicare payment = MS-DRG allowance − $1,132 Medicare Part A deductible)	
Patient's responsibility	$1,132
Hospital write-off	$1,700

Although the Medicare MS-DRG allowance is less than the itemized hospital bill, the insured is legally obligated to pay only the $1,132 Part A 2011 deductible.

EXAMPLE 2 Medicare MS-DRG allowance exceeds itemized billed amount.

Hospital bill	$ 8,700
DRG allowance	$10,000
Medicare payment	$ 8,868
Patient's responsibility	$ 1,132

Even though the Medicare payment exceeds the itemized hospital bill, the insured is still legally obligated to pay the $1,132 Part A 2011 deductible.

ACTIVITY #6

Computing Hospital Write-offs

Directions: Compute the hospital write-off amount for the following scenario.

Hospital bill	$ 9,500
DRG allowance	$ 7,500
Medicare payment	$ 6,368
(Medicare payment = MS-DRG allowance − $1,132 Medicare Part A 2011 deductible)	
Patient's responsibility	$ 1,132
Hospital write-off	$ _____

Directions: Compute the patient's responsibility amount for the following scenario.

Hospital bill	$ 5,000
DRG allowance	$ 7,500
Medicare payment	$ 6,548
Patient's responsibility	$ _____

Medicaid

Medicaid is a joint federal–state medical assistance program for certain categories of low-income people. The federal Medicaid program was established under Title XIX of the Social Security Act of 1965. The purpose of this program is to provide the needy with access to medical care. The Medicaid program is administered by each individual state, using federal and state funding.

Each state administers its Medicaid program, and the name of the program may vary from state to state. Medi-Cal is the name of California's Medicaid health care program. This program pays for a variety of medical services for those eligible for and enrolled in the program.

Medicaid Eligibility

The regulations governing eligibility under this program are extremely complex. Individuals may be entitled to coverage because of medical, family, or financial situations. The fact that the individual has private insurance does not preclude eligibility for Medicaid benefits.

Most Medicaid recipients belong to one of two classes: the categorically needy and the medically needy. **Categorically needy** recipients usually earn less than the poverty level every month. They may or may not be working, and they may or may not have other health insurance. Coverage for some programs may be limited to pregnant women or their children.

Medically needy recipients are those whose high medical expenses and inadequate health care coverage (often a result of catastrophic illnesses) have left them at risk of being indigent. Many disabled and elderly persons fall into this category.

For a claimant's services to be covered under Medicaid, the claimant must be a Medicaid beneficiary and the provider must be an approved Medicaid provider. To be an approved provider, the provider of services must agree to accept Medicaid's determination of approved amounts as binding. That is, similar to Medicare's approved amount on assigned claims, the provider is not allowed to bill the patient for any amount not approved by Medicaid. In recent years, many providers have dropped out of the Medicaid program because their allowances and payments are extremely low, even lower than those provided by Medicare.

Medicaid Covered Services

Medicaid providers must accept the Medicaid allowance as payment in full for service(s) rendered. Providers are forbidden to balance bill patients for amounts not paid by Medicaid. In most states Medicaid eligibility is determined by a state-designated organization. Covered benefits under Medicaid include these:

- Inpatient hospital care
- Outpatient hospital services
- Provider services
- Laboratory and x-ray services
- Screening, diagnosis, and treatment of children under age 21
- Immunizations
- Home health care services
- Family planning services
- Outpatient hospital services
- Early and Periodic Screening, Diagnosis, and Treatment (EPSDT) services

EARLY AND PERIODIC SCREENING, DIAGNOSIS, AND TREATMENT. The **Early and Periodic Screening, Diagnosis, and Treatment (EPSDT) Program** is a preventive screening program designed for the early detection and treatment of medical problems in welfare children (known in California as the Child Health and Disability Prevention [CHDP] program).

EPSDT includes such things as medical histories and physical examinations of children, immunizations, developmental assessments, and screening for dental problems, hearing loss, vision problems, and lead poisoning. If problems are found, states may be required to provide services and treatment. To indicate that EPSDT services were rendered, use block 24H on the CMS-1500 form. If billing for EPSDT services, indicate an E in block 24H, and if billing for family planning services, indicate an F in block 24H.

Additional benefits may be offered in various states, such as these:

- Ambulance charges
- Emergency room care
- Podiatry services
- Psychiatric services
- Dental services
- Chiropractic services
- Private duty nursing
- Optometric services (eye care)
- Eyeglasses and eye refractions
- Intermediate care
- Care in a clinic setting
- Prosthetic devices
- Diagnostic and screening services
- Preventive and rehabilitative services (e.g., physical therapy)
- Treatment for allergies
- Dermatologic treatments
- Some medical cosmetic procedures (often reconstructive)
- Prescription drugs

You can obtain further information from your state's Medicaid agency.

Medicaid Eligibility Verification

When billing for services for Medicaid recipients, you must have a copy of the Medicaid eligibility card for the month the services are rendered because a patient may be eligible one month and not the next. Medicaid recipients will have an **eligibility card** to show that they are eligible for Medicaid.

The guidelines for determining eligibility for Medicaid recipients differ from state to state. It is important that you become familiar with these guidelines by reviewing the manuals that are provided by your state.

Some Medicaid-covered services require the Medicaid beneficiary to pay a copayment, a small fee for services. The services that require copayments vary from state to state.

In most states, Medicaid claims must be submitted within sixty days of the end of the month for which services were rendered. Some general exceptions apply to this rule (and these services must be billed within one year of the date of service):

1. Dental bills
2. Obstetric care
3. Treatment plan completion
4. When the patient has other insurance coverage
5. Retroactive eligibility
6. If the patient did not inform the provider that there was Medicaid coverage

Reimbursement from Medicaid

By law, Medicaid is always secondary to private group health care plans. Therefore, if the patient has other coverage through an employer or any other insurance carrier, that carrier should be billed first. Once payment has been received, Medicaid should be billed and a copy of the EOB from the other carrier attached to the claim.

If Medicaid inadvertently pays primary, it will exercise its right of recovery and seek reimbursement from the private plan or directly from the provider. The private plan or provider is required to process Medicaid's request for reimbursement and pay back the monies Medicaid paid.

The Medicaid program does not process its own claims. Medicaid contracts with an organization to act as the fiscal intermediary, as Medicare does. The intermediary processes the claims according to specifications set forth by the Medicaid program.

The rates under this program are based on the results of reimbursement studies conducted by the U.S. Department of Health and Human Services. Reimbursement for hospital inpatient services is based on each facility's "reasonable cost" of services as determined from audit cost reports and annual limitations on reimbursable increases in cost.

Providers are not allowed to bill or submit a claim to the Medicaid beneficiary for any service included in the program's scope of benefits except to collect money from a patient's private health care coverage prior to billing Medicaid, or to collect the patient's "share of cost."

Some Medicaid systems collect a small **share of cost** payment or fixed copayment from the patient. A share of cost payment or copayment is the amount the patient is responsible for paying for services rendered. This amount will not be printed on the Medicaid recipient's eligibility card. The amount collected should be indicated in block 10d of the CMS-1500 form. You should always ask about any share of cost when you contact Medicaid to verify the patient's eligibility.

MEDICAID REMITTANCE ADVICE. A **Medicaid Remittance Advice (MRA)** is issued to providers for claims submitted to Medicaid over a certain period of time. Payment for claims submitted during this time period is made in a lump sum payment. This MRA provides information about claims that were paid, adjusted, voided, and denied. Some intermediaries send the MRA separately from the claims payment; others combine the claims payment with the MRA. The Medicaid Remittance Advice is very similar to the Medicare Remittance Notice.

POSTING MEDICAID PAYMENTS. As with Medicare, Medicaid payments will probably be lower than the actual billed charges. Because Medicaid recipients are not financially responsible for the balance, an adjustment to the patient's account will have to be made. When the remittance advice is received from Medicaid, each patient ledger will need to be pulled and the payments recorded. The adjustments should be made on the next corresponding entry line on the ledger card if using a manual system. The payment amount should be subtracted from the billed amount and the difference should be written off. If the patient's eligibility for Medicaid is terminated at the time services are rendered, the patient becomes financially responsible for the charges. At that time, the patient should be billed directly.

MEDICAID APPEALS. If a Medicaid claim payment is not satisfactory to the provider of services, the provider has the option to file an appeal. An appeal must be made to the fiscal intermediary within ninety days of the action causing the grievance. The appeal must be submitted in writing. Copies of the appeal letter, claim, and any additional documentation should be included with the submission.

THE MEDICAID CLAIM FORM. Medicaid Claim Forms must be filled out when submitting claims to Medicaid. Many states now use the CMS-1500 form for billing, but with the mandatory requirement of most states of electronic billing, this form may soon become obsolete. Additional information on completing the CMS-1500 is given in Chapter 14.

PRACTICE **PITFALLS**

The following suggestions will help with properly completing Medicaid billing forms and complying with Medicaid guidelines:

1. Type the claim rather than write it.
2. Use capital letters only when typing claims.
3. Do not strike over to correct errors.
4. Do not use "N/A"; leave the space blank.
5. Be as complete and accurate as possible.
6. Code accurately and to the greatest possible number of digits, using the ICD-9-CM and CPT.
7. Use all appropriate modifiers, and list them in order of importance.
8. Be sure diagnosis codes substantiate the services provided.
9. If a claim is unusual, it may be better to send it manually rather than electronically, if you are permitted to do so. Electronic claims do not allow for the addition of medical reports or additional data to substantiate services.
10. Because Medicaid pays secondary to Medicare, claims for patients who are eligible for both programs should first be billed to Medicare. Medicare will automatically forward the claim to the Medicaid carrier after payment. Medicare often pays more than the Medicaid-allowed amount, and no payment will be forthcoming unless the patient has a deductible that has been met.
11. If the patient is over age sixty-five but is not eligible for Medicare, indicate this on the claim in the Remarks section, along with the reason. For example, if the patient is an alien, "over 65 and not eligible for Medicare—ALIEN."

Many states' Medicaid forms are read by computer, so it is important to complete them correctly. It is important to follow the proper Medicaid billing requirements for your state in order to receive correct reimbursement from Medicaid.

Medicaid as Secondary Payer

Federal regulations require Medicaid to be the **payer of last resort.** This means that all third parties, including Medicare, TRICARE, workers' compensation, and private insurance carriers, must pay before Medicaid pays. In addition, providers must report any such payments from third parties on claims filed for Medicaid payment.

If the Medicaid-allowed amount is more than the third-party payment, Medicaid will pay the difference up to the Medicaid-allowed amount. If the insurance payment is more than the Medicaid-allowed amount, Medicaid will not pay an additional amount.

Medicaid is not responsible for any amount for which the recipient is not responsible. Therefore, a provider cannot bill Medicaid for any amount greater than what the provider agreed to accept from the recipient's private plan. If the recipient is not responsible for payment, then Medicaid is not responsible for payment.

Certain Medicaid programs are considered "primary payers." When a Medicaid recipient is entitled to one or more of the following programs or services, Medicaid pays first (this is not an all-inclusive list):

- Vocational Rehabilitation Services
- Division of Health Services for the Blind
- Maternal and Child Health Delivery Funds

Treatment Authorization Request

In many cases, prior authorization is required before services are rendered. A Treatment Authorization Request (TAR) form is completed to obtain authorization for specific services (Figure 5-12 ●, form may vary by state). This form must be completed and sent to the appropriate agency for authorization to be given before services can be rendered. The prior authorization number should be indicated in block 23 of the CMS-1500 form. Please check with

Verbal Control No. *1	Type of Service Requested *2 ☐ ☐ Drug Other	Is Request Retroactive? ☐ ☐ YES NO *3	Is Patient Medicare Eligible? ☐ ☐*4 YES NO	Provider Phone No. *5	Patient's Authorized Representative (IF ANY) Enter name and address: *6

Provider Name and Address *7		Provider Number *8	FOR STATE USE Provider, your request is: *9

Name and Address of Patient
Patient Name (Last, First, MI)   *10 | **Medicaid Identification Number** *11

☐ Approved as Requested
☐ Approved as Modified
(items marked below as authorized may be claimed)

Street Address | **Sex** *12 | **Age** *13 | **Date of Birth** | *14 |

☐ Denied

City, State, Zip Code | **Patient Status** *15 ☐ Home ☐ Board & Care

☐ Deferred

By: _____
Medi-Cal Consultant

Phone Number *16 | ☐ SNF/ICF ☐ Acute

Comments/Explanation

Diagnosis Description *17 | **ICD-9 CM** *18 **Diagnosis Code**

Medical Justification *19

*20

Line No.	Authorized Yes | No	Approved Units	Specific Services Requested	Units of Service	NDC/UPC or Procedure Code	Quantity	Charges
1	☐ ☐	*21	*22	*23	*24	*25	*26
2	☐ ☐						
3	☐ ☐						
4	☐ ☐						
5	☐ ☐						
6	☐ ☐						

To the best of my knowledge, the above information is true, accurate and complete and the requested services are medically indicated and necessary to the health of the patient.

*27

_____ _____ _____
Signature of Physician or Provider   Title   Date

Authorization is valid for services provided *28⬚
From   Date   To   Date
| | | |

Office | Sequence Number *29⬚

FIGURE 5-12

State Treatment Authorization Request Form

your state's Medicaid fiscal intermediary for prior treatment authorization guidelines. The following are some of the services that require a TAR:

- Inpatient hospital services
- Home health agency services
- Hearing aids
- Chronic hemodialysis services
- Some surgical procedures

INSTRUCTIONS FOR COMPLETING THE TAR. Each State's Medicaid agency has a form for requesting authorization for treatment of Medicaid patients. This form must be completed before the rendering of services. An explanation of how to complete the sample form is provided here.

1. *Verbal Control Number.* This number is given when there is insufficient time to request a Treatment Authorization Number for the services provided. Once a Verbal Control Number is given, you must complete and submit a TAR immediately.
2. *Type of Service Requested.* Place an X in the appropriate box.
3. *Request Is Retroactive.* Place an X in the appropriate box.
4. *Is Patient Medicare Eligible?* Place an X in the appropriate box.
5. *Provider Phone Number.* Enter the area code and phone number for the provider.
6. *Patient's Authorized Representative (If Any)/Enter Name and Address.* When the patient has an authorized representative, enter the name and address of that representative here.
7. *Provider Name and Address.* Enter the name and address of the provider.
8. *Provider Number.* Enter the provider's Medicaid-assigned number.
9. *For State Use.* Leave this area blank. This is where the Medicaid consultant will indicate if the services requested are approved, approved but modified, denied, or deferred. If the TAR is approved but modified, denied, or deferred, the consultant will give an explanation in the Comments/Explanation section. The reviewing consultant must sign and date the TAR, or it is not valid.
10. *Name and Address of Patient.* Enter the patient's last name, first name, and middle initial. Enter the patient's address and telephone number on the following lines.
11. *Medicaid Identification Number.* Enter the patient's Medicaid identification number as it appears on the eligibility label or ID card.
12. *Sex.* Enter "M" for male or "F" for female.
13. *Age.* Enter the age of the patient.
14. *Date of Birth.* Enter the patient's date of birth in an eight-digit format (i.e., 01/01/CCYY).
15. *Patient Status.* Place an X in the appropriate box.
16. *Phone Number.* Enter the patient's telephone number.
17. *Diagnosis Description.* Enter the description of the diagnosis.
18. *ICD-9-CM Diagnosis Code.* Enter the ICD-9-CM diagnosis code for these services. Diagnosis descriptions and codes must relate to the services requested in the section below.
19. *Medical Justification.* Enter the medical justification (attach consultation report or other medical documentation if necessary) for the medical consultant to determine medical necessity. Enter the hospital name and address on the first line of this section. If the patient is inpatient in a skilled nursing or intensive care facility, enter the name and address of the facility in this section.
20. *Authorized Yes/No.* Leave blank. The Medicaid consultant will check these boxes if some services are approved but others are denied.
21. *Approved Units.* Leave blank. The Medicaid consultant will enter the approved number of units.
22. *Specific Services Requested.* Enter the name of the procedure or service requested. Up to six services may be requested on each TAR.
23. *Units of Service.* Enter the means for determining units of service (e.g., 15 minutes for treatments that are calculated per 15-minute blocks).
24. *NDC/UPC or Procedure Code.* Enter the procedure (CPT) code or the drug code for the procedure or drug for which you are requesting authorization. (The code on the TAR and the claim submitted must be the same.)
25. *Quantity.* Enter the number of times the service or procedure is to be performed.

26. *Charges.* Enter the usual and customary fee for the requested services.
27. *Signature of Provider or Provider.* The signature of the provider of services or authorized representative must appear in this space. Enter the title of the person signing the TAR and the date.
28. *Authorization Is Valid for Services Provided.* This section will be completed by the state agency reviewing the TAR. The authorized services must be completed within the dates specified. If the TAR is for a hospitalization, the claim submitted cannot have a date of service earlier than the "From Date" on the TAR.
29. *Sequence Number.* The TAR control number is preprinted on the form at the time of production. The consultant may add additional numbers or letters. (This number must be entered as the TAR control number on the claim when submitted to Medicaid.)

PRACTICE **PITFALLS**

Because Medicaid eligibility is usually determined periodically, eligibility must be verified monthly to ensure that the patient is eligible for coverage. A provider rendering services to a Medicaid patient must accept the Medicaid payment as payment in full and cannot balance bill the patient. Medicaid claims are paid directly to the provider of services; therefore, no assignment of benefits is necessary.

Medicaid Billing Guidelines

When billing Medicaid, the provider must complete the appropriate billing forms. Most Medicaid charges are billed on the CMS-1500 form. Special requirements on the CMS-1500 for Medicaid claims are as follows:

- *Blocks 4 and 7.* Enter the primary insurance policyholder's name and address (if different than the patient).
- *Blocks 9–9d.* Enter information if Medicaid is the secondary payer. If Medicaid is the primary insurer leave 9–9d empty.
- *Block 10d.* Enter the share of cost as follows "SOC 2249"—no sign or decimal points are used. This block is used only by a few state programs.
- *Block 12.* Leave blank.
- *Block 13.* Leave blank.
- *Block 20.* Enter an X in the "No" box. Medicaid law forbids billing for services rendered by another provider.
- *Block 23.* Enter the prior authorization number if applicable.
- *Block 24A.* Enter the date in the MM DD YY format in the "From" column. Do not enter a date in the "To" column (no date ranging is allowed on Medicaid claims).
- *Block 24H for EPSDT.* If EPSDT service is provided, indicate with a capital "E"; if family planning services are provided, indicate with a capital "F."
- *Block 24I (EMG).* If services rendered are for emergency hospital services provided at the hospital, indicate by marking an X.
- *Block 24J (COB).* Enter an X if the patient has other insurance; also attach the EOB.
- *Block 27.* Enter an X in the "Yes" box.
- *Block 29.* Enter the amount paid by the other carrier if Medicaid is the secondary payer; otherwise leave blank.
- *Block 30.* Enter the balance due if Medicaid is the secondary payer; otherwise leave blank.

Children's Health Insurance Program

The State Children's Health Insurance Program (SCHIP), now known more simply as the Children's Health Insurance Program (CHIP), is a federal government program administered by the U.S. Department of Health and Human Services. The program's intent has always been to try to provide coverage for uninsured children in families with incomes too high to qualify for Medicaid. On February 4, 2009, the Children's Health Insurance Reauthorization Act was signed into law. This Act expanded the health care program to cover an additional four million children and pregnant women, including legal immigrants, without a waiting period.

Like Medicaid, CHIP is a partnership between federal and state governments. Each state individually runs its program according to the requirements set forth by the federal Centers for Medicare and Medicaid Services.

CHAPTER REVIEW

Summary

- Medicare and Medicaid billing guidelines change frequently. It is essential for the medical biller to keep abreast of all the changes that occur.
- Medicare intermediaries send out bulletins on a regular basis. The medical biller should read through these bulletins as soon as possible to become familiar with any updates or changes in the billing procedures.
- Medicaid was established under Title XIX of the Social Security Act of 1965 to provide the needy with access to medical care. The Medicaid card must be used when billing for Medicaid services.
- It is important to remember that providers who accept Medicare patients are not allowed to bill the patient for any amounts that Medicare does not cover. If the patient is covered by other insurance, the other insurance carrier is primary to Medicaid and should be billed first.
- Each state's Medicaid program dictates the appropriate guidelines to use for billing. If the correct guidelines are not used, Medicaid may not accept the claim for payment.

Review Questions

Directions: Answer the following questions without looking back into the material just covered. Write your answers in the space provided.

1. What is Medicare? _____

_____

_____

2. On what three criteria is Medicare eligibility based? _____

_____

_____

3. Medicare _____ is considered the basic plan or hospital insurance and

Medicare _____ is the medical insurance that covers providers' services.

4. Briefly explain how to file an appeal on a Medicare claim. _____

_____

_____

_____

_____

5. What does it mean if a provider accepts assignment of benefits with regard to Medicare?

_____

_____

_____

_____

6. What is the purpose of the Medicaid program? _____

_____

_____

7. (True or False?) By law, Medicaid is always primary to private group health insurance plans. _____

8. In what situation are providers allowed to bill or submit a claim to the Medicaid beneficiary?

_____

9. Once Medicaid pays, is the doctor allowed to balance bill the patient for any amount Medicaid did not cover? _____

_____

10. In order for a claimant's services to be covered under Medicaid, the claimant must be a _____ and the provider must be an _____.

If you are unable to answer any of these questions, refer back to that section in the chapter, and then fill in the answers.

Activity #7: Word Search

Directions: Find and circle the words listed below. Words can appear horizontally, vertically, diagonally, forward, or backward.

1. Carrier
2. Clean claim
3. Downcoding
4. Intermediary
5. Medicaid
6. Medicare
7. Medicare fraud
8. Medicare HMO
9. Medigap
10. Part B
11. Part D
12. Share of cost
13. Supplements

```
D S C G C R V W P N E K Y
U U H A N Y E M M R A R D
A P M A R I D H A D A A I
R P E L R R D C P I R A A
F L D U Z E I O D X P S C
E E I U X D O E C A L I I
R M G Q E N M F R N J Q D
A E A M T R B T C C W K E
C N P W E A B Q T O V O M
I T D T R A P E B H S B D
D S N M E D I M E D I T Q
E I M E D I C A R E H M O
M I A L C N A E L C J D R
```

Activity #8: Locating the Key Terms

Directions: Complete the crossword puzzle by filling in a word from the key word(s) that fits each clue.

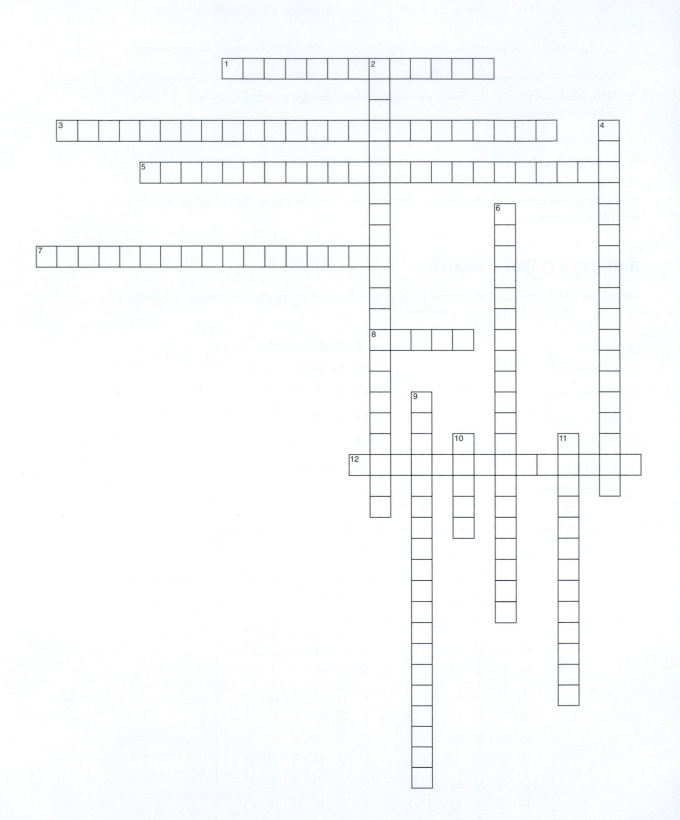

Across

1. A period that begins with the first day of admission to the hospital and ends after the patient has been discharged from the hospital or skilled nursing facility for a period of sixty consecutive days (including the day of discharge)

3. The most common reason for denial of claims by Medicare for services that are considered not medically necessary

5. Equipment that can withstand repeated use, is primarily and customarily used to serve a medical purpose, is generally not useful to a person in the absence of an illness or injury, and is appropriate for use in the home

7. Means that all third parties, including Medicare, TRICARE, workers' compensation, and private insurance carriers, must pay before Medicaid pays

8. Medicare's basic plan or hospital insurance

12. A patient whose high medical expenses and inadequate health care coverage (often a result of catastrophic illnesses) have left him or her at risk of being indigent

Down

2. Providers who agree not to practice balance billing, or charging patients for more than the Medicare allowed amount

4. People who usually make less than the poverty level every month

6. A condition that occurs when a person's kidneys fail to function

9. Separate plans written exclusively for Medicare participants that pay for amounts that Medicare does not pay

10. Medicare's Advantage portion, and includes coverage in an HMO, PPO, and so on.

11. It is quite similar to Medicare fraud except that it is not possible to establish that abusive acts were committed knowingly, willfully, and intentionally

Activity #9: Matching Key Terms

Directions: Match the following terms with the proper definition by writing the letter of the correct definition in the space next to the term.

1. _____ Advanced Beneficiary Notice

    a. A number assigned to providers/suppliers in Medicare Part B for the practice location(s) where they provide services to beneficiaries

2. _____ Medicaid Remittance Advice

    b. When Medicare pays secondary to employer-sponsored group insurance, individual policies carried by the employee, workers' compensation insurance, beneficiary entitled to Black Lung benefits, automobile or no-fault insurance, and third-party liability

3. _____ Medicare Summary Notice

    c. A standard unique health identifier for providers consisting of nine numbers plus a check digit in the tenth position

4. _____ Nonparticipating providers

    d. The redetermination letter issued by the Appeals Department that contains all the information necessary to request the next level of appeal

5. _____ Provider Identification Number

6. _____ Resource-Based Relative Value Scale

7. _____ Centers for Medicare and Medicaid Services

8. _____ Early and Periodic Screening, Diagnosis, and Treatment

9. _____ Medicare Remittance Notice

10. _____ National Provider Identifiers

11. _____ Unique Provider Identification Number

12. _____ Medicare secondary payer

13. _____ Diagnosis-related group

14. _____ Medicare Health Insurance Claim Number

15. _____ Durable Medical Equipment Regional Carriers

16. _____ Medicare Redetermination Notice

e. Provides information about claims that were paid, adjusted, voided, and denied

f. A number for identifying the provider ordering or referring services

g. One of four regional Medicare carriers responsible for the processing of durable medical equipment claims

h. An explanation of benefits sent to the Medicare beneficiary, detailing the processing of claims submitted for payment

i. A unique identification number assigned to Medicare beneficiaries that normally consists of a Social Security number followed by a letter of the alphabet and possibly another letter or number

j. Under DRG, a flat-rate payment based on the patient's diagnosis instead of the hospital's itemized billing

k. The organization that oversees the Medicare and Medicaid programs

l. An explanation of benefits issued to providers (who accept Medicare assignment) for claims submitted to Medicare for a certain period of time

m. A preventive screening program designed for early detection and treatment of medical problems in welfare children

n. Providers who treat Medicare patients but who decide whether to accept assignment on a case-by-case basis

o. A standardized provider's payment schedule; payments for services determined by the resource costs needed to provide them

p. A written notice a provider gives a Medicare beneficiary before rendering services, which informs a patient that a particular procedure may not be considered medically necessary by Medicare, and that if payment is denied by Medicare, the patient will be responsible for paying for the procedure

Workers' Compensation

After completion of this chapter you should be able to:

Describe the eligibility and basic benefits of workers' compensation.

List situations or places that would be covered by workers' compensation if an accident were to occur.

List the types of claims for which workers' compensation provides coverage.

Describe the three disability levels for workers' compensation claims.

Describe the benefits provided by workers' compensation coverage.

Describe what a medical service order is and what it is used for.

Describe how to handle patient records for workers' compensation cases.

Describe the Doctor's First Report of Illness/Injury and how it is used.

State the information that should be included in a Doctor's First Report and Progress Reports.

Key Words and Concepts you will learn in this chapter:

Death benefits

Doctor's First Report of Injury/Illness

Lien

Medical–legal evaluation

Medical service order

Nondisability claims

Permanent disability claims

Provider's Final Report

Rehabilitation benefit

Subjective findings

Temporary disability claims

Treating provider/physician

Treatment plan

Workers' compensation (WC)

List the factors that may delay the close of a workers' compensation case.

State the guidelines for billing services related to workers' compensation.

Explain how to handle delinquent claims.

List signs to look for that may indicate fraud or abuse of a workers' compensation case.

Describe how third-party liability on a workers' compensation case can affect the medical biller.

Properly complete lien documents.

Explain how to handle a claim that is reversed or denied by the workers' compensation board (WC Appeals Board).

▶ **CRITICAL THINKING QUESTION:** Are all employers required to offer workers' compensation? If so, why?

Workers' compensation (WC) is a separate medical and disability reimbursement program that provides 100 percent coverage for job-related injuries, illnesses, or conditions arising out of and in the course of employment. The employer, by law, is responsible for the benefits due to an injured worker for work-related injuries and illnesses. WC insurance includes benefits for medical care expenses, disability income, and death benefits.

When a patient first enters the office for treatment of an accident, it is important to obtain a statement of exactly what happened so it can be determined whether a claim is covered by WC or by the patient's regular insurance. Job-related injuries include any injuries that happen during the performance of work-related duties, whether they are inside or outside of the office (Figure 6-1 ●). Occupational illnesses are considered to be any disorders, illnesses, or conditions that arise at work or from exposure to factors at work. Occupational illnesses may be caused by inhaling, directly contacting, absorbing, or ingesting the hazardous agent. Some occupational illnesses may take years to develop or may remain latent for a number of years before flaring up. For this reason, some states have WC laws that cover workers for years after they cease active employment in a field. For example, construction workers who have dealt repeatedly with asbestos may develop asbestosis years after exposure.

Federal WC programs cover federal workers, coal miners (Black Lung Program), longshoremen, harbor workers, and energy employees. State WC laws cover everyone else. States set up their own guidelines, with the federal government mandating a minimum level of benefits.

Each state's WC Board has the sole authority to oversee the rights and benefits of an injured or ill worker. It is through this board that injured workers not finding resolution with their employer's workers' compensation insurance can appeal.

As a general limitation, most insurance plans specify that the claimant will not be entitled to payment for "bodily injury or disease resulting from and arising out of any employment or occupation for compensation or profit."

Most personal insurance plans will investigate claims that could be a work related injury, illness, or condition. Because the resolution of a WC case usually takes one to two years, private plans are obligated to pay the benefits for which the member is entitled and then to file a lien with the member and the WC Board to recover their losses when the case is settled.

Once the WC carrier has accepted liability for the claim(s), the private insurance plan will discontinue providing benefits for medical care. At that point, the claim would be denied on the basis that it is work related.

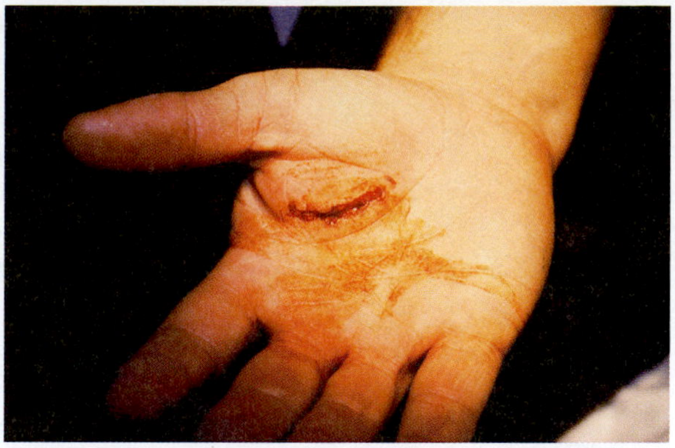

FIGURE 6-1

A possible job-related injury: laceration of the hand

© Michal Heron/Pearson Education

Intent of the Workers' Compensation System

Before WC, injured workers were responsible for their own care, regardless of whether they were hurt on the job or at home. Injured workers had to seek and pay for their own medical care and then attempt to collect from their employer if they felt the company was at least partially responsible for their injury. Many times, the only way to collect was by bringing a lawsuit against the employer, thus creating hard feelings between the employer and the injured worker. Employers who accepted blame for an accident and agreed to cover medical expenses would often choose the medical provider based on price rather than quality of service. In addition, employers were not encouraged to stress safety in the workplace, as the damages awarded in an accident often had more to do with the injured worker's injury than with the amount of negligence on the part of the employer.

Since the implementation of WC and the inclusion of the WC insurance agency, both the employer and the injured worker have a third party to whom they may address grievances and that assists with the rehabilitation of the injured worker.

WC has the following benefits:

1. The employer must provide a choice of at least two providers through which the employee can seek care.
2. It allows injured workers and employers to understand the rights and responsibilities of workers injured on the job. This eliminates many lawsuits and the animosity they entail. It also allows the injured worker to be reimbursed quickly, without waiting for the lawsuit to settle, and to gain a higher portion of the award since there are no attorney's fees and court costs involved.
3. It allows the injured worker to continue to receive income during a disability.
4. It relieves the employer of liability for workplace injuries, except in cases of gross negligence.
5. It relieves hospitals, providers, and public charities of the obligation to cover the costs of caring for those injured workers who are unable to pay for services, especially in the case of an accident that causes permanent disability.
6. It allows for compilation of reports that allow studies of workplace accidents. This provides additional information that can be used to reduce preventable accidents and to assist employers with upgrading workplace safety.
7. It allows special provisions for coverage of minors under age eighteen (or age twenty-one in some states).
8. It allows coverage for all injured workers, regardless of the wealth of the employer or the type of business.

More information can be found at the Department of Labor website and the OSHA website.

Employee Activities

The following section contains some general guidelines as to what constitutes an injury or illness as recognized by a WC Board in most states based on the type of activity, not injury.

Company Activities

Company activities can be defined as the following:

1. An injury sustained while attending an activity sponsored by an employer for the purpose of obtaining some business gain (e.g., company party for morale purposes; sporting activity for which the injured worker is provided transportation or the company gains advertisement by virtue of having the injured worker wear a company "athletic shirt")
2. An injury sustained by an injured worker for which the company provides remuneration
3. An injury sustained while in the course of a person's occupation

Use of Company Vehicles

Most WC laws provide coverage for an injury sustained while driving or as an authorized passenger in a company vehicle. This is true whether the injury is incurred in the course of the person's occupation or the vehicle is provided as part of the injured worker's benefits to use for transportation to and from work.

The law's interpretation of "in the course of employment" is very different from most laypeople's interpretation. For instance, someone injured while eating lunch at a company-sponsored event may be considered covered by WC. Therefore, always undertake investigations and let the appeal to the WC Board handle the final determination. An investigation also should be undertaken to determine if benefits may be payable under automobile insurance coverage.

Business Trips

Most WC laws provide coverage for a person who is on a business trip. This coverage is applicable as long as the person is engaged in employment duties. Of course, there are always exceptions to this rule.

Company Parking Lot

Most WC laws provide that if an injured worker is injured in a parking lot that is owned or maintained by the employer and furnished to the injured worker free of charge, the injured employee may be covered under WC. In addition, coverage would extend, in some instances, to an injury sustained by the injured worker while on neutral ground between the parking lot and the place of employment. An exception would be if such incidents were specifically excluded in the WC law, or if the injuries were sustained from willful or negligent actions on the part of the injured worker.

Usually, WC is not liable for injuries sustained in a parking lot that is owned by the employer and for which a rental fee is charged for the parking space. In such instances, the injured worker has a free choice to park elsewhere, which would relieve the employer of any and all responsibility.

Occupational Disease

Most of the time, coverage will extend to injured workers who contract a disease that develops by working within a certain industry. For instance, most states provide compensation for individuals working with asbestos material over a period of years who then develop asbestosis or silicosis. Likewise, individuals can develop dermatitis from working with certain chemicals, such as in the exterminating industry.

Sometimes, a claimant may have an occupational illness claim that is submitted to the WC Board and a concurrent nonoccupational illness claim for which reimbursement may be made under the plan. In such instances, a separate billing should be completed by the provider, indicating those charges that were solely for the treatment of the nonoccupational disability.

Time Limits

Injured workers must report their injury or illness to their employer within a reasonable period of time, which in many states is thirty days. If an individual was to file within the state's established time frame and the injury later recurs, the individual may be able to file for additional benefits within two years of the original claim.

If a patient is being treated for a work-related injury, be sure that the employer of the injured person has been notified. If not, encourage the patient to do so immediately since WC benefits may be denied if an injury is not reported within a specified period of time. Also, let the patient know that many states will refuse to pay anything for claims if the injury is not reported in a timely manner.

ACTIVITY #1

Online Research: Understanding State Workers' Compensation Laws

Directions: To see how the various laws of workers' compensation vary from state to state, have each student in the class pick a different state to research online. Then discuss and share as a class the information discovered on each of the individual state Web sites.

Fraud and Abuse

Unfortunately, fraud and abuse occur frequently in the WC system. Many injured workers, employers, providers, and insurance carriers find it easy to defraud the system and reap significant financial rewards.

In the past, there has been little deterrent to abusing the system. It frequently was possible to find a doctor who was willing to testify that injuries were more serious than was first thought. Likewise, numerous lawyers stepped in and set up relationships with doctors to produce claims where no actual injury or illness existed. This is especially true when work-related stress became a popular diagnosis for any one of a number of ailments. Many of these lawyers would locate people in the unemployment office and convince them that they could get better reimbursement through WC than they could through unemployment.

It is important for the medical biller to realize that committing fraud or abuse of the WC system is a felony in most states. In addition, not reporting suspected or known cases of fraud or abuse is also illegal in many states. Although most claims are legitimate, the medical biller should recognize what constitutes fraud. The following are some signs of fraud or abuse:

- An injured worker who cannot clearly describe the pain or injury, or whose description changes each time details of the incident are related
- An injured worker who is overly dramatic regarding an injury
- An injured worker who complains of an injury that cannot be substantiated by medical evidence (This may include soft tissue injuries that cannot be seen on an x-ray or a patient who insists that there is a serious injury even when there is medical evidence to the contrary.)
- An injured worker who delays the reporting of an injury, especially an injury that is reported on a Monday when the injured worker claims it happened on Friday
- An injured worker who reports the injury to an attorney or regulatory agency before reporting the injury to the employer
- An injured worker who changes providers frequently, or shows up for the first treatment but seems unhappy with the diagnosis and changes providers (The patient may be seeking a provider who will grant additional time off work or will testify to a greater degree of injury.)
- An injured worker who is a short-term worker or who was scheduled to terminate employment just after the injury occurred
- An injured worker who has a history of curious or excessive WC claims
- An injured worker who complains of a severe injury and an inability to perform certain tasks but is seen using the injured limb or body part while in the waiting room
- An employer who refuses to accept that an injury occurred on the job when there is evidence to the contrary
- An employer who refuses to complete the necessary paperwork and instead attempts to pay for medical services through the company
- A medical provider who orders or performs unnecessary procedures or tests
- A medical provider who inflates the severity of the injury to qualify for higher reimbursement (e.g., lists a fracture as open rather than closed, bills for a high-complexity exam rather than a moderate-complexity exam, etc.)

- A medical provider who charges for services that were never performed or adds additional procedures onto existing claims
- A medical provider who makes multiple referrals to a lab, clinic, or hospital and receives a referral fee from these organizations
- A medical provider who states that an injury exists and needs treatment when no injury is actually present
- A medical provider who sends in duplicate billings with information changed (e.g., dates) to make it appear that services were performed more than once
- A medical provider who files many claims with subjective injuries (e.g., pain, strain, emotional disturbance, inability to perform certain functions)
- A medical provider who files claims for several injured workers of the same company that show similar injuries (e.g., injuries for which reports or x-rays may have been duplicated)
- An attorney who pressures a provider to give additional treatment or to increase the severity of the diagnosis
- An attorney who encourages a provider to charge for services not rendered, stating that the insurance carrier will cover it
- An attorney who refers numerous clients to a specific provider, which suggests that the attorney and provider may be in collusion with each other

These examples suggest signs that a medical biller should look for. If a biller suspects fraud, it should be reported to the appropriate authority immediately. If a biller becomes aware of fraud by the employing provider, he or she should seek the help of an attorney. Billers can be considered guilty of fraud if they knew of the fraud and did nothing to prevent it. This is true even if the biller receives no money from the fraud.

Types of Workers' Compensation Benefits

Workers' compensation provides the following five types of benefits to injured workers.

Nondisability Claims

Nondisability claims are for minor injuries that will not require the patient to be kept from the job. The patient is able to continue working despite the injury. On the first visit to the provider, the provider should complete a Doctor's First Report of Occupational Injury/Illness (First Report), discussed later in this chapter. This form and a copy of the bill should be submitted to the WC carrier. These types of claims include medical expenses such as medical services, hospital treatment, surgery, medications and prosthetics or appliances, and durable medical equipment (Figure 6-2 ●).

Temporary Disability Claims

Temporary disability claims are submitted when the patient is not able to perform job requirements until he or she recovers from the injury involved. When a provider sees a patient in this situation, a first report will be submitted and ongoing reports will be issued every two to three weeks until the patient is discharged to return to work.

Each state has a waiting period before temporary disability becomes effective, usually three to seven days (except in the Virgin Islands, where the waiting period is one day). During temporary disability the injured worker is paid a partial salary as a tax-free benefit. Payments are based on the injured worker's salary and the length of the disability. Temporary disability ends when the patient is able to return to work, even with limitations or to a different department, or when the patient's condition ceases to improve and the patient is left with a permanent disability.

Permanent Disability Claims

Permanent disability claims usually commence after temporary disability when it is determined that the patient will not be able to return to work. The provider will prepare a discharge report stating that the patient is "permanent and stationary." This means that nothing more can be done and the patient will have the disability for the rest of his or

FIGURE 6-2

An injury to the eye may not prohibit the individual from returning to work.

© Michal Heron/Pearson Education

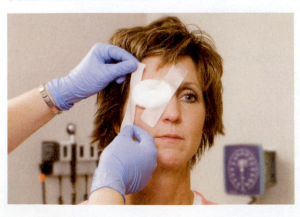

her life (Figure 6-3 ●). The case will be reviewed by the WC Board and, if the disability is determined to be permanent, a compromise and release will be issued. This is a settlement from the insurance carrier for a payment to the injured party.

The amount of the settlement is based on the age of the disabled worker, the amount of money he or she was making at the time of the injury, and the severity of the injury. The older an employee is, the higher the disability rating. This is based on the idea that a younger patient has a better chance than an older worker would of finding other employment or of being retrained for another job. In addition, death benefits and rehabilitation benefits may be provided. Permanent disability payments, either in the form of weekly or monthly payments or as a lump sum distribution, are made to the injured worker.

Death Benefits

Death benefits compensate the family of a deceased injured worker for the loss of income that the injured worker would have provided to the family. Some states also provide a burial benefit to assist with the funeral and burial expenses for the injured worker.

Rehabilitation Benefits

If an injured worker is found to have a permanent disability, some states allow for a rehabilitation benefit. A **rehabilitation benefit** is a benefit provided to retrain the injured worker in a physical ability that will help in seeking future employment (e.g., proper use of a wheelchair, use of the left hand when a person loses their right hand, etc.).

Some states participate in a vocational rehabilitation program, wherein injured workers are provided therapy that strengthens their abilities to perform work-required tasks so they can return to work on full duty. Often, injured workers in such a program will be returned to work on a limited or restricted basis. Providers, therapists, employers, insurance carriers, and all others concerned with the injured worker's case must keep in constant communication to ensure that the patient is not returned to work either sooner or later than possible, and that the injured worker will continue to receive adequate benefits that do not encourage them to cease work (Figure 6-4 ●).

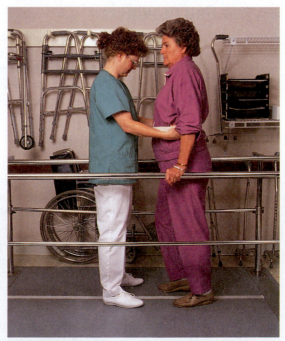

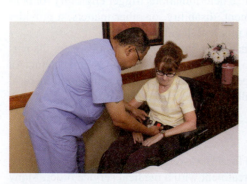

FIGURE 6-3

A permanent disability where the individual is wheelchair bound

© Pat Watson/Pearson Education

FIGURE 6-4

A physical therapist working with a patient who has had a leg injury

© aceshot1/Shutterstock.com

Many states also allow for vocational rehabilitation or retraining in a different job field when the injured worker is unable to return to his or her former position. This can include courses in colleges and vocational schools, or on-the-job training programs. Often, injured workers are paid a weekly allowance (as in the case of temporary disability) while they are attending school and for a limited time after graduation. The time allowed after graduation provides time to locate a job. The injured worker is then considered to be off temporary disability and having returned to work. Vocational rehabilitation can also include job guidance, résumé preparation, and job placement services.

Insurance carriers will often attempt to get the injured worker retrained and back to work as soon as possible, especially because the longer a person is off work, the higher the likelihood that he or she may never return to full-time employment.

ACTIVITY #2

Testing Your Knowledge—Defining the Five Types of Workers' Compensation Benefits

Directions: List and define the five types of workers' compensation benefits.

1. _____

   _____

2. _____

   _____

3. _____

   _____

4. _____

   _____

5. _____

   _____

Treating Providers

A **treating provider (TP)** is used to initially establish the employee's eligibility for workers' compensation benefits. The role of the TP is to provide care and treatment to the injured worker. Treating providers share the same provider–patient relationship as they would with any other patient. The TP may be an employer-selected provider or may be selected by the injured worker, depending on the circumstances.

Medical–Legal Evaluations

Within the workers' compensation system, medical determinations trigger eligibility for benefits. However, when disputes arise over treatment, disability, or other matters, a provider other than the TP may be called on to perform a **medical–legal evaluation**.

The term *medical–legal* means that the evaluation provides medical evidence for the purpose of proving or disproving medical issues in a contested workers' compensation claim. An evaluating provider (also referred to as an independent medical examiner, qualified medical evaluator, or agreed medical evaluator) may be called in when a party objects to the TP's report.

Medical Service Order

The first indication that a patient is being treated for a work-related injury is usually when the injured worker enters the provider's office for treatment with a medical service order. Many employers have a standard medical service order. A **medical service order** is a form stating that the patient is being referred to the provider in regard to a work-related injury and that the employer is responsible for coverage of services. A sample of a medical service order is shown in Figure 6-5 ● and may vary from state to state.

**EMPLOYER
MEDICAL SERVICE ORDER**

ON LETTERHEAD

To Dr./Hospital/Clinic _____
Address _____

We are requesting treatment for _____(name)_____,
in accordance with the workers' compensation statutes for the state of XX. Please submit any necessary reports to the State Compensation Insurance Fund as soon as possible. Compensation cannot be paid without the completion of the proper reports.

Thank you,

Employer Representative _____
Title _____

If the injured worker is unable to return to work immediately, please so indicate by signing and dating this form below. If the injured worker is able to return to work with limitations or restrictions, please describe any limitations on the reverse of this form. This form should be returned to the injured worker for forwarding to the employer.

Dr. _____
Signature _____
Date/Time _____

FIGURE 6-5

Sample Medical Service Order

If the patient does not arrive with a medical service order, the biller should contact the employer immediately and request that one be faxed over. If the employer does not have a medical service order, the provider should fax one to the employer and ask the company representative to complete it and fax it back immediately. This form can assist with the collection of a claim in case of a dispute, and a copy should be attached to any claims when they are submitted for payment.

To preserve the original signatures for your records, a photocopy should be made of the medical service order before the doctor completes it. The original should be kept for your records. The copy should be signed by the doctor, if necessary, and a photocopy made of the front and back for the records. The copy that was signed by the doctor should then be returned to the patient.

If the patient must be referred to an additional facility for testing or treatment, authorization should be obtained from the employer before transferring the patient. The medical biller should call the employer and specify the reason for the transfer or referral, the name and address of the facility to which the patient is being transferred, and the treatment needed at the facility. The employer should then fax an authorization for transfer or referral. If verbal authorization is given, the date and time, and the name and title of the person giving the authorization, should be recorded. The authorization (whether by faxed copy or the verbal information) should be placed directly on or attached to the transfer or referral order and a copy retained for your records.

Patient Records in a Provider's Office

If a patient is being treated for a work-related injury, all records relating to the injury and treatment should be kept separate from the patient's regular medical records. Because employers are covering the costs of treatment, privacy guidelines are somewhat different from the normal privacy agreement between patient and provider. In WC cases, the agreement is actually between the provider and the employer, not the injured worker. The employer may request to see records regarding the injury, and these records may be subpoenaed. So that confidentiality between the provider and the patient is not breached for non-work-related treatments and conditions, no information pertaining to the injured worker's non-work-related treatment should be made part of this file. Many providers place work-related injury records in a colored file so that it can be clearly identified as different from the patient's routine medical file.

If the provider finds a non-work-related condition during an injury-related examination (e.g., during the exam the provider discovers the patient has a heart condition), the WC agreement would be in force for all treatment relating to the injury, and the patient and his normal insurance carrier would be responsible for treatment of the non-work-related condition. It is important to clarify this with the patient and, if possible, to treat the two conditions at separate times. At no time should the doctor bill twice for the same examination. The examination should be charged according to the main activity of treatment (i.e., was most treatment related to the work-related injury or to the non-work-related injury?).

Doctor's First Report of Injury/Illness

Regardless of the type of workers' compensation claim or benefits, the doctor must file a **Doctor's First Report of Injury/Illness** (Figure 6-6 ●), a form that may vary depending on the state. This form requests basic information on the date, time, and location of the injury/illness and treatment; the patient's subjective complaints, and the provider's objective findings; the diagnosis; and the treatment rendered. The description of how the accident or exposure happened should be supplied by the patient if possible.

Subjective findings are those findings that cannot be discerned by anyone other than the patient (e.g., pain, discomfort). The provider should give an opinion as to the extent of pain, a description of activities that produce pain, and any other findings. A **treatment plan**, or schedule of procedures and appointments designed to restore, step by step, the health of a patient, should also be indicated.

If the provider chooses to send a narrative report along with the standard report, the following information should be included:

- History of the accident, injury or illness
- Diagnosis
- Any connection between the primary injury and any subsequent injuries, especially if the interrelating factors between the primary and secondary injuries are not immediately discernible
- Subjective and objective findings

Providers must make a report of injury, disability, or death within a specified time period. This varies from immediately upon knowledge of the incident to within thirty days. Different states set different time limits and different requirements for reporting. There also may be different limits for different levels of injury (e.g., injury, disability, death).

The original form should be submitted to the WC insurance agency, a copy of the form sent to the employer and one kept in the patient's medical record.

The Doctor's First Report of Injury/Illness is an extremely important document. It may be a major factor in the decision of the employer or insurance company to accept or contest the workers' compensation claim. Care should be taken to complete this form properly.

Many First Report forms contain a space for the occupation of the patient. It is important to list the patient's actual job so that the insurance carrier can determine if the injured worker was engaged in normal work activity at the time of injury. This also allows the carrier to ensure that the employer listed job titles and normal work activities accurately. Some employers attempt to list workers in less hazardous jobs (e.g., office worker rather than cutting machine operator), as insurance premiums are based on the hazards the injured worker may encounter in the job.

If the First Report requests the time the patient was examined, it is important to list the date and time of the examination as well as the date and time of the injury. This lets the insurance carrier know how much time elapsed between the injury and the patient seeking treatment for the injury.

Be sure to indicate the provider's complete address and telephone number on the bottom of the form. This is the address to which payment will be sent. The provider's title (e.g., M.D., D.C.) should be included, as well as his or her complete license number.

Make the required number of copies of the First Report before signing them, and then have the provider sign each copy in ink. Stamped signatures are unacceptable. In addition, the preparer should place his or her initials in the lower left-hand corner.

STATE OF CONFUSION

DOCTOR'S FIRST REPORT OF OCCUPATIONAL INJURY OR ILLNESS

Within 5 days of your initial examination, for every occupational injury or illness, send two copies of this report to the employer's workers' compensation insurance carrier or the insured employer. Failure to file a timely doctor's report may result in assessment of a civil penalty. In the case of diagnosed or suspected pesticide poisoning, send a copy of the report to Division of Labor Statistics and Research, P.O. Box 555555, Anytown, USA 12345-6789, and notify your local health officer by telephone within 24 hours.

	PLEASE DO NOT USE THIS COLUMN
1. **INSURER NAME AND ADDRESS**	
2. **EMPLOYER NAME**	Case No.
3. Address: No. and Street City Zip	Industry
4. Nature of business (e.g., food manufacturing, building construction, retailer of women's clothes)	County
5. **PATIENT NAME** (first name, middle initial, last name) 6. Sex ☐Male ☐ Female 7. Date of Mo. Day Yr. Birth:	Age
8. Address: No. and Street City Zip 9. Telephone number ( )	Hazard
10. Occupation (Specific job title) 11. Social Security Number - -	Disease
12. Injured at: No. and Street City County	Hospitalization
13. Date and hour of injury Mo. Day Yr. Hour _____ a.m. _____ p.m. or onset of illness 14. Date last worked Mo. Day Yr.	Occupation
15. Date and hour of first Mo. Day Yr. Hour _____ a.m. _____ p.m. examination or treatment 16. Have you (or your office) previously treated patient? ☐Yes ☐No	Return Date/Code

Patient please complete this portion, if able to do so. Otherwise, doctor please complete immediately; inability or failure of a patient to complete this portion shall not affect his/her rights to workers' compensation under the California Labor Code.

17. **DESCRIBE HOW THE ACCIDENT OR EXPOSURE HAPPENED.** (Give specific object, machinery or chemical. Use reverse side if more space is required.)

18. **SUBJECTIVE COMPLAINTS** (Describe fully. Use reverse side if more space is required.)

19. **OBJECTIVE FINDINGS** (Use reverse side if more space is required.) A. Physical examination B. X-ray and laboratory results (State if none or pending.)

20. **DIAGNOSIS** (If occupational illness specify etiologic agent and duration of exposure.) Chemical or toxic compounds involved?   ☐ Yes   ☐ No
ICD-9 Code ___ ___ ___ - ___ ___

21. Are your findings and diagnosis consistent with patient's account of injury or onset of illness?   ☐Yes   ☐No   If "no," please explain.

22. Is there any other current condition that will impede or delay patient's recovery?   ☐Yes   ☐No   If "yes," please explain.

23. **TREATMENT RENDERED** (Use reverse side if more space is required.)

24. If further treatment required, specify treatment plan/estimated duration.

25. If hospitalized as inpatient, give hospital name and location.   Date admitted   Mo.   Day   Yr.   Estimated stay

26. WORK STATUS -- Is patient able to perform usual work?   ☐Yes   ☐No
If "no," date when patient can return to: Regular work ____/____/____
Modified work ____/____/____   Specify restrictions _____

Doctor's Signature _____   License Number _____
Doctor Name and Degree (please type) _____   IRS Number _____
Address _____   Telephone Number _____

FORM 5021 (Rev. 4)

Any person who makes or causes to be made any knowingly false or fraudulent material statement or material representation for the purpose of obtaining or denying workers' compensation benefits or payments is guilty of a felony.

FIGURE 6-6

Sample of a Doctor's First Report of Injury/Illness

ACTIVITY #3

Completing a Doctor's First Report of Injury/Illness Form

Directions: Utilizing Figure 6-6, complete the Doctor's First Report of Injury/Illness for the following case. Refer to the Patient Data Table in Appendix A for additional information.

Patient:	Bobby Brumble
Job Title:	Waiter/Host
Provider:	Joanne Jones, M.D.
	1029 Jonathan Lane
	Anytown, USA 12345
	(765) 555-0987
License:	A1234567
EIN:	11-0987654

Incident: Patient states that at 5:10 p.m. on 10/16/CCYY, he was carrying a dessert tray. He slipped on some soda that was spilled on the floor and landed on his back, striking his head on the floor. The dessert tray turned upside down and landed on him. The patient is complaining of headache and difficulty breathing through his nose.

Injuries: Concussion (no fracture, no apparent brain damage), foreign matter (chocolate mousse) in both eyes, foreign body (cherry) lodged in nose. Patient treated at Provider Medical Center from 10/16/CCYY to 10/19/CCYY.

Procedures Performed: Physical examination and history, new patient, moderate complexity ($70); X-ray of the skull, 2 views ($45); removal of foreign body from nose ($85); irrigation of eyes ($18).

Treatment Plan: Bed rest for two days, wake patient every hour during first twenty-four hours to ensure no LOC, limited activity for two weeks, re-check in ten days. Patient estimated able to return to work 10/30/CCYY.

Signed: Joanne Jones, M.D., 10/19/CCYY, 6:05 p.m.

Progress Reports

Following the Doctor's First Report, the provider should follow up with progress reports (sometimes called supplemental reports) after every visit (Figure 6-7 ●; form may vary depending on the state). Many states have forms for subsequent progress reports; however, they also may allow a narrative report to be filed, rather than completion of the specified form. Retain a copy for your files and provide the insurance carrier with its required number of copies (usually three or four). Subsequent reports also should be sent at the end of a hospitalization, even if the patient is expected to be readmitted later. This report serves both as a report on the patient's condition and as a bill.

If the patient's condition changes significantly, a reexamination report, or a detailed progress report, should be filed with the insurance carrier.

Provider's Final Report

The WC carrier often will wait until the provider indicates that the patient's condition is permanent and stationary before finalizing a claim. The provider should then notify the WC carrier that no further treatment is needed (or that no further treatment will significantly alter the patient's condition) and that the patient has been discharged. This is called the **Provider's Final Report**. Some states require the final report to be submitted on a specified form, and some states use the same form for both subsequent and final reports. The Provider's Final Report should indicate that the patient has been discharged; the level of the patient's permanent disability, if any; and the balance due on the patient's account (usually provided as a patient's statement showing services, dates of service, charges, and any payments rendered). Once this information is received, the WC carrier will establish the level of permanent disability, if any; medical and other expenses will be paid; and the case will be closed.

Additional pages attached ☐

STATE OF CONFUSION
Division of Workers' Compensation

PRIMARY TREATING PHYSICIAN'S PROGRESS REPORT (PR-2)

Check the box(es) indicating why you are submitting a report at this time. If the patient is "Permanent and Stationary"

(i.e., has reached maximum medical improvement), do not use this form, You may use DWC Form PR-3.

☐ Periodic Report (required 45 days after last report)   ☐ Change in treatment plan   ☐ Released from care

☐ Change in work status   ☐ Need for referral or consultation   ☐ Response to request for information

☐ Change in patient's condition ☐ Need for surgery or hospitalization   ☐ Request for authorization   ☐ Other:

Patient:

Last_____First_____M.I. _____Sex_____

Address_____City_____State_____Zip_____

Date of Injury_____ Date of Birth_____

Occupation _____SS # _____-_____-_____ Phone (_____)_____

Claims Administrator:

Name_____ Claim Number _____

Address_____ City_____ State_____Zip_____

Phone (_____)_____ FAX (_____)_____

Employer name: _____ **Employer Phone (_____)** _____

The information below must be provided. You may use this form or you may substitute or append a narrative report.

Subjective complaints:

Objective findings: (Include significant physical examination, laboratory, imaging, or other diagnostic findings.)

Diagnoses:

1. _____ICD-9-CM _____

2. _____ICD-9-CM _____

3. _____ICD-9-CM _____

FIGURE 6-7

Sample Progress Report

Treatment Plan: (Include treatment rendered to date. List methods, frequency, and duration of planned treatment(s). Specify consultation/referral, surgery, and hospitalization. Identify each physician and non-physician provider. Specify type, frequency, and duration of physical medicine services (e.g., physical therapy, manipulation, acupuncture). Use of CPT® codes is encouraged. Have there been any changes in treatment plan? If so, why?

Work Status: This patient has been instructed to:

☐ Remain *off* work until _____.

☐ Return to *modified* work on _____ with the following limitations or restrictions.

   (List all specific restrictions re: standing, sitting, bending, use of hands, etc.

☐ Return to full duty on _____ with no limitations.

Primary Treating Physician: (original signature, do not stamp)   Date of exam: _____

I declare under penalty of perjury that this report is true and correct to the best of my knowledge and that I have not violated Labor Code § 139.3.

Signature: _____   Lic. _____

Executed at: _____   Date: _____

Name: _____   Specialty: _____

Address: _____   Phone: _____

FIGURE 6-7 (*Continued*)

PRACTICE PITFALLS

If the provider chooses to submit a narrative report, the following information should be included:

- Complete identification of the patient, including WC case number, name and address of the patient
- Date and description of all examinations and treatment procedures performed since the last report was submitted
- Progress of the condition since the last report
- Any proposed changes in the treatment plan
- Any lab tests, function tests, or other items that show any change in the patient's condition
- Status of the patient's disability, including an estimated time that the patient can return to work, or any estimated permanent disability (If this changes from the doctor's report of first injury, it should be brought to the attention of the insurance carrier so that it may adjust funding to cover the new situation.)
- Treatment plan including a description of the planned course, scope, frequency, and duration of treatment and an estimated date of completion

Billing for Workers' Compensation Services

When billing WC claims, it is important to follow all guidelines and regulations provided by the state WC board and the WC insurance agency. Using incorrect forms or not following procedures can cause delays in claims or difficulty in collecting for procedures performed. Following are general guidelines regarding billing WC cases:

1. As mentioned, services rendered in a WC case are the responsibility of the employer, not the injured worker.
2. Some states pay WC cases according to a fee schedule, whereas others may use amounts based on Medicare's allowed amounts. A fee schedule limits the amount providers can charge for services. Each service is given a different allowed amount based on the difficulty of the procedure, the time involved, the risk to the patient, and other factors. Fee schedules prevent doctors from overcharging for services. The amount paid under a fee schedule is considered payment in full for the services, and the biller should write off any amounts not covered.
3. If any unusual factors affect the amount the provider has charged, documentation should be sent with the claim to substantiate the increased fees charged. The insurance carrier will then determine if the fees are warranted.
4. If any procedures are listed as "By Report" (BR) on the fee schedule, a complete report of the procedure, initialed by the doctor, should accompany the claim. This report will allow the insurance carrier to determine the appropriate payment for the procedure. Be sure to attach any lab reports, x-rays, or other data that support either the excess fees or the BR procedure.
5. As a biller, always remember to ask if a case is work related when a patient first visits for treatment of an injury, illness, or condition. This prevents billing the wrong party and having to go through costly adjustments and reimbursements. If the case is work related, the patient should be instructed to provide the doctor's office with the case number as soon as it is obtained.
6. Because WC cases often go before a jury, every contact with the patient, the patient's employer or attorney, or anyone else related to the case should be documented and placed in the file. This includes contacts in person, by phone, or through a third party. Be sure to include the date and time of the contact, the full name of the person contacted, who initiated the contact (e.g., patient called, carrier called, etc.), and the details of the contact.
7. Be sure to use the proper CPT and ICD-9-CM or ICD-10-CM codes and complete all boxes on all forms. Incomplete information is one of the main causes of delay in closing a case.
8. In WC cases, all materials and drugs should be itemized in detail and charged at cost.
9. If a patient is injured in one state and then seeks treatment in a different state, the laws of the state where the claim occurred would cover the injured worker. This situation occurs most often in cities that straddle a state line or in rural areas where the nearest hospital is in a neighboring state.

    The WC carrier should be contacted before treatment, if possible, as some states have restrictions on treatment. If treatment is approved, be sure to get a written authorization for the patient record. Be sure to ask for all necessary forms for provider's first report of illness/injury, progress reports, provider's final reports, and any other reports needed. Also ask about billing requirements. Some states require billing on a CMS-1500 or other form, some states will accept an itemized patient statement or superbill, and other states require electronic billing.
10. Be sure to file claims for workers' compensation services as soon as possible. Many states have time limits on when you can submit a claim to the insurance carrier (e.g., six months after treatment). If you are past the time limit, some WC carriers will reduce the benefit payment and others may completely refuse to pay the claim.

If you have questions regarding the payment of a particular claim, call the WC insurance carrier and ask to speak with the adjuster in charge of the case. Answers to general questions regarding the state's WC benefits, rules, and legislation can be obtained from your state's WC Appeals Board.

Third-Party Liability

It is possible to have third-party liability in a WC case. For example, George works at a restaurant and is taking trash out to the trash bin behind the building. A plumber had been visiting the restaurant. On leaving, the plumber backed up without looking and ran over George's leg.

Because George was clearly injured in the normal performance of his duties, the accident would be covered by WC. The WC insurance carrier would be required to pay all benefits to which George is entitled. However, as the accident was clearly the plumber's fault, the WC insurance carrier may encourage George to sue the plumber for damages. Automobile insurance and personal liability insurance may be involved if George wins the case against the plumber, in which case the WC insurance carrier has a right to collect all monies it has paid out for George's benefits.

PRACTICE PITFALLS

When billing for services rendered to an injured worker, the provider must complete the appropriate billing forms. Some insurance carriers require a specific billing form or method for submission of workers' compensation claims. However, most workers' compensation charges are billed on the CMS-1500 form. Special requirements on the CMS-1500 for workers' compensation claims are as follows:

- **Header.** Enter the name and address of the workers' compensation insurance company.
- **Block 1a.** Enter the patient's WC claim number if available. If not, enter the employer's policy number.
- **Block 4.** Enter the name of the patient's employer.
- **Block 6.** Enter an X in the "Other" box.
- **Block 7.** Enter the address of the patient's employer.
- **Block 8.** Enter an X in the "Employed" box.
- **Block 9-9d.** Leave empty unless claim has not been declared WC.
- **Block 10a.** Enter an X in the "Yes" box.
- **Block 10b.** Only check "Yes" if the accident happened while the patient was performing work-related activities.
- **Blocks 11–11c.** Leave empty.
- **Block 12.** Leave empty.
- **Block 13.** Leave empty.
- **Block 14.** Enter the date of injury or illness in the MM DD YY format.
- **Block 16.** Enter the dates the patient is unable to work if applicable in the MM DD CCYY format.
- **Block 17.** Enter the SSN or EIN of the employer.

Any fees that exceed the payment made by the workers' compensation insurance company may not be billed to or collected from the patient. Providers must accept the workers' compensation payment as reimbursement in full.

Liens

In permanent disability, a compromise and release will be issued by the insurance carrier for the injuries to the patient. If the provider has been seeing the patient and there are unpaid medical expenses, a lien should be filed for payment of services rendered. A **lien** is a legal document that expresses claim on the property of another for payment of a debt (Figure 6-8 ●; form may vary depending on the state). A lien is completed and then submitted to the attorney representing the injured party to be paid on monetary settlement of the WC claim.

A lien should be sent along with the bill for the initial visit. Whenever additional services are rendered, a copy of the bill should be submitted to the attorney so that all concurrent care will be included in the lien. All services must be for the care of the injury covered under the WC claim. Many states have a special lien form for WC purposes. These forms can be obtained through the local Division of Industrial Accidents. (A sample copy of a lien is shown in Figure 6-9 ●; form may vary depending on the state.) Complete the lien form and send copies to the WC Appeals Board, the patient's employer, the patient, and the WC insurance carrier. A copy also should be kept for the files.

TO: Attorney_____

_____

_____, Confusion

RE: Medical Reports and Insurance Carrier Lien

FOR_____

I do hereby authorize the above insurance carrier to furnish you, my attorney, with a full report of any records and resultant payments of myself in regard to the accident in which I was involved.

I hereby authorize and direct you, my attorney, to pay directly to said insurance carrier such sums as may be due and owed for payment of medical services rendered me or the provider of services both by reason of this accident and by reason of any other bills that are due, and to withhold such sums from any settlement, judgment, or verdict as may be necessary to adequately protect said insurance carrier. And I hereby further give a lien on my case to said insurance carrier against any and all proceeds of any settlement, judgment, or verdict which may be paid to you, my attorney, or myself as the result of the injuries for which I have been treated or injuries in connection therewith.

I fully understand that I am directly and fully responsible for reimbursement of any payments for all medical bills submitted for services rendered and that this agreement is made solely for said insurance carrier's additional protection and in consideration of its awaiting payment. And I further understand that such payment is not contingent on any settlement, judgment, or verdict by which I may eventually recover said fee.

Dated: _____   Patient's Signature:_____

The undersigned being attorney of record for the above patient does hereby agree to observe all the terms of the above and agrees to withhold such sums from any settlement, judgment, or verdict as may be necessary to adequately protect said insurance carrier named above.

Dated: _____   Attorney's Signature:_____
Mr./Ms. Attorney: Please sign, date, and return one copy to our office at once.

Keep one copy for your records.

FIGURE 6-8

Sample lien letter

If a lien is not filed, all monies recovered at the close of the case officially belong to the patient. It is then the patient's responsibility to cover the medical expenses. If any liens are filed, the patient must first pay the liens and then pay any other resultant expenses. Therefore, if the lawyer files a lien and the legal fees exhaust most of the money, little or nothing will be left for other expenses. If at all possible, patients should be persuaded to pay for medical services before settlement of the claim.

If a lien is filed, the biller should have the provider's copy of the lien letter signed by the patient and the patient's attorney. This makes the attorney responsible for payment of the provider's bills. If the attorney does not remit the necessary funds from the patient's settlement, the attorney must cover the medical expenses.

WORKERS' COMPENSATION APPEALS BOARD

STATE OF CONFUSION

CASE NO. _____

NOTICE AND REQUEST FOR ALLOWANCE OF LIEN

_____
LIEN CLAIMANT   ADDRESS
VS.

_____
INJURED WORKER   ADDRESS

_____
EMPLOYER   ADDRESS

_____
INSURANCE CARRIER   ADDRESS

The undersigned hereby requests the Workers' Compensation Appeals Board to determine and allow as a lien the sum of

_____ dollars ($_____) against

any amount now due or which may hereafter become payable as compensation to _____
                                                                                    INJURED WORKER

on account of injury sustained by him/her on _____.
                                                          DATE

This request and claim for lien is for: (Mark appropriate box)
- ❑ The reasonable expense incurred by or on behalf of said injured worker for medical treatment to cure or relieve from the effects of said injury; or
- ❑ The reasonable medical expense incurred to prove a contested claim; or
- ❑ The reasonable value of living expenses of said injured worker or of his dependents, subsequent to the injury, or
- ❑ The reasonable living expenses of the wife or minor children, or both, of said injured worker, subsequent to the date of injury, where such injured worker has deserted or is neglecting his family; or
- ❑ The reasonable fee for interpreter's services performed on _____.
                                                                     DATE

NOTE: ITEMIZED STATEMENTS MUST BE ATTACHED
The undersigned declares that he delivered or mailed a copy of this lien claim to each of the above-named parties on

_____
ATTORNEY FOR LIEN CLAIMANT   DATE

_____
ADDRESS OF ATTORNEY FOR LIEN CLAIMANT   LIEN CLAIMANT

INJURED WORKER'S CONSENT TO ALLOWANCE OF LIEN

I consent to the requested allowance of a lien against my compensation.

_____
ATTORNEY FOR INJURED WORKER   INJURED WORKER

DEPARTMENT OF INDUSTRIAL RELATIONS
DIVISION OF INDUSTRIAL ACCIDENTS

FIGURE 6-9

Sample lien form

A lien should have a specified time limit on it; this often is a period of one year. If settlement has not been reached by that time, or charges on the patient's account relating to the WC injury are ongoing, an amended lien should be filed. The subsequent lien should state the balance of the patient's account, and should have the word "AMENDED" stamped across the top or below the WC Appeals Board case number.

The biller should place all files with liens in a special section and hold them until the cases have been settled. It is illegal to continually bill or harass the patient when a lien agreement has been signed.

In effect, the lien acknowledges the provider's agreement to wait for reimbursement until the case has been settled. The biller should contact the patient's attorney at least once every quarter for an update on the case and to determine when settlement is expected to occur. The attorney also should be contacted within two weeks after the date settlement is expected to find out the results of the case and ask when payment can be expected.

In some states, the law allows the provider to be paid prior to the attorney or patient collecting any monies from the settlement. Statutes in the relevant state should be checked to protect the provider. If your state has such a provision, attorneys may not collect their fee and then state that insufficient funds were recovered to cover the provider's total bill. Some states also allow the provider to bill the patient for any funds that were not received from the settlement. Once again, check the laws of the relevant state to determine if patients can be billed or if any amounts not collected should be written off.

Liens are an inexpensive way of ensuring that the provider will be reimbursed for services provided. The cost is much lower than suing the patient and ensures that payment will be received when the dispute between the patient and the WC insurance carrier is settled. A lien is a legal document that will be recognized by the court and will provide protection in the event of litigation.

ACTIVITY #4

Completing a Lien Letter and a Lien Form

Directions: Complete a lien letter and a lien form for the following case. Refer to the Patient Data Table and Provider Data Table in Appendix A for additional information.

Bobby Brumble states that on 9/11/CCYY, as he walked down the stairs into the reception area to pick up a fax his office had received, he slipped on a banana peel, causing him to injure his back.

Case Number:	54321B
Lien Claimant:	Paul Provider
Injured Worker:	Bobby Brumble
Employer:	Blue Corporation
Insurance Carrier:	Ball Insurance Carrier
Lien Sum:	$31,792.00
Date of Injury:	09/11/CCYY
Attorney for Lien Claimant:	Faren Ekual, Esq., 9354 Doublemint Place, Anytown, USA 12345
Attorney for Injured Worker:	Idee Fendu, Esq., 4345 Justiceville Place, Anytown, USA 12345

Delinquent Claims

If payment is not received within forty-five days of billing the WC insurance carrier, the biller should contact the adjuster in charge of the case to determine the reason for the delay. Often, the proper forms have not been received from one party or another. If this is the case, ask which form is missing and who is responsible for sending it. If completion of the form is required by another person (e.g., the employer) contact that person and request that the form be completed as soon as possible so you may receive payment.

If the employer or other party has not completed the necessary item within thirty days of contacting them, send a letter to the WC Board or OSHA Agency in your state. The letter should state that you are requesting help in securing the necessary items from the party. Be sure to include the case number; the name, address, and phone number of the party who should provide the item; the patient's name and address; the date of the injury; and the name and address of the insurance carrier or other person to whom the item should be sent. Also list the patient's balance due.

Delay of Adjudication

When a patient is released to work, all benefits have been paid, and the case is closed, the claim is said to have been adjudicated. Often adjudication occurs within two to eight weeks after the provider submits the report stating that the patient has been discharged and is able to return to work.

If the patient suffers a permanent disability, adjudication can take much longer, especially if the amount of permanent disability is protested and a lawsuit ensues. Additional factors that may delay the close of a case include the following:

1. Confusion or questions on any of the reports submitted by the employer, injured worker, or provider (This can include conflicting information from one or more parties; vague or ambiguous terminology, especially by the provider; or illegible items.)
2. Omitted information on a report, including incomplete forms, boxes not filled in, or signatures not included
3. Incorrect billing or questions on the billing provided by the provider
4. Insufficient progress reports to update the insurance carrier on the status of the patient

Workers' Compensation Appeals

If you disagree with a decision made on a workers' compensation claim, you may appeal that decision. During an appeal, the facts of the case are reviewed, including any new information that is provided. An appeal usually can only be filed by an injured worker or employer.

For most states, there are two levels of appeal. The first level is a request for review of an adjudicator's claim decision. This appeal is usually forwarded to a hearing officer or an administrative law judge.

The second-level review is an appeal of the first-level review to a workers' compensation tribunal or workers' compensation board. This level of review is usually final.

Reversals

Occasionally, an accident that was thought to be WC will turn out not to be. This can happen when a patient hides or omits facts regarding when and how the accident occurred. It also can be found that there is a nonindustrial, underlying condition that caused the accident. For example, a patient may have epilepsy and suffer a seizure at work; any injuries directly received on the job site could be considered WC, but the treatment of the underlying epileptic condition would not be WC.

In some cases, the injured worker may be found to be negligent in his or her actions, or willfully not abiding by established workplace rules. In such cases, injuries sustained as the result of negligence by an injured worker may not be considered an industrial accident. For example, if the injured worker is told to refrain from wearing hoop earrings but chooses to do so anyway, the worker may be considered liable if the earrings are caught on machinery and ripped from the ear.

In such cases, the WC Appeals Board would deny payment on the claim. All claims for treatment should then be sent to the patient's regular insurance carrier with the denial notice from the WC Appeals Board. A letter should also be sent to notify the injured worker that the claim was denied and that their regular insurance is being billed for the charges.

CHAPTER REVIEW

Summary

- WC insurance is a separate medical insurance program that covers work-related injuries, disabilities, and death. A wide range of activities may be covered under WC laws.
- WC provides nondisability claims, temporary disability claims, permanent disability claims, death benefits, and rehabilitation benefits to injured workers.
- Vocational rehabilitation or training in a different job field is allowed by many states.
- The information provided on the Doctor's First Report of Injury/Illness is a major factor in the decision of the employer or insurance company to accept or contest the workers' compensation claim. The basic information contained on the form includes the date, time, and location of the injury/illness; and the treatment rendered.
- The Provider's Final Report is usually the last report the provider submits, stating that the patient has been discharged.
- The provider must notify the WC carrier that no further treatment is needed.
- Using incorrect forms or not following procedures can cause a delay in your claim. It is extremely important to follow all guidelines and regulations. The claim is said to be adjudicated when all the benefits have been paid and the patient is released to work.
- Some factors that may delay the close of a case are confusion or questions on any of the reports, omitted information on a report, incorrect billing or questions on the billing, and insufficient progress reports.

Review Questions

Directions: Answer the following questions without looking back into the material just covered. Write your answer in the space provided.

1. What is workers' compensation? _____

_____

_____

2. What items are likely to cause a delay in adjudication of a case?

_____

_____

_____

3. What do you do if a patient states he or she incurred a WC injury but has nothing from the employer to prove it? _____

_____

_____

_____

4. What is a lien? _____

_____

_____

5. Why should you file a lien? _____

_____

6. What signatures should you get on a lien? _____

_____

7. Define *temporary disability*. _____

_____

_____

8. Define *permanent disability*. _____

_____

_____

9. What is a nondisability claim? _____

_____

10. If an injured worker is injured while at a company-sponsored game, is it considered a WC case? _____

_____

If you are unable to answer any of these questions, refer back to that section in the chapter, and then fill in the answers.

Activity #5: Locating the Key Terms

Directions: Complete the crossword puzzle by filling in a word from the key words that fits each clue.

Across

6. This is a separate medical and disability reimbursement program that provides 100 percent coverage for job-related injuries, illnesses, or conditions arising out of and in the course of employment.

Down

1. The doctor must file this report regardless of the type of workers' compensation claim or benefits. This form requests basic information on the date, time, and location of the injury/ illness and treatment; the patient's subjective complaints; the provider's objective findings; the diagnosis; and the treatment rendered.

2. A benefit provided to retrain an injured worker in a physical ability that will help them to seek future employment

3. Minor injuries that will not require the patient to be kept from his job

4. An evaluation that provides medical evidence for the purpose of proving or disproving medical issues in a contested workers' compensation claim

5. Compensates the family of a deceased injured worker for the loss of income that the injured worker would have provided to the family

7. The report notifying the WC carrier that no further treatment is needed (or that no further treatment will significantly alter the patient's condition) and that the patient has been discharged. The report should indicate that the patient has been discharged, the level of the patient's permanent disability, if any, and the balance due on the patient's account.

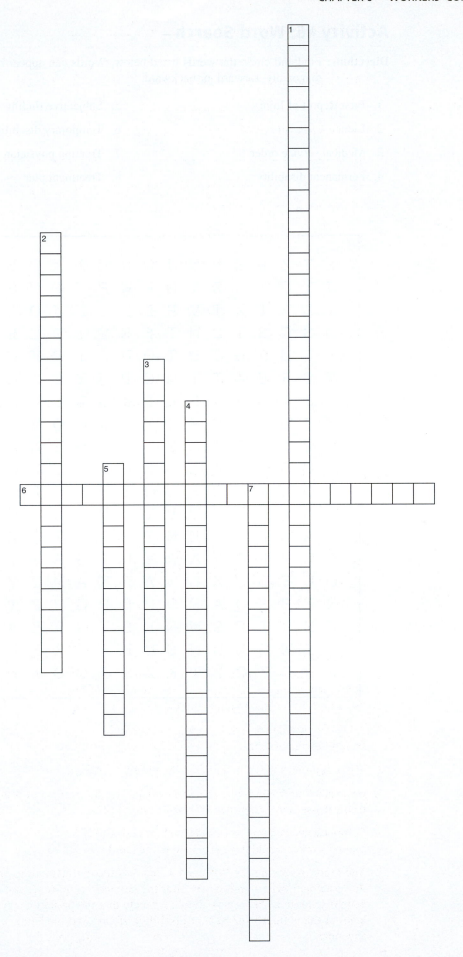

Activity #6: Word Search

Directions: Find and circle the words listed below. Words can appear horizontally, vertically, diagonally, forward, or backward.

1. First Report of Injury
2. Lien
3. Medical service order
4. Permanent disability

5. Subjective findings
6. Temporary disability
7. Treating physician
8. Treatment plan

```
X Y Z P Z S W J O R E I K D E P D R Y
J T Q L S Z I M K W F M P W S T R R W
Y L R I X T V H L F I F J Q Z W U Z F
D S G N I D N I F E V I T C E J B U S
V F M J D J D T O U C I P K N C B H X
F T R E A T I N G P H Y S I C I A N X
P S R A V R F L P K G Z F M S Q B T J
M J L X L D M Y Y D K O Q V T X I K G
Y T I L I B A S I D T N E N A M R E P
M E D I C A L S E R V I C E O R D E R
Z O L J G E P E O I W B C P X M J K A
B L C N Y W T P Y N R R D S U W N W L
N A L P T N E M T A E R T Q Z J K P C
T E M P O R A R Y D I S A B I L I T Y
Q N F L T X L M A F K A M Y Y I T R J
N F E S Q A E O U B R G H F T T Z V D
H M R I E S W E E S I S A E A M L X G
T I W G L N N E M K F K K H A V W X A
F H D K G X T K Z S J O O W K H E X Z
```

Managed Care

After completion of this chapter you should be able to:

List the reasons for rising health care costs.

Describe ways that insurance carriers decrease costs.

Describe the main types of managed care organizations and their function.

List the common Health Maintenance Organization (HMO) benefits.

Describe the various types of Preferred Provider Organizations (PPOs) and their function.

Explain the purpose of the membership card and eligibility rosters.

Explain the difference between reporting patient encounters on a CMS-1500 and billing on a CMS-1500.

Describe how risk for expenses is shared between groups/Independent Practice Associations (IPAs) and Managed Care Plans (MCPs).

Key Words and Concepts you will learn in this chapter:

Active member roster

Capitation

Complaints

Disenrollment

Eligibility roster

Exclusive provider organization (EPO)

Grievances

Independent Practice Association (IPA)

In-network providers

Managed care

Management Service Organization (MSO)

New member roster

Out-of-network provider

Provider Hospital Organization (PHO)

Preferred Provider Organization (PPO)

Primary Care Provider (PCP)

Reinsurance

Self-insurance

Social Health Maintenance Organization (S/HMO)

Stop-loss

Terminated member roster

Withhold

Explain how providers are reimbursed in a capitation agreement.

Describe the proper handling of the patient's medical record.

Properly handle authorizations, referrals, and second-opinion referrals using a given scenario.

List the steps in the second-opinion process.

List the steps to be taken in the case of a member grievance or complaint.

Properly complete a grievance log.

State the reasons why a member may be disenrolled and the information that must be documented in a disenrollment.

Describe the standard provisions for continuing care when a provider terminates his or her agreement with an MCP.

Properly complete a patient population record.

Properly generate a payment to an outside provider using a given scenario.

Properly complete a denial notice.

Describe stop-loss and the procedures for obtaining stop-loss reimbursement from an HMO.

> Managed care contracts were created in an attempt to bring health care costs under control by having providers share some of the financial risks of health care with the patient and the insurance carrier.

Rising Health Care Costs

The cost of health care in America is rising for numerous reasons. Following are some of the most common causes:

1. The higher costs of doing business, including rising rents, employee salaries, and so on
2. The rising costs of education for medical professionals
3. Little or no competition among providers (It is not customary for doctors to advertise their prices. In addition, the American consumer often does little comparison shopping on the basis of cost when trying to find a provider, especially when insurance carriers cover most of the cost of services.)
4. Little or no control by traditional plans on the utilization of care (These plans normally pay on claims with little or no restrictions.)
5. Greater number of lawsuits, causing ever-increasing malpractice insurance premiums (In addition, many doctors are ordering more tests and trying more treatments to protect themselves against possible lawsuits.)
6. Higher utilization of medical services (Some people visit the doctor for even the most insignificant reason.)
7. The cost of new medical technology (Patients like to see doctors who have the latest technology and equipment. Unfortunately, this equipment costs a tremendous amount of money. Some medical equipment can cost over $500,000.)
8. More people living longer, and those over sixty-five using more medical services than any other age group
9. Millions of people not having health insurance (These people utilize services and then are unable to pay, or they pay on a delayed timetable. The costs associated with treating the uninsured are often passed on to those patients with insurance.)
10. More catastrophic illnesses in the world today

▶ **CRITICAL THINKING QUESTION:** What solutions might you suggest to address the issues that the United States health care system is experiencing?

ACTIVITY #1

Researching Health-Care Challenges in Other Countries

Directions: Rising health care costs present a challenge for the United States. What challenges might other countries be facing when it comes to health care? To learn about the challenges that other countries face regarding their health care systems, select a country and conduct research utilizing the Internet or your school or local library. Write a one-page report outlining the type of health care coverage being offered in the selected country and the types of issues that are currently being faced in that country.

Managed Care

Managed care is a system for organizing the delivery of health services so that the cost of care is reduced and the quality of care is maintained or improved. There are many different types of managed care organizations, including health maintenance organizations, preferred provider organizations, gatekeeper PPOs, exclusive provider organizations, provider hospital organizations, and management service organizations.

Health Maintenance Organizations

Health Maintenance Organizations (HMOs) are one of the most common forms of managed care. Many other managed care models may start with an HMO base and modify it based on the needs of the members. HMOs are organizations or companies that provide both the coverage for care and the care itself. See Figure 7-1 ● for an overview of an HMO. A **Social Health Maintenance Organization (S/HMO)**, also known as a Medicare HMO, is an organization that provides the full range of Medicare benefits offered by standard HMOs plus additional services.

Under an HMO setup, members pay a set amount each month and the HMO agrees to provide all their care, or to pay for the covered care they cannot provide. The HMO hires providers and sets up hospitals (or contracts with existing providers and hospitals). Members choose a specific provider for their care (commonly called a **primary care provider** or primary care physician [PCP]).

Health Maintenance Organizations are so named because of the underlying belief that health care costs could be controlled by providing services that maintained and encouraged the health of HMO's members. By adding benefits such as low-cost provider visits and annual checkups, the HMOs sought to encourage members to seek medical attention for minor medical problems before they became serious medical emergencies.

There are several different types of HMOs. The most common include the staff model, group model, independent practice association, and network model.

STAFF MODEL. The staff model is the original concept for HMO services. Providers are hired to work at the HMO's facility, are usually paid a salary, and may receive additional bonuses. Providers work only for the HMO and do not see outside patients.

GROUP MODEL. A group model HMO contracts with providers or provider groups to render services. These providers agree to provide care only for HMO members, but they do so at their own facilities. In the group practice model, care is often provided at a centrally located facility. The HMO may have several facilities in the region it services, or just a few, depending on the size and diversity of the population served.

Some HMOs will own one or more hospitals that provide the inpatient services that members need. All providers and other personnel are on staff and paid a salary by the HMO. Any specialists needed to treat the patients are provided by the HMO.

Other HMOs contract with hospitals for a specified number of beds, or for a wing of an existing hospital, rather than operate its own facilities due to the increased costs associated with building a new hospital and the decreased utilization of hospitals. Sharing a facility can be a good way to provide an HMO the resources and treatment options needed, while at the same time increasing hospital revenue. HMO personnel normally provide care to HMO patients at these facilities.

FIGURE 7-1

Overview of an HMO

PATIENTS

- Choose an HMO and contract with that HMO to provide all medical care for a set monthly premium,
- Choose a provider who has contracted with the HMO as his or her primary care physician, and
- Visit the chosen primary care physician for all medical needs unless an emergency situation exists, and pay a copayment for each medical visit.

HMOS

- Collect premiums from patients,
- Contract with providers to provide certain services, and
- Oversee quality of care, and authorize and pay for services not covered by the doctor's capitation plan.

PROVIDERS

- Provide all capitated care for patients,
- Refer patients to specialists when needed,
- If specialist services are not covered by capitation, obtain authorization for referral from HMO, and
- If specialist services are covered by capitation, provide reimbursement (payment) to the specialist from the capitation amount.

GROUPS/IPA

- Contract with providers to join a group so they have greater bargaining power with the HMOs, and
- Contract with the HMOs to provide care for HMO patients in a specified region.

SPECIALISTS

- Treat patients referred by the provider and authorized by the provider or HMO, and
- Bill provider or HMO for services, and may sign a contract with the provider or HMO to limit charges for services to managed care patients.

INDEPENDENT PRACTICE ASSOCIATIONS. An **Independent Practice Association (IPA),** sometimes called an Individual Practice Organization or IPO, is a legal entity comprising a network of private practice providers who have organized to negotiate contracts with insurance companies and HMOs.

This type of organization has two arms. The HMO arm acts as an insurer, oversees the program, enrolls members, collects premiums, and handles the claims. The IPA organizes providers and contracts with the HMO for discounted rates on services. The medical group as a whole is paid a capitation amount for each member, and the group oversees the care of the members and attempts to control costs. **Capitation** is the practice of paying a provider a set amount per month to provide treatment to Managed Care Plan (MCP) members and for performing other administrative duties.

The individual providers (who are members of the medical groups) agree to see patients in their own offices along with their regular fee-for-service clients. The providers are able to easily gather a large number of patients by joining the IPA, and at the same time they retain their autonomy and freedom, unlike the traditional HMO providers who are hired by the HMO and placed on salary.

This type of arrangement allows the HMO to add numerous providers, which allows patients a wider freedom of choice. Because providers are paid a capitation amount according to the number of members they see, the HMO incurs no additional cost for adding numerous additional providers.

NETWORK MODEL. In a network model, the HMO contracts with several providers in a given area, allowing some overlap in a geographic region. This allows more choice for subscribers and allows an HMO to increase its subscriber base without worrying about unduly overloading a single provider. In the network model, providers see not only the HMO members but also continue to see their regular fee-paying patients as well.

HMO COVERAGE. Most HMOs offer a higher level of coverage than traditional indemnity plans. For example, not only do HMOs cover provider visits and necessary testing but also treatment by a specialist (when the patient is referred by a PCP) is often covered. HMOs also tend to cover prenatal care, emergency care, home health care, skilled nursing care, drug and alcohol abuse treatment, physical therapy, allergy treatment, and inhalation therapy, often to a higher degree than coverage provided by indemnity plans. Most provider visits require a small copayment from the member or patient.

Hospitalization is usually covered in full by most HMO plans. However, many plans require a per-day inpatient copayment and if a patient is seen in the emergency room (ER) a separate copayment is often required.

In addition, HMOs often cover preventive services. Preventive coverage provides for services such as an annual physical, routine cancer screening (Pap smears, mammograms, etc.), flu shots, immunizations, and well-baby care. Many HMO plans also cover health education, cessation of smoking classes, nutrition counseling (especially for diabetics and those needing weight control), or exercise classes. Traditional indemnity plans either limit or restrict coverage of such services.

Eye exams for both children and adults are covered by most HMOs; however, additional vision services (glasses, contacts, etc.) may not be covered.

For those plans that cover prescription drugs, a small copayment is often required from the member for each prescription. Prescriptions are often limited to a thirty-day supply, but many HMOs have no limit to the number of prescriptions that may be filled in a month.

Mental health treatments often require a higher copayment than provider visits and are often limited to short-term care. The number of visits per year is usually limited.

Physical therapy (Figure 7-2 ●) is often covered for brief periods and only if significant improvement is expected for the patient.

Controversial or experimental procedures (e.g., temporomandibular joint [TMJ] surgery, laser surgery, gastric stapling) often are not covered. Cosmetic procedures, unless deemed medically necessary, are almost never covered.

Those HMOs that are federally qualified must provide the following minimum benefits:

1. Preventive care
2. All hospital inpatient services with no limits on costs or days
3. Hospital outpatient diagnosis and treatment services, including rehabilitative services, with some limitations
4. Skilled nursing home and home health care services
5. Short-term detoxification treatment for drug and alcohol abuse
6. Medical treatment and referral for substance abuse

Preferred Provider Organizations

A **Preferred Provider Organization (PPO)** is the second most common managed care alternative. It is, in essence, a hybrid of an HMO and a traditional plan.

In a PPO, the insurance carrier contracts with providers to provide services at a contracted rate. These providers, called **in-network providers**, agree to provide services at a reduced fee in exchange for

FIGURE 7-2

A physical therapist works with a patient

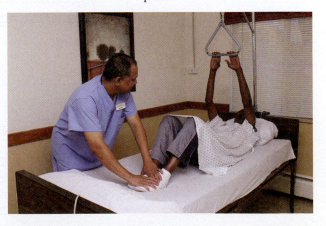

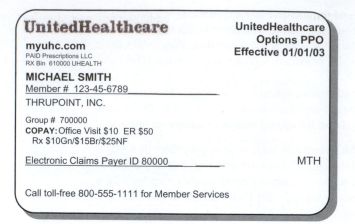

FIGURE 7-3

An example of a PPO insurance card

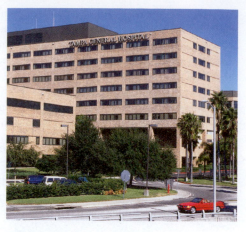

FIGURE 7-4

A general hospital
© Michal Heron/Pearson Education

referrals from the carrier. In addition the carrier agrees to reimburse providers in its network at a higher percentage than providers outside its network.

In a PPO, the insurance carrier contracts with a group of hospitals or providers to provide services at a set fee for each service (Figure 7-3 ●). Some services may be covered by a capitation amount. Those fees that are not covered by the capitation amount will be billed on a discounted basis to the carrier.

Many services will be covered by the insurance carrier in full. Other services will have a standard coinsurance percentage (e.g., 80 percent).

Patients may choose to go to an in-network provider or to a provider who has not contracted with the insurance company (**out-of-network provider**). However, if a patient chooses to visit an out-of-network provider, the benefits may be reduced.

In addition, when a patient visits an in-network provider, the provider is usually contractually obligated to handle the claims submission paperwork for the patient.

EXCLUSIVE PROVIDER ORGANIZATION. Basically an **Exclusive Provider Organization (EPO)** is a much smaller PPO. In an EPO, the patient must select a PCP and can use only those providers who are part of the network or who are referred by the PCP. EPOs usually do not provide coverage for care performed outside of the EPO's network or facilities. EPO providers are paid as services are rendered.

PROVIDER HOSPITAL ORGANIZATION. A **Provider Hospital Organization (PHO)** is an organization of providers and hospitals (Figure 7-4 ●) that band together for the purpose of obtaining contracts from payer organizations. The PHO bargains as an entity for preferred provider status with various payers. The organization members also refers clients to each other.

ACTIVITY #2

Demonstrating Your Understanding of PPOs

Directions: List the four types of preferred provider organizations and describe the structure of each.

1. _____
   _____

2. _____
   _____

3. _____
   _____

4. _____
   _____

MANAGEMENT SERVICE ORGANIZATION. A **Management Service Organization (MSO)** is a separate corporation set up to provide management services to a medical group for a fee. Individual and group providers contract with the MSO for services. An MSO may be owned by a single hospital, several hospitals, or investors.

Self-Insurance

Many employers are turning to a concept called **self-insurance**. Instead of paying monthly premiums to an insurance carrier, they place the money in an escrow account. An employee who receives medical attention submits the claim to the employer and is reimbursed according to the terms of the employer's contract.

This idea works well for employers with many employees but not as well for those with few employees. For example, a company with only ten employees that pays $1,000 a month in health care premiums would have $12,000 in its account for use each year. One employee with a catastrophic illness could wipe out this account within a few weeks of treatment.

However, if the employer has 1,000 employees, with premiums of $100,000 a month, the account would accumulate a total of $1,200,000 during the year, which is more than enough to handle most claims.

These companies, in essence, create their own small insurance company. They must hire employees to oversee the collection of premiums from employees (if any), the accounting of the department, the processing of claims, and all other aspects an insurance company covers, perhaps with the exception of a marketing department. These extra employees generate additional costs.

To help manage these costs, some companies hire administrative services only (ASO) companies or third-party administrators (TPAs) to handle the processing of claims. The employee sends any claims directly to the ASO and may not even know that the plan is self-funded by the employer. This often happens in the case of large insurance carriers that have an ASO arm, such as Blue Cross/Blue Shield. The ASO handles the paperwork, processes the claims, and pays benefits out of the escrow account.

Companies who elect to be self-insured run the risk that their employees may utilize more care than the premiums they would have paid. They could then lose money. However, by tightening controls or altering benefits, they can keep costs under control.

One reason this strategy works is that employees tend to be healthier, as a whole, than the general population. There are no elderly, and most of the people are well enough to show up to work on a regular basis.

Many self-insurance plans purchase **reinsurance**, also known as stop-loss insurance. Reinsurance is an insurance policy that protects the company against catastrophic medical costs levied against its plan, either by a single employee or by all employees as a whole. This protects the employer in case of a company disaster (e.g., plant collapsing and injuring numerous workers, fire, chemical poisoning, etc.), a non-work-related disaster (e.g., earthquake, flood, tornado, with numerous injuries to employees and their families), a generally unhealthy year, or when the payment amount exceeds a certain dollar threshold.

▶ **CRITICAL THINKING QUESTION:** With the knowledge you now have regarding HMOs, PPOs, and self-insurance, which type of coverage would you prefer and why?

Billing Managed Care Plans

Providers who treat patients covered by MCPs create the same bills they would for any other insured patient. The main difference is in preapprovals and in the patient's choice of providers.

Billing MCPs

MCPs, however, have specific rules and regulations that must be followed regarding the keeping of patient charts, determining member eligibility, and all other pertinent data. These rules will be set forth in a policies and procedures manual, which will be given to each provider/group/IPA on the signing of a contract with the MCP. It is important that all office staff understand the rules and regulations contained within this manual.

Disobeying any of the rules could result in substantial loss of revenue to the provider or in termination of their contract with the MCP.

The Membership Card

On enrollment, each MCP member is issued a membership card. This card shows the member's name and will contain a record number or other means of identifying the patient. Often a magnetic strip on the back of the card will have additional information encoded on it.

The membership card also may list a plan number or type that will indicate the benefits covered for this individual. The reverse of the card may show contact numbers for authorization of emergency treatment.

If an MCP member transfers from one medical group to another, or changes benefits, the MCP may issue a new membership card.

PRACTICE **PITFALLS**

Whenever a member seeks treatment, the provider should check the identification card to verify eligibility and to ensure that the correct patient chart has been pulled. If necessary, the provider may request an additional piece of identification to ensure that the person using the card is actually the member to whom it was assigned.

Eligibility Rosters

Because the membership card is retained by the patient and remains unchanged from month to month, many MCPs may maintain an **eligibility roster** to assist the provider in determining who is eligible for treatment. These rosters list those patients who have chosen the provider as their PCP. Several different rosters are commonly used.

The **active member roster** lists those patients whose coverage has continued into the next month. This usually means that the insured or the employer has paid the monthly premium to continue coverage for another month.

The **new member roster** shows those patients who have signed up for MCP coverage and have chosen the provider as their PCP. In addition to members who have just begun coverage, the new member roster shows those existing patients who have recently chosen this provider as their PCP.

The **terminated member roster** shows those members whose coverage has been terminated or who have chosen to terminate this provider as their PCP. For those whose eligibility has terminated, this list is most accurate for those whose coverage is handled by the employer. In such a case, the employer will notify the MCP that the employee is no longer with the company and that any benefits are being terminated.

Some patients will not be included on any of the rosters. This may be because they have not formally terminated their coverage but have not paid their monthly premium prior to the time the rosters were created. If the name of a patient seeking treatment does not show up on any of the rosters, contact the MCP to verify that he or she is still eligible for coverage before providing services. See "Supplemental Capitation" later in this chapter and follow the guidelines presented there to ensure that the provider receives the capitation amount for patients who are still eligible for coverage.

The roster also may contain information in addition to the patient's name. This may include identifying information such as Social Security number, date of birth, gender, insurance information such as covered benefits, employer group number, plan effective date, and other data.

Member rosters are the primary means of identifying eligibility for a patient. The medical group should verify eligibility every time the member seeks treatment. If services are provided without verifying eligibility, the provider is at financial risk for the services provided and may not receive reimbursement from the MCP.

PRACTICE **PITFALLS**

Be sure to verify the following before the provider renders services: that the member is eligible for service for the month, that the member has chosen this provider as the PCP, the amount of copayment, and the correct group or plan number.

Copayment Amounts

MCPs have very few deductibles that must be satisfied each year. The primary form of patient contribution by the member is a copayment, a fixed amount a member must pay for a covered service.

The eligibility roster, or the group designation chart, will identify the services covered by the capitation amount. It also will identify the copayment amount that should be collected from the patient for each visit. This copayment is per provider visit. Therefore, if a patient sees one provider in a medical group and is referred to a different provider within that group, the group should collect the copayment twice, once for each visit with each provider (Figure 7-5 ●). If this money is not collected at the time of the visit, the provider must absorb the loss of this amount.

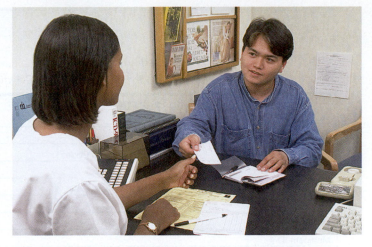

FIGURE 7-5

Collecting payment from a patient at the time of service
© Michal Heron/Pearson Education

Copayment amounts may vary for different services. For example, the member may have a $25 copayment for outpatient visits and a $50 copayment for inpatient stays. For this reason it is important to check the contract for each of the services performed.

For purposes of copayments, services are often divided into the following five categories:

- **Outpatient services**, including provider office visits, outpatient lab and radiology, outpatient surgery, durable medical equipment, home health services, and so on
- **Inpatient services**, including facility charges, drugs, anesthesia, inpatient laboratory and radiology, emergency services, and so on
- **Pharmacy and prescription services**
- **Vision care services**
- **Dental care services**

Some contracts may not cover some of these services (e.g., vision and dental care), and some contracts may not cover items that are listed under a specific type of service (e.g., durable medical equipment).

Occasionally, two copayment amounts may be designated because different types of services were performed in a single visit. In such a case, only one copayment should be collected from the member. Most provider groups/IPAs will collect the higher of the two amounts.

ACTIVITY #3

Testing Your Knowledge on the Categories of Copayments

Directions: List the five categories of copayments.

1. _____
   _____
2. _____
   _____
3. _____
   _____
4. _____
   _____
5. _____
   _____

Patient Encounter Forms

Some MCPs require that all patient encounters (i.e., visits) be reported to the MCP. This reporting is often done using an encounter form. The MCP may specify the use of a designated form for reporting encounters or may use the CMS-1500. Samples of these forms are shown in Figures 7-6 ● and 7-7 ●.

Encounter Form

Date:

Paul Provider, M.D.
5858 Peppermint Place ● Anytown, USA 12345 ● (765) 555-6768

Provider Information

Name:

Address:

City: State: Zip Code:

Telephone #:

Fax #:

Tax ID #:

Medicaid ID #:

Medicare ID #:

Provider's Signature:_____ Date: _____

Patient Information

Name:

Address:

City: State: Zip Code:

Telephone #:

Patient Account #:

Date of Birth:

Gender:

Relationship to Guarantor:

Marital Status:

SSN #:

Insurance Type: ☐ Private   ☐ Medicare   ☐ Medicaid   ☐ Workers' Compensation   ☐ Other _____

Appointment Information

Appt. Date: Time:

Request Next Appt. Date: Time:

Date of First Visit:

Date of Injury:

Referring Physician:

Guarantor Information

Name:

Insurance ID #:

Insurance Plan Name:

Insurance Plan Group #:

Employer Name:

Employer Address:

City: State: Zip Code:

SSN #:

Authorization

☐ Authorization to Release Information
☐ Authorization for Assignment of Benefits
☐ Authorization for Consent for Treatment
☐ I understand that my insurance will be billed as a courtesy to me but that there may be a patient responsibility remaining on account.

Signature:_____ Date: _____

Clinical Information

	Date of Service	Place of Service	CPT Code/Description	ICD-9 Code/ Description	Fee
1.					
2.					
3.					
4.					
5.					
6.					
7.					
8.					

Billing Instructions

Notes:

Special Instructions:

Statement of Account Information

Previous Balance:	$	Payment:	$
Today's Fee:	$	Received by:	
Copay:	$	☐ Cash	
Adjustment:	$	☐ Check	
		☐ Credit Card	
New Balance:	$	☐ Other	

FIGURE 7-6

Sample Encounter Form

SAMPLE

1500

HEALTH INSURANCE CLAIM FORM

APPROVED BY NATIONAL UNIFORM CLAIM COMMITTEE 08/05

| | PICA | | | | | | | | | | | PICA | |

| 1. MEDICARE | MEDICAID | TRICARE CHAMPUS | CHAMPVA | GROUP HEALTH PLAN | FECA BLK LUNG | OTHER | 1a. INSURED'S I.D. NUMBER | (For Program in Item 1) |
| (Medicare #) | (Medicaid #) | (Sponsor's SSN) | (Member ID#) | (SSN or ID) | (SSN) | (ID) | |

2. PATIENT'S NAME (Last Name, First Name, Middle Initial)

3. PATIENT'S BIRTH DATE   MM   DD   YY   SEX   M   F

4. INSURED'S NAME (Last Name, First Name, Middle Initial)

5. PATIENT'S ADDRESS (No., Street)

6. PATIENT RELATIONSHIP TO INSURED   Self   Spouse   Child   Other

7. INSURED'S ADDRESS (No., Street)

CITY   STATE

8. PATIENT STATUS   Single   Married   Other

CITY   STATE

ZIP CODE   TELEPHONE (Include Area Code)   ( )

Employed   Full-Time Student   Part-Time Student

ZIP CODE   TELEPHONE (Include Area Code)   ( )

9. OTHER INSURED'S NAME (Last Name, First Name, Middle Initial)

10. IS PATIENT'S CONDITION RELATED TO:

11. INSURED'S POLICY GROUP OR FECA NUMBER

a. OTHER INSURED'S POLICY OR GROUP NUMBER

a. EMPLOYMENT? (Current or Previous)   YES   NO

a. INSURED'S DATE OF BIRTH   MM   DD   YY   SEX   M   F

b. OTHER INSURED'S DATE OF BIRTH   MM   DD   YY   SEX   M   F

b. AUTO ACCIDENT?   YES   NO   PLACE (State)

b. EMPLOYER'S NAME OR SCHOOL NAME

c. EMPLOYER'S NAME OR SCHOOL NAME

c. OTHER ACCIDENT?   YES   NO

c. INSURANCE PLAN NAME OR PROGRAM NAME

d. INSURANCE PLAN NAME OR PROGRAM NAME

10d. RESERVED FOR LOCAL USE

d. IS THERE ANOTHER HEALTH BENEFIT PLAN?   YES   NO   **If yes**, return to and complete item 9 a-d.

READ BACK OF FORM BEFORE COMPLETING & SIGNING THIS FORM.

12. PATIENT'S OR AUTHORIZED PERSON'S SIGNATURE I authorize the release of any medical or other information necessary to process this claim. I also request payment of government benefits either to myself or to the party who accepts assignment below.

SIGNED_____ DATE _____

13. INSURED'S OR AUTHORIZED PERSON'S SIGNATURE I authorize payment of medical benefits to the undersigned physician or supplier for services described below.

SIGNED_____

14. DATE OF CURRENT: MM   DD   YY   ◄ ILLNESS (First symptom) OR INJURY (Accident) OR PREGNANCY(LMP)

15. IF PATIENT HAS HAD SAME OR SIMILAR ILLNESS. GIVE FIRST DATE   MM   DD   YY

16. DATES PATIENT UNABLE TO WORK IN CURRENT OCCUPATION   MM   DD   YY   FROM   TO   MM   DD   YY

17. NAME OF REFERRING PROVIDER OR OTHER SOURCE

17a.

17b. NPI

18. HOSPITALIZATION DATES RELATED TO CURRENT SERVICES   MM   DD   YY   FROM   TO   MM   DD   YY

19. RESERVED FOR LOCAL USE

20. OUTSIDE LAB?   YES   NO $ CHARGES

21. DIAGNOSIS OR NATURE OF ILLNESS OR INJURY (Relate Items 1, 2, 3 or 4 to Item 24E by Line)

1. |___.___|
2. |___.___|
3. |___.___|
4. |___.___|

22. MEDICAID RESUBMISSION CODE   ORIGINAL REF. NO.

23. PRIOR AUTHORIZATION NUMBER

24. A. DATE(S) OF SERVICE		B. PLACE OF SERVICE	C. EMG	D. PROCEDURES, SERVICES, OR SUPPLIES (Explain Unusual Circumstances)		E. DIAGNOSIS POINTER	F. $ CHARGES	G. DAYS OR UNITS	H. EPSDT Family Plan	I. ID. QUAL.	J. RENDERING PROVIDER ID. #
From	To			CPT/HCPCS	MODIFIER						
MM DD YY	MM DD YY										
1										NPI	
2										NPI	
3										NPI	
4										NPI	
5										NPI	
6										NPI	

25. FEDERAL TAX I.D. NUMBER   SSN EIN

26. PATIENT'S ACCOUNT NO.

27. ACCEPT ASSIGNMENT? (For govt. claims, see back)   YES   NO

28. TOTAL CHARGE $

29. AMOUNT PAID $

30. BALANCE DUE $

31. SIGNATURE OF PHYSICIAN OR SUPPLIER INCLUDING DEGREES OR CREDENTIALS (I certify that the statements on the reverse apply to this bill and are made a part thereof.)

SIGNED_____ DATE _____

32. SERVICE FACILITY LOCATION INFORMATION

a. NPI   b.

33. BILLING PROVIDER INFO & PH #   ( )

a. NPI   b.

NUCC Instruction Manual available at: www.nucc.org

OMB APPROVAL PENDING

FIGURE 7-7

CMS-1500 Form

Groups/IPAs

Most MCPs require the group or independent practice association (IPA) to include a certain number of providers in varying specialties—for example, a general practitioner or internist, a pediatrician, an obstetrician/gynecologist, and a cardiologist. This allows the group to treat all aspects of the patient's care and to provide appropriate services to all members who choose that group/IPA as their PCP.

PRACTICE PITFALLS

Some MCPs have their providers or groups/IPAs report patient encounters on a CMS-1500. If services that a provider renders are not covered by the capitation amount, the amount for these charges should be placed in block 24F. If the charges are covered by a capitation amount, and there is no charge for the service, $0 would be listed in block 24F. The total charges and the balance due would be indicated as charged if not covered under the capitation amount, or as $0 if there are no total charges or balance due.

Some MCPs may have providers or groups/IPAs submit charges that are the MCP's responsibility on a separate claim form from those that are covered under capitation. Thus, two claim forms for the same provider, patient, and dates of service may be necessary.

MCP TO GROUP/IPA RISK. MCPs often use existing providers to deliver care to their patients by signing the providers to contracts. They introduce a mechanism for financial risk sharing by providing cost incentives to providers in order to contain their expenditures (e.g., the provider is paid a set amount, regardless of the services provided to the patient).

In many MCP situations, the risk for patient services is shared between the group/IPA and the MCP. The contract between the MCP and the group/IPA will outline who is responsible for what services and any conditions or limitations that apply to those services.

Risk determinations are usually considered as follows:

- *No risk.* The MCP collects and keeps the monthly capitation amount, and merely pays providers on a fee-for-service basis for the treatment rendered to members. This is similar to a regular insurance carrier setup, except that the member pays only the copay amount, no deductibles or copayment percentage. This arrangement is almost never seen.
- *Partial risk.* The MCP is responsible for most services; however, the capitation covers basic services.
- *Shared risk.* The MCP and the group/IPA share the responsibility for services. A contract will designate which services or treatments are covered by the MCP and which are covered by the provider.
- *Full risk.* The group/IPA is responsible for most, if not all, of the services. The MCP is just in the business of selling policies and writing contracts with groups/IPAs.

Most MCP contracts with providers are on a shared-risk basis. The MCP will provide a list to the group/IPA of all possible services (often indicated by CPT codes and descriptions), and an indication of who is responsible for those services (Figure 7-8 ●). A letter code will often designate who is responsible for payment for that service (e.g., G = Group/IPA responsibility, H = MCP/HMO responsibility, etc.).

This document also will list any services that are denied and the appropriate copayment amount for many of these services. It is important to note that, if the plan is an S/HMO, any services that normally are covered by Medicare should be covered services under the S/HMO contract

---

PRACTICE PITFALLS

If an MCP offers numerous types of policies (e.g., group coverage, individual coverage, Medicare HMO coverage, etc.), then each of these plans may be listed on the same sheet. It is important for the biller to look at the correct procedure code and the correct plan to determine who is financially responsible for a service.

Covered Services	MEDICARE		COMMERCIAL						
	Standard	Medi-Medi	AMG	Rocky	CAT	MIPC	CAIT	SBA	RICE
Abortion - Elective (CPT 59840 - 59841) Note: Refer to Super Panel contracts for financial responsibility for specific procedures	G/P¹	G/P²	G/P²	G/P¹	G/P²	G/P²,³	G/P⁴	G/P⁴	G/P⁴
Abortion - Therapeutic (CPT 59812 - 59857) If the life of the mother could be endangered if the fetus is carried to term, or in cases of fetal genetic defect.	-	G	G	G	G	G	G	G	G
Acupuncture	-	-	-	-	-	-	-	-	G
Acute Care • Facility Component	P	P	P	P	P	P	P	P	P
• Hospital-Based Physicians, including clinical and anatomical pathologist (CPT 80002 - 83999), radiologist (CPT 70010 - 76499), anesthesiologist (CPT 00100 - 01999, 99100 - 99140)	P	P	P	P	P	P	P	P	P
• Professional Component, including consultations and follow-up care visits (CPT 99217 - 99239, 99251 - 99275)	G	G	G	G	G	G	G	G	G
• Closed-panel physicians under contract with a hospital for test reading (e.g. EKG)⁵	P	P	P	P	P	P	P	P	P
• Special services and reports, miscellaneous (CPT 99000 - 99090, 99175 - 99199)	G	G	G	G	G	G	G	G	G

¹Not covered except in cases of rape or incest, or when the life of the mother would be endangered if the fetus were brought to term.
²Covered for the first thirteen (13) weeks of pregnancy only.
³Copay for HIPC is the same as for inpatient hospitalization.
⁴Covered through the second trimester (24 weeks) of pregnancy only.
⁵Plan to confirm closed panel status.

Legend: G = Medical Group Responsibility; P = Plan/HMO Responsibility; G/P = Shared Responsibility; -- = Not Covered

This chart shows a sampling of CPT codes and the party that bears responsibility for covering costs for each procedure under numerous different plans. It is important to check the correct column for the plan being processed to determine if services are covered or not.

FIGURE 7-8

Distribution of responsibility

(regardless of whether the group, MCP, or HMO has financial responsibility). Therefore, if Medicare determines that it will begin covering a specific type of treatment, then the S/HMO also must begin covering that type of treatment.

GROUP/IPA TO PROVIDER RISK. In addition to the MCP transferring all or part of the risk to the group/IPA, the group/IPA may transfer some or all of its risk to an individual capitated provider as well. The levels of risk transferred to the capitated provider include the following:

- *No risk.* The group/IPA keeps the entire capitation payment and providers are paid on a fee-for-service basis. There are usually no withholds or bonuses as part of the provider's contract. However, a fee schedule will often be incorporated as part of the contract agreement, so the amount that the provider receives for services will be determined by the fee schedule.
- *No referral risk transferred.* All or part of the payment to the provider involves risk, but that risk is not tied to referrals. Only the capitation amount, bonuses, and withholds are at risk (e.g., the provider may perform more services than the capitation, withholds, and bonuses cover). Under this arrangement, *referral* means any service not provided for by the provider. Essentially, it is expected that the capitation, withholds, and bonuses are the only payments for any and all care that the provider renders to the member. The provider is not responsible for paying for referrals, and the amount of money paid to the provider is not affected by the decision of the provider to make referrals to other providers.
- *Referral risk is transferred, but not substantial.* Part of the payment to the provider is dependent on the decisions the provider makes to refer patients to other providers. However, that part of the payment is not substantial (e.g., is under 25 percent). Therefore, if this type of provider makes too many patient referrals to other providers, up to 25 percent of his or her capitation amount may be withheld.
- *Substantial risk for referrals is transferred, but stop-loss protection is in place.* If more than 25 percent of total payments to the provider are at risk for referrals, the medical group/IPA must have aggregate or per-patient stop-loss protection in place. **Stop-loss** protection means that if the costs to the provider exceed a specified amount, the provider will be reimbursed by the group/IPA for at least 90 percent of expenditures over that amount.

In general, the higher the risk that is transferred to the provider, the higher the capitation amount. If less risk is transferred to the provider, the group/IPA keeps a higher percentage of the capitation amount to cover its expenses.

Capitation Payments

When a contract is signed between an MCP and a provider, an agreement is made regarding a capitated fee. This fee often is dependent on the type of plan under which the patient is covered. Varying factors such as the gender and age of the patient and their overall health also may be considered. The provider and MCP will also agree which services are covered by the capitation amount.

Often, capitation amounts pay for all the basic treatment the patient needs during the month. If the patient does not see the provider that month, the provider keeps the fee. If the patient becomes ill and requires treatment, the provider is expected to provide the necessary services without additional compensation by the MCP. Usually, the amount saved and the extra amount spent balance out.

The capitation amount for each provider is determined by those who are included on either the active or new member roster. The PCP usually receives capitation payments for the previous month. The amount of the capitation payment will vary according to the coverages or plans that have been selected. Additional amounts may be provided for patients who have entered a hospice or skilled nursing care facility, as well as those who have been diagnosed with specific diseases (e.g., HIV or ESRD) (see "Additional Capitation Amounts").

The MCP may retain a portion of the monthly capitation amount to protect the HMO from inadequate patient care or financial management by the PCP. This amount is called a **withhold**. The MCP also may withhold a portion to ensure the quality of care given to patients and promptness of payments to outside providers. This amount is outlined in the contract signed by the group and the MCP.

For example, consider a primary care provider with 1,000 members from 123 MCP. The capitation rate is $25 per member per month, so the provider earns $25,000 per month (1,000 members

× $25 each), regardless of how many or how few patients are seen from 123 MCP. The MCP withholds 3 percent ($750) from the payment for insolvency and unpaid claims and an additional 5 percent ($1,250) for its Medical Management Incentive Program. The provider actually receives $23,000 per month. The MCP sets the $1,250 withhold aside in a fund until the end of the year for the Medical Management Incentive Program. At that time the withhold may be paid, based on criteria such as those described above. The provider may be paid some or all of the $750 held for insolvency and unpaid claims when and if the contract with 123 MCP is terminated.

PRACTICE **PITFALLS**

To cover financial insolvency and unpaid claims by the group/IPA, 123 MCP withholds 3 percent of the capitation amount. If all obligations have been met, this amount will be returned when the group terminates its contract with the MCP. In addition, 123 MCP will withhold 5 percent of the capitation for its Medical Management Incentive Program. This program stipulates that the 5 percent will be reimbursed to the group/IPA if the following guidelines are met:

- 25 percent of the withheld amount will be reimbursed if the provider/group/IPA has submitted less than the budgeted amount of hospital expenses covered by the HMO.

- 10 percent of the amount will be reimbursed for customer satisfaction. The MCP will randomly survey patients to determine their satisfaction with the provider and the services rendered. If the provider is above average in customer satisfaction, he or she will receive this amount.

- 10 percent of the withheld amount will be reimbursed for low disenrollment. If the provider/group maintains less than 2 percent disenrollment (those terminating MCP coverage or transferring to another provider), then they will receive this amount.

- 40 percent of the withheld amount will be reimbursed for quality of care. This will be determined by a review of medical records by the MCP. If the medical review panel agrees with the treatment given at least 80 percent of the time, the provider will receive this amount.

- 15 percent of the withheld amount will be reimbursed for protocol compliance. This is calculated as follows:
  - 5 percent for compliance with all facility requirements as determined by an audit of the facility
  - 5 percent for timeliness of claim payments
  - 5 percent for timeliness in submission of all contractually required statements to the MCP

Upon meeting all the stipulations outlined, the provider will keep the 5 percent quality care amount.

You can see how the things you do as a biller may affect the amount the provider receives in his or her monthly capitation check. If you are rude to a patient and a complaint is made, or if a member chooses to transfer to another provider, it could cost the group/IPA. If you do not process claim payments promptly, submit statements to the MCP on time, or let the providers in the group know that they are near the limit on their hospital costs, additional amounts will be withheld. It is important that the biller understand all factors that can cause withholding from the provider's capitation amounts and do their best to see that the goals are met for compliance with HMO guidelines.

Supplemental Capitation

On occasion, an eligible member will not appear on the eligibility rosters. The biller should keep a list of all eligible patients seen by the provider (Figure 7-9 ●). If at any time a patient does not show up on an eligibility roster, the biller should contact the MCP to determine the reason.

There may be a legitimate reason a name is not on a roster (e.g., the patient has transferred to another PCP, but the transfer paperwork has not yet been received), or the patient may have been inadvertently left off the list. If you discover a patient who should be on the roster and is not, contact the HMO to determine the correct procedure for having the patient's name placed on the roster. Also ask what paperwork is required to receive the capitation amount for this patient.

Provider Medical Group

Supplemental Capitation Request

TO: _____   FROM:_____
Provider Network Manager   Medical Group Name and Number

Date Submitted: _____   For Eligibility Month/Year:_____

Member Name	Plan Type	Member Number	DRG/Diagnosis

FIGURE 7-9

Supplemental Capitation Request Form

In addition, many patients who sign up for MCP coverage do not immediately choose a PCP. These people may not choose a PCP until they feel the need for treatment. At that time they will choose a provider and will be added to that provider's new member roster.

The billing office should contact all new members as soon as possible to determine how long they have been a member and what precipitated their decision to choose a particular provider as their PCP. If they have been an MCP member for a while but simply had not requested a specific provider, the MCP has been keeping the capitation amounts for that patient and not assigning them to a specific provider. The contract between the provider and the MCP, or the MCP and the member, may stipulate that the MCP will assign a PCP to any enrollee who does not choose one within a specified time. If this is not being done, the provider/group should be notified that they may want to contact the MCP regarding the matter. They may be due additional patients (and capitation amounts) because of new members who should have been assigned to a PCP.

Additional Capitation Amounts

Many MCPs will pay an amount in addition to the regular capitation amount for those patients who have been diagnosed with certain illnesses or whose illness or condition has required them to enter a hospice or skilled nursing facility.

It is the responsibility of the provider to inform the MCP of changes in the patient's status in order to receive the additional reimbursement. The biller should consult the MCP's policies and procedures manual to determine which conditions allow for additional reimbursement and which form to file to obtain this reimbursement. The biller should then make a list of those conditions that qualify for additional reimbursement and the time limits and other conditions for applying for the reimbursement.

As with supplemental capitation, usually specific forms must be used and explicit deadlines met for a provider to receive the additional capitation. For example, if the deadline for submitting the paperwork is not met, the MCP may refuse to add the additional capitation amount until the following month and the provider may forfeit the additional capitation for the current and preceding months.

Billing for Services

Although the monthly capitation amount covers most services, some services will be reimbursed on a fee-for-service basis. This means that the provider will bill the MCP for these services when they are performed. Most agreements between a provider and an MCP will have a list of those services that are covered by the capitation amount or those that are considered to be on a fee-for-service basis. Fee-for-service procedures are usually billed on a CMS-1500 form the same as non-MCP services, or they may be electronically billed if required.

Medical billers should familiarize themselves with those services that are covered by the capitation amount and those that are billed before treating a patient. They also should collect the copayment amount from the patient before treatment is rendered by the provider.

Appointment Scheduling

The MCP will usually dictate the maximum amount of time a patient must wait for an appointment (e.g., the appointment must be scheduled within four weeks of the patient's request for an appointment). Different time frames may be given for routine appointments than for urgent care appointments. Table 7-1 ● illustrates the maximum time that a patient may have to wait to get an appointment. It is important that these time frames be met. Failure to do so could result in sanctions against the provider. Numerous sanctions could result in the provider losing the contract with the MCP.

Many MCPs require a certain number of appointments to be set aside for emergencies. This allows a patient to be seen within twenty-four hours if an emergency situation arises. All decisions regarding whether a patient should be seen immediately are the responsibility of the provider. At no time should a medical biller attempt to determine the emergent nature of the patient's condition.

TABLE 7-1 **Maximum Time for a Patient to Wait for an Appointment**

Appointment Type	Maximum Time
Urgent Care	Same day
New patient, routine	Two weeks
Established patient, annual physical	Four weeks
Problem-oriented visit	Two days

If the provider is unable to meet the patient's request for an appointment within the allotted time, the provider should refer the patient to another appropriate provider who can see the patient within the allotted time. The charges for this appointment will be the responsibility of the provider.

If you are scheduling elective surgery, whether inpatient or outpatient, you should avoid the ending and the beginning of the month so that eligibility may be cleared. In addition, many MCPs will insist that the surgical procedure be performed on the first day of admission. Any necessary preadmit testing should be done on an outpatient basis the day before surgery. If this is not possible, the documentation to substantiate the need for an overnight stay before surgery should be attached to the Treatment Authorization Request (TAR). The MCP is part of the RVU. Refer to Chapter 4 to review this information.

Missed Appointments

Each time a patient misses an appointment, the provider must review the patient's chart and determine the appropriate follow-up activity. This decision should be documented in the patient chart and initialed and dated by the provider. The following are appropriate follow-up activities:

- No follow-up needed. Wait for patient to call for a new appointment.
- Send a letter advising the patient to call to reschedule an appointment.
- Telephone the patient to reschedule the appointment.

If the appropriate follow-up was a letter, the letter should contain the member's name, the date and time of the missed appointment, the reason for the appointment, the provider's name and address, and a phone number that the patient can call to reschedule their appointment.

If the appropriate follow-up is a phone call to reschedule the appointment, record any phone calls or attempts to contact the member in the patient record. This should include the date and time of the call, name and title of the person making the call, and outcome of the call (e.g., new appointment scheduled, left message, no answer, etc.).

If the provider notes that the patient should be seen as soon as possible, the biller should attempt to contact the member the same day as the missed appointment. The member should then be scheduled for the first available emergency appointment.

If there is no telephone number, or if there has been no contact after three attempts, a letter should be sent asking the member to call the office to reschedule the appointment. A copy of this letter should be placed in the patient chart.

If any correspondence sent to the patient is returned by the postal service as undeliverable, it should be date stamped and filed in the patient's chart. The doctor should be informed, and a notation of his or her decision regarding follow-up placed in the patient's chart.

▶ **CRITICAL THINKING QUESTION:** What should you do if a patient becomes extremely agitated when he or she is telephoned about continuously missing appointments?

Authorizations, Referrals, and Second Opinions

It is important for the medical biller to be familiar with the agreement between the MCP and the provider. Often the MCP will require a second surgical opinion (SSO) or preauthorization for treatment. If the patient is to be admitted to the hospital, precertification may be required. These "precertifications" will often have time limits on when treatments are to be performed. For example, precertification must often take place at least five days before a scheduled inpatient admission and emergency treatments require notification to the MCP within forty-eight hours of admission.

With precertification and preauthorization, the MCP will evaluate the proposed treatment and inform the provider and patient as to whether or not they will cover the services. If the MCP decides that the services are not necessary, they will deny payment. The provider and patient must then decide whether they will abandon the treatment, seek authorization for an alternate treatment, or go ahead with the treatment with the understanding that the patient is completely responsible for the charges.

Preauthorization

It is important to obtain preauthorization for services that are the responsibility of the MCP. If these services are performed without preauthorization, the group/IPA may be responsible for payment of services. Each MCP may have its own specific Treatment Authorization Request (TAR).

Often a TAR approval will be valid for a limited time, usually thirty days. If services are not performed within that time, an additional TAR must be completed and another preauthorization received. In the case of ongoing treatments (e.g., chemotherapy, dialysis, etc.), monthly authorizations of services covered by the MCP may be needed.

If authorization has not come back from the MCP within ten to fifteen days, the MCP should be contacted. If the TAR was never received, it may be necessary to reschedule the patient and to resubmit a new TAR. For this reason, it is best to choose a date that is several weeks in the future. However, every attempt should be made to avoid the beginning and ending of the month because the patient's eligibility may change and the MCP will insist that all routine follow-up care or hospital stays be included in the one authorization.

TARs often are three- or four-part forms. If not, you should make a copy of the TAR for your records before sending it to the MCP. Any additional documentation that is necessary to substantiate the need for services should be included with the TAR and firmly attached to it.

If it is not possible to reschedule the patient's surgery due to the nature of the treatment, many MCPs have an emergency request procedure that allows faxing of the TAR and overnight approval. If it is not prudent for the patient to wait for this approval, he or she should be instructed to go to the ER, where the hospital will call the MCP and request approval for an emergency admission.

If a specific date of surgery is listed on the TAR, surgery must be performed on that date. TARs may not be valid for any dates other than the date listed. In surgery is not performed on the approved date, the group/IPA or provider may be responsible for payment of services, not the MCP.

The MCP also will indicate the number of days of hospitalization allowed (if it is an inpatient admission). If it becomes necessary for the patient to remain in the hospital longer (e.g., as a result of complications), then as soon as possible the group/IPA should submit a request and documentation to the MCP to substantiate the need for additional inpatient days.

Utilization Review

As noted in Chapter 4, utilization review (UR) is a process whereby insurance carriers review the treatment of a patient and determine whether or not it will cover the costs. Many insurance carriers began creating UR departments in an effort to control costs and avoid unnecessary procedures. Although this process was started with traditional insurance carriers, managed care carriers have taken the concept a step further, creating complete UR departments and reviewing every outside procedure that may require additional costs and every referral to a specialist.

Many providers dislike the UR process. They feel the UR committee cannot always make an effective decision based on the data provided in the medical report. They dislike being second-guessed by a committee that is not familiar with the patients and their problems. Many providers have found a need to hire an additional office person just to review medical information over the phone with the insurance companies in order to get their procedures approved (Figure 7-10 ●).

However, insurance carriers insist that the process has prevented numerous unnecessary surgeries and helped providers to consider alternate forms of treatment that may be as or more beneficial to the patient.

In addition, UR committees are becoming more selective in the items and providers they choose to review. Some procedures are nearly always allowed (e.g., cystourethroscopy), whereas more questionable procedures (e.g., MRIs of the knees) are nearly always reviewed. In addition, some insurers are tracking the records of providers. Those who are known for ordering tests or procedures that are nearly always necessary are less closely watched than those who have a history of ordering questionable procedures.

Specialist Referrals

If a member requests to see a specialist, the provider must discuss the request with the member. If the request is denied, the procedures for denial of services must be followed, including sending a denial letter to

FIGURE 7-10

Obtaining a referral over the telephone

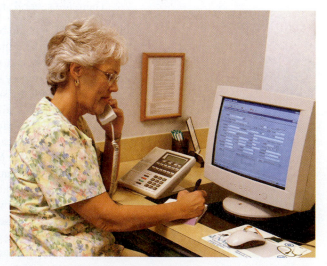

the member. If the provider agrees with the member's request, or recommends that the member see a specialist, an appropriate referral form should be completed and approved. The decision to refer or not to refer a member is a medical decision that should be made by the provider.

The group/IPA must provide a written notice of its decision to the member. If the request is approved, the notice must advise the member of the name, address, and phone number of the consultant and either state an appointment time or inform the member about how to schedule an appointment.

The group/IPA is required to have contracts with its specialists. They must maintain contracts with a sufficient number of specialists so that members are not inconvenienced by excessive appointment waiting times. The provider's office also should keep a Specialist Referral Log listing all patients referred to a specialist. This log should include the following:

- The name of the member or patient
- The request date
- The appointment date
- The referring provider
- The consulting provider or specialist
- The problem or reason for the referral
- The date the report was received from the specialist
- Any comments

This log can help the practice keep track of patients who have been seen by a specialist and whether or not the results of that referral have been received from the specialist.

Denial of Services to Members

If a member requests a specific treatment and the provider/group/IPA determines that the treatment or service is not medically necessary, would be detrimental to the patient, or would provide no medical benefit to the patient, the service may be denied (i.e., performing of the treatment refused). The provider should discuss with the patient why it is believed these services would not be beneficial. A patient who wishes to pursue the request can ask for a second opinion or for the provider to reconsider the treatment.

Second Opinions

Many MCPs have a second-opinion policy designed to resolve differences of opinion regarding proposed treatment among providers, members, consultants, or the MCP. Second opinions are often provided in the following instances:

- At the request of the member before a surgical or other invasive procedure
- If the provider's opinion is contrary to the member's expressed expectations, even after the provider has counseled the member
- If the opinion of the provider differs substantially from the recommended treatment plan of the specialist on the case
- At the request of the MCP

There are several steps to the second-opinion process:

1. A request is made by the provider, member, consultant, or MCP for a second opinion. This request may be either verbal or in writing.
2. The patient's chart is documented with the request.
3. An internal review is performed. This is a second opinion performed by another provider affiliated with the same group/IPA as the provider.
4. If the member is still dissatisfied, or if the two opinions differ substantially, an external review may be performed. This is an opinion provided by a provider who is not a member of the group/IPA to which the member belongs. Any member who is still dissatisfied should contact the MCP to request the external review. The MCP reviews the records and—if it deems an external review necessary—will inform the provider and the member. The MCP may send the member to a provider of its choosing.
5. All records are forwarded to the MCP's chief medical officer, who makes a determination of the proper course of treatment. The provider will then be informed of the decision. It is then the provider's responsibility to carry out the proposed treatment plan. This may mean treating the patient or referring the member to a specialist for treatment.

Financial responsibility for second opinions is usually shared among the group/IPA and the MCP as follows:

1. The provider/group/IPA is responsible for the internal review.
2. The MCP is responsible for the external review unless the provider/group/IPA failed to document the internal review, the provider/group/IPA did not properly complete a TAR and obtain authorization before sending the member for an external review, or the opinion of the external review provider differs substantially from the provider/group/IPA decision.

All activities regarding the second opinion process must be thoroughly documented in the patient's record. Any time that the MCP must bear financial responsibility for any services, including the external review, a TAR must be completed and the treatment preauthorized.

Because of member complaints and substantial delays in receiving authorizations or referrals, some MCPs are now allowing members to refer themselves for a second opinion. However, self-referring members are limited to obtaining a second opinion from another provider who is affiliated with the same MCP, and the number of times they may refer themselves for a second opinion is limited (e.g., once every six months).

Denials of Service After a Second Opinion

Once the member has exhausted the second-opinion process or chooses not to proceed with the process (i.e., accepts the decision of the internal review), the provider/group/IPA must send a denial letter to the member. A copy of this letter also must be sent to the MCP along with any supporting documentation. This letter must state the patient's name, the date services were requested, the services that were requested, and the reason for the denial of services.

The MCP often will keep a log of these denials. If it thinks a provider/group/IPA is denying too many treatments, it may ask for a review of the record to monitor the quality of care given to the patients.

Member Appeals of Denied Services

Members may appeal any decision that involves the denial of services that they believe should have been performed or covered. This includes the right to appeal decisions both before and after the service has been performed. It also applies to the proposed termination of treatment that the patient is currently receiving (e.g., termination of a hospital stay or continued plan of treatment).

To file an appeal, the member must contact the MCP, usually in writing, and include the following items:

- Patient name
- Member name (if different from patient)
- Member identification number
- Member address
- Phone number
- Name of provider/group/IPA
- Name of provider
- Date service was rendered if previously done
- Complete description of the problem or why it is believed the services should not have been denied
- Member signature

Members who wish to deliver this appeal to the provider/group/IPA should be told to mail it to the MCP; otherwise the provider/group/IPA may be required to accept the appeal and mail it to the MCP themselves.

The MCP will review the appeal and all appropriate supporting evidence. It also will look up the denial and supporting evidence that was filed by the provider/group/IPA. This is why it is so important that the group/IPA file its notices of denial in a timely manner with all necessary supporting documentation.

Within a specified time limit (usually thirty days), the MCP will make a decision regarding the denial of services. If it determines that the services should have been covered or performed, it will instruct the provider/group/IPA to do so. If it upholds the decision of the provider/group/IPA that the services were correctly denied, it will inform the member by letter. A copy of this letter also will be forwarded to the provider/group/IPA and should be placed in the patient's record.

For services that have not yet been rendered, some MCPs have an expedited appeal process in which the MCP is required to make a decision within a few days. It is a requirement that this expedited appeal process be available to Medicare members, but it also may be available to other members.

Member Grievances and Complaints

Grievances are written complaints made by members regarding quality of services, access to care, interpersonal communication, or any other aspect of their care or relationship with their provider. **Complaints** are verbal expressions regarding such dissatisfactions. Members may file a grievance or complaint with the provider, the group/IPA, or the MCP.

If the member files the grievance or complaint with the provider or the group/IPA, the following steps should be taken:

1. The provider or group/IPA should attempt to resolve the issue through patient counseling, whether in person or over the phone.
2. If the provider or group/IPA is unable to resolve the grievance or complaint, or it is outside his or her scope of responsibility (e.g., the member is dissatisfied with the MCP contract), the provider must refer the grievance to the MCP. A time limit is usually associated with this procedure. Often the provider must refer the grievance within one working day of receiving it if it is unable to resolve it. For this reason, it is imperative that all provider/group/IPA members and staff take complaints from MCP members very seriously.
3. If the grievance or complaint has been resolved at the provider level, the provider/group/IPA must send a letter confirming the resolution of the issue to the member. A copy of this correspondence and any supporting documentation also must be mailed to the MCP.
4. If the provider is unable to resolve the complaint within a specified time limit (e.g., thirty days), the member must be given the opportunity to file a written complaint with the MCP.
5. If the grievance or complaint concerns any aspect of medical care, it must be reviewed by the provider/group/IPA medical director.

Grievance Logs

Often, provider/group/IPAs are required to keep a log of all grievances in addition to documenting all grievances in the patient chart. Some MCPs require that a copy of this log be forwarded to them at set intervals (e.g., every thirty days). If a copy of the log is required but no grievances or complaints have been received, the provider/group/IPA must submit a log with the words No Grievances printed on it.

The following items are often required on a grievance log:

1. Member name
2. Member identification number
3. Date of grievance or complaint
4. Type of grievance or what the grievance was about
5. Date of resolution letter or date referred to MCP

If numerous grievances or complaints are received, the MCP may withhold a portion of the monthly capitation amount or may terminate its relationship with the provider/group/IPA.

Transfers

A member may transfer from one provider to another at any time. Often, the MCP will require the patient to complete a request for transfer. There will then be a waiting period while the MCP verifies that the member is eligible for coverage and has chosen a provider who is contracted under the member's plan. The transfer will become effective at the beginning of the next month. Because capitation amounts are paid month to month, this eliminates the need to split a capitation amount between two or more providers.

Usually, if one member of a family chooses to transfer to another medical group as a provider, then all members of the family must transfer to the same medical group. However, each family member may see a different provider within that medical group. This often is the reason that a medical group will be required to have providers of different specialties within their group (e.g., general practitioner, pediatrician, cardiologist, etc.).

Any member requesting a transfer must complete a transfer request form. This form also must be completed if a patient chooses to transfer from one provider to another within the same medical group. On receipt of the transfer form, the medical group must forward a copy of the patient's medical records to the MCP. The MCP will then forward them to the new provider. If no chart is available (e.g., the patient has never visited the provider), then the original provider must inform the MCP of that.

If the provider has a need for a copy of the patient chart, a copy should be made prior to sending the chart to the MCP. The fact that the patient has been transferred to another facility should be noted on the copy, along with the date, and then the entire duplicate file should be placed in an "inactive" file. A medical biller who receives a notice that a patient is transferring into the medical group is responsible for ensuring, before that patient is treated, that the group has received a copy of the patient's medical record.

Disenrollment

When a patient transfers his or her care from a provider, it is considered **disenrollment** from that provider. A patient may disenroll from a provider at any time by requesting a transfer to another provider. A patient also may disenroll from an MCP program by stopping payment of premiums or by seeking other insurance coverage.

Because an MCP is responsible for all care given to a patient, there is often no secondary insurance coverage under an MCP. Many MCPs will include a provision in their contract with the patient stating that if the patient enrolls in another MCP or obtains other insurance coverage, the policy with the MCP will be immediately terminated.

MCP-Initiated Disenrollment

The MCP may disenroll a member for various reasons. These reasons must have been previously stated in the contract with the member and verified by documentation from the provider or the MCP.

The reasons for disenrollment can include but are not limited to the following:

1. The member disregards the enrollment agreement by habitually seeking covered services, other than emergency care, from a provider who is not a contracted provider.
2. The patient/provider relationship has deteriorated. This can be evidenced by a pattern of broken appointments and refusal to follow provider advice or orders. The MCP may require that the member be referred for psychiatric evaluation prior to initiating this type of disenrollment to ensure that the patient can be held mentally competent and legally responsible for his or her actions.
3. A pattern of physical or verbal abuse of the provider or his or her staff has occurred. This often must be documented and a police report filed. The MCP also may require these members to be sent for psychiatric evaluation before initiating disenrollment.
4. The member moves out of the service area covered by the MCP.
5. The member fails to pay the required monthly premium.

Each pattern of missed appointments, abusive behavior, or failure to follow medical advice must be carefully documented by the provider and made a part of the patient's record. Once a provider has documented a habitual problem, disenrollment of the patient may be requested. This is often accomplished by filing a request for disenrollment form. These forms vary from one MCP to another but usually contain only basic patient information. The request must then be substantiated with documentation. This documentation should include the following:

1. Documentation in the patient record or progress notes showing dates of visits or missed appointments, or a listing of these (There should be a sufficient pattern shown to document the "habitual" nature of the offense.)
2. Documentation in the patient record or progress notes or in a grievance log showing the date, time, and subject of any counseling the member received from the provider/group/ provider's staff in an effort to prevent or repair the breakdown in the relationship
3. Explanation of why the problem cannot be resolved
4. Documentation that a discussion of why a change to another provider is not appropriate or has not been done
5. Copies of any correspondence sent to the member in an effort to resolve the situation, or to assist the member in understanding the plan procedures (e.g., when to use the ER, need for prior authorization, importance of keeping medical appointments, etc.)

6. Evidence that the member has demonstrated a total lack of cooperation with the plan, has continued to misuse services, or has been physically or verbally abusive after receipt of the correspondence or other written attempts to correct the problem (In many cases, a police report will meet this requirement.)

7. Evidence that the noncompliant or abusive member has been referred to a psychiatrist, or evidence showing the reason why this action was not appropriate

The provider will be required to continue treating the patient until officially notified by the MCP that the member has been disenrolled.

Continuing Care

There are times when a provider or group chooses to terminate the contractual obligation with the MCP. If a provider terminates the contract with the MCP or the group, the remaining members of that group continue to be responsible for the treatment that provider's patient. Members are assigned to a group, as well as to a provider within that group, and that relationship will continue regardless of whether one provider leaves the group or not.

However, if an entire group/IPA terminates its contract with the MCP, a need may arise for continuation of coverage for members who were being treated by the terminating group. Continuation of coverage exists when a specified treatment was begun by the terminating group/IPA and must be continued by the newly assigned provider or group/IPA. For continuing care coverage to exist, the following rules often apply:

- The patient must be involved in a specific treatment plan that has been previously authorized by the medical director of the terminating group/IPA.
- The treatment has a clearly identifiable termination. (Ongoing treatments for a condition that has no cure [e.g., diabetes] would not be reimbursable under continuing care rules.)
- Medical care was terminated as a result of the group/IPA situation rather than through any fault of the member.
- If the patient is pregnant, specific rules may apply regarding the length of the gestation and time left to the termination of treatment.

In such cases, the newly assigned group may be allowed additional compensation for the continuing care treatment that is provided to these patients. For example, the provider may be reimbursed by the MCP for each treatment provided in relation to continuing care at the normally contracted rate. The regular capitation amount will apply for all treatments that are provided for a reason other than the continuing care.

Specific rules must be followed to obtain the proper reimbursement, and the policies and procedures manual should be checked before rendering services. For example, to qualify for an additional reimbursement under continuing care rules, the provider may need to seek preauthorization for all treatments.

It is often the responsibility of the group/IPA that receives the member to identify the need for continuing care coverage. These members should be identified as quickly as possible so that proper rules and reimbursement can be applied.

FIGURE 7-11

Minor outpatient surgery being performed

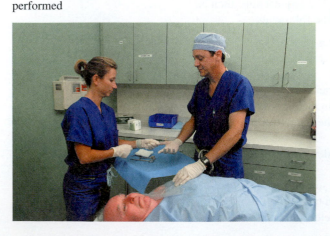

Miscellaneous Services

Certain rules can apply to select types of services under an MCP agreement. These services can include, but are not limited to, outpatient surgery, ER services, durable medical equipment, and prescriptions.

Outpatient Surgery

Some MCPs will provide a list of surgeries that must be performed in an outpatient setting (Figure 7-11 ●). This is most often done in a shared-risk contract when the group/IPA is financially responsible for outpatient services and the HMO is responsible for inpatient services.

It is important to know which surgeries must be performed on an outpatient basis. If these guidelines are not followed, the group/IPA may be financially responsible for all inpatient costs in relation to the surgery.

Emergency Room Services

If the provider/group/IPA is considered financially responsible for ER services, then it is responsible for managing the member's utilization of ER services and for paying for the cost of these services (Figure 7-12 ●). The provider/group/IPA must provide written information to its members on how to access these services. The provider/group/IPA must have procedures for the authorization of these services. Payment may not be denied based on lack of notification or lack of authorization for these services.

Durable Medical Equipment

All durable medical equipment (DME) must be ordered and prescribed by the provider for the patient's use. If the financial responsibility for DME lies with the provider/group/IPA, it is imperative that authorization be obtained as soon as possible. Requests and prescriptions for DME must include a specified time period. Often MCPs will authorize the rental of DME only for a month at a time. Thus, the authorization must be requested each and every month for patients with chronic conditions (e.g., a glucometer for a diabetic). Also, each request for DME must be on a separate prescription or authorization request form. Thus, it is possible for one patient to have several outstanding DME authorizations (e.g., oxygen, bed, wheelchair, and such). Each specific DME request will be assessed based on member eligibility and medical necessity. Therefore, it may be necessary to include a copy of the documentation with each DME request (Figure 7-13 ●).

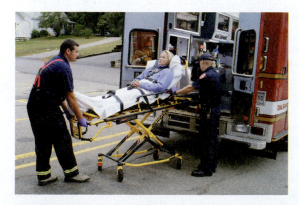

FIGURE 7-12

Ambulance transport is typically covered under emergency room services
© Michal Heron/Pearson Education.

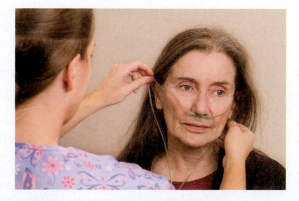

FIGURE 7-13

Placing oxygen on a patient

Prescription Coverage

When an MCP offers prescription coverage to a member, limitations often apply:

1. The member must purchase the drugs from an MCP-contracted facility. If prescriptions are obtained from a noncontracted pharmacy, the member will bear the cost of the pharmacy services. There may be exceptions to this rule for emergency situations, or situations in which the patient is outside the service area, or the prescription is not available from a contracted pharmacy.
2. Drugs and medications may be limited to a thirty-day supply.
3. Only prescription drugs are normally covered. Over-the-counter medications are usually not covered.
4. Only oral and topical drugs may be covered. Injectable drugs often are not covered under the pharmacy benefit; they may, however, be covered under the medical benefit, and this is especially true for injectable medications that the patient needs for survival (e.g., insulin for a diabetic).
5. The generic equivalent of a prescribed drug may be required if it is available. If there is no generic equivalent, the MCP will often cover the brand name at the standard copayment amount. However, if there is a generic equivalent, the MCP may only cover the cost of the generic equivalent. Thus, the member will be charged the standard copay, plus the difference between the generic and the brand name medication.

Some generic drugs are not the same as their brand name counterparts. They may have a similar, but different, active ingredient, or they may be in a different dosage amount from the brand name drug. In such a case they are not considered to be therapeutically equivalent. For these drugs, the MCP may require the provider to prescribe the generic drug, or it may allow the full benefit for the brand name drug.

Sanctions

If a provider/group/IPA fails to meet the quality standards, reporting requirements, or any other provisions of its contract with the MCP, the MCP may impose sanctions on the provider/group/IPA or the individual provider. These sanctions usually include the withholding of specified amounts or disallowing any new members to be enrolled to that provider/group/IPA.

It is not uncommon for sanctions to escalate for additional offenses. Therefore, an MCP may impose a $1,000 (or 5 percent of capitation) sanction for the first offense, $3,000 (or 10 percent of capitation) for the second offense, and $10,000 (or 15 percent of capitation) for the third offense. The provider/group/IPA or the individual provider may be terminated for additional offenses.

Because of potential sanctions, it is important that all reports, forms, or claim payments be properly completed in a timely manner and all rules be expressly followed.

Claim Payments

If an MCP is deemed to be responsible for payment of services, then the provider/group/IPA must either provide these services or pay for provision of these services. Often groups/IPAs will attempt to sign a wide variety of providers to their group/IPA so that they do not need to refer patients to outside providers. This often means that they will enter into a contractual agreement with a specific provider (e.g., a chiropractor) in their area to provide services for their patients at a specified rate. This specified rate may be on a fee-for-service basis or on a capitation basis.

Clean Claims

A *clean claim* is defined as one that can be paid as soon as it is received because it is complete in all aspects, including patient information, coverage information, coding, itemization, dates of services, billed amounts. There usually are time limits on how long a provider may take to pay a clean claim.

If a claim is submitted without a piece of information, omission of this information alone will not make it an unclean claim. For example, if preauthorization was required, simply leaving off an authorization number should not make the claim unclean. In addition, the need for medical review of a claim to determine appropriateness of services does not make it an unclean claim.

When a claim is unclean (it does not contain all the information necessary for processing), the group/IPA must send a written notice to the provider regarding the information needed to process the claim. Many providers have a standard form letter for this purpose.

If you do not receive a response within thirty days, send a denial notice stating that the services were denied. A copy of a denial notice is shown in Figure 7-14 ●.

Group/IPA Payment Responsibility

When a claim is received from a provider outside the group, or is paid on a fee-for-service basis, the following steps need to be taken:

1. Date-stamp the claim and any supporting documents. This helps to prove the timeliness of your claim payments. State and federal laws govern how soon a claim should be paid (usually within thirty days). In addition, the MCP may require that the claim be paid within a specified time or the provider may forfeit a portion of his capitation amount (see "Capitation Payments").

Date:

Member Name
Address
City, State Zip

File # _____

Dear:

We have received your request for the specific service or referral described below.

Service/Referral Requested: _____
_____

This Service/Referral request is being denied for the reason(s) shown below:
_____   Services are not a covered benefit with your plan.
_____   You have exhausted the benefit for this particular service.
_____   Service/Referral request denied because _____
_____
_____
_____

If you believe this determination is not correct, you have the right to request a reconsideration. You must file the request in writing within 60 days of the date of this notice. File the appeal with: Your HMO, Attn: Member Services, Address, City, State, Zip.

In addition to the complaint process described above, you may also contact the Department of Corporations (DOC). The DOC is responsible for regulating health care service plans in this state. The DOC has a toll-free number (1-800-XXX-XXXX) to receive complaints regarding health plans. If you have a grievance against the health plan, you should contact the plan and use the plan's grievance process. If you need the DOC's help with a complaint involving an emergency grievance or with a grievance that has not been satisfactorily resolved by the plan, you may call the DOC's toll-free number.

Please include your name and date of birth on all correspondence. If you have any questions about this notice, please call YOUR HMO at 1-800-XXX-XXXX.

Sincerely,

Name of Medical Group/IPA

cc: Member Services
     Quality Assessment
     Primary Care Provider

FIGURE 7-14

Sample denial notice

2. Notify the provider in writing if the claim is incomplete, improperly completed, or additional reports or documentation are needed. Attach a copy of this notification to the claim.
3. Complete eligibility verifications and any internal review (e.g., were treatments authorized or allowed, or did the member choose independently to see the provider?).
4. Prepare a proper remittance advice or denial notice for denied claims.
5. Determine the proper payment amount.
6. Prepare and mail a check. For timeliness guidelines, a claim is usually considered paid when the check is placed in the mail.

In addition, the provider/group/IPA is required to provide a check voucher or remittance advice to any fee-for-service provider showing the patient information, service rendered, date of service, amount billed, disposition of copayment (if any), amount group/IPA is paying, and a reason code for any denied services or amounts.

If the provider is paid on a capitated basis, the group/IPA must provide a count of members listed by plan, a payment amount for each plan, and copies of the member rosters. In essence, the same type of document that the group/IPA receives from the MCP when paid its monthly capitation amounts must be provided.

Determining the Proper Payment Amount

If no contract is in place between the provider and the provider/group/IPA before services are rendered, the provider/group/IPA has no legal basis for discounting payment to a provider. The provider/group/IPA must pay the full amount of the bill, minus any copayment amounts that should have been collected from the patient.

Legally, if a member has met all contractual obligations (e.g., seeking preauthorization or emergency authorization for treatment), he or she has no responsibility for payment for services other than the copayment amount stipulated in the contract. Therefore, the provider/group/IPA must pay a provider's billed amount, minus any copay. A statement should accompany payment to the provider stating that the copayment is the only amount that may be collected from the patient.

If there is a contracted amount for services, the terms in the contract should be adhered to. Usually, a fee schedule will accompany contracted terms. This fee schedule may be different for each provider with whom the provider/group/IPA contracts. The proper contract should be pulled and the correct allowed amount determined. The member's copayment amount should then be subtracted from this amount and the remainder paid to the provider. A notice should accompany the check voucher or remittance advice stating that this is the contracted amount for this service and no amounts other than the copayment may be collected from the member. It is the responsibility of the provider/group/IPA to ensure that neither the member nor the MCP incurs any financial responsibility for claims that are contractually deemed to be the responsibility of the provider/group/IPA.

For services rendered to seniors who are covered by Medicare HMOs, the fee schedule may indicate that fees are limited to the Medicare Fee Schedule. Under this arrangement, Medicare participating providers are limited to the allowed amount as determined by the most recent Medicare Fee Schedule. Nonparticipating providers would be paid the nonparticipating fee amount; the nonparticipating fee equals 95 percent of the participating fee amount. The maximum amount a nonparticipating provider or supplier will receive is the Medicare limiting charge, which is equal to 115 percent of the allowable charges, with the beneficiary paying for charges above the 95 percent. In either case, if the fee is limited by contractual agreement with the provider, a copy of the contract and the accompanying fee schedule should be attached to the claim when it is filed.

Claim Files

Claims are usually filed in a separate claim file, along with all documentation submitted by the provider, and a copy of the explanation of benefits (fee-for-service providers) or member rosters and capitation amounts (capitated providers). In addition, a copy of the claim or some documentation showing the services rendered should be placed in the patient chart. If any of the documentation supporting the claim payment is pertinent to further treatment of the patient, this information should also be copied and filed in the patient chart. At no time should any information regarding capitation payments be placed in the patient chart. This information is part of the contract between the provider and the group/IPA and should be considered privileged information.

Denial of a Claim or Service

If a claim or service is denied, a denial letter must be included with a remittance advice indicating the reason for the denial. The denial notice also must include a statement that the provider has the right to appeal the denial within sixty days as well as the address of where to file an appeal.

If the claim is for emergency services, the member or provider is requested to notify the MCP within forty-eight hours of the initiation of care. However, some MCPs may limit the ability of a provider/group/IPA to deny claims based on the lack of notification within this forty-eight-hour period.

If it is believed that these services were not medically necessary, or were not true emergency services, then the claim must be sent through a medical review process. The medical reviewer should use the presenting diagnosis rather than the discharge diagnosis as the basis for decision making, and must consider the member's understanding of the medical circumstances that led to the emergency service.

If this medical review determines that the services were not medically necessary or were not true emergency services, then a specific denial letter is required for these claims. This denial letter must meet federal requirements. The MCP often will provide a copy of an appropriate denial letter in its policies and procedures manual. In such a case, this letter should be used verbatim and the wording left unaltered.

All denial notices must contain an explicit reason, in layperson's terms, of why the service(s) are being denied. If the MCP provides a list of denial reasons, then the appropriate denial reason should be written on the denial letter. No code may be used unless the meaning of that code is indicated in the denial letter. In addition, all denial letters must meet the following criteria:

1. The decision to deny must be correct and based on approved medical practices.
2. The denial reason must be clear to the member and must use CMS-approved denial reasons.
3. The denial letter must include mandated appeals language and the correct health plan address.
4. The denial letter must be sent to the appropriate parties (the provider, the member, or both).
5. The denial notice must be issued within required time frames.

There are additional guidelines that mandate which items must be included and what size the type used must be. The MCP should furnish all providers with copies of appropriate denial letters, and these should be used by the provider.

If the member is not covered by the provider/group/IPA, then certain steps must be taken before the claim can be denied. First, call the MCP to determine if the member was covered at the time services were rendered, and who the assigned provider was at that time. If the member was not covered at all, then the claim may be denied for that reason. If the member was not eligible under the provider/group/IPA, but was a covered member under the MCP, then the claim must be forwarded to the MCP.

In addition, any claims that have been denied by the provider/group/IPA must be sent to the MCP with a copy of any contact or denial letters that were sent to the member or provider. Many MCPs also require the use of a denied claim log that includes the following information:

- Current month and year
- Group name
- Contact person
- Phone number
- Member name
- File/member number
- Provider name
- Whether the provider was contracted or noncontracted
- Date of service
- Reason for the denial
- Date the claim was received
- Date the notice was sent to the member
- Date the notice was sent to the provider

A copy of this log should be forwarded to the MCP on a regular basis. If there are no denials for the month, a copy of the log should still be forwarded to the MCP with the words No Denials on the first line of the log.

Appeals

Any member or provider has the right to appeal a denied claim. All denial letters, by law, must include a statement saying that the receiver has the right to appeal the decision and whom to contact to begin the appeal process.

If a member or provider appeals a denied claim, the MCP will review the claim and make a determination of whether to uphold or reverse the denial. If the MCP determines that the services should have been covered, it will inform the provider/group/IPA of its decision and will instruct the provider/group/IPA to pay the claim.

The payment should be generated immediately, and a copy of the proof of payment should be sent to the MCP. If the MCP does not receive proof of payment in a timely fashion, it has the right to pay the claim and deduct the payment from the provider/group/IPA's capitation amount. The MCP may have a fund set up under the provider's name in which it has withheld a portion of the provider/group/IPA's monthly capitation amount (e.g., 3 percent). If so, the claim will be paid from this fund.

If the MCP processes the claim and makes payment to the provider, it not only goes against the provider's record but also the MCP has the right to charge an administrative fee for processing the claim. This fee usually ranges from $100 to $250.

Medical billers should be aware of the appeals process and should routinely appeal all claims in which services performed by their provider were denied. If possible, additional information substantiating the need for the services or the urgent nature of the services should be included with the appeal.

MCP Responsibilities

If the provider/group/IPA determines that the MCP is responsible for payment of a claim, it must forward the claim to the MCP. The following steps should be completed:

1. Determine which services, if any, are the responsibility of the provider/group/IPA, and process these claims according to the guidelines given in this chapter.
2. Indicate on the remittance advice or write a letter stating which services are the responsibility of the MCP, and indicate that the claim is being forwarded to the MCP for payment.
3. There is usually a transmittal form that must be sent with any claims. A copy of this form is shown in Figure 7-15 ●.

Reinsurance/Stop-loss

Stop-loss is an attempt to limit payments by an insured person, or a provider/group/IPA in the case of a catastrophic illness or injury to a member. Many MCP contracts have a stop-loss or reinsurance clause included in them. This clause may state that the provider/group/IPA will be financially responsible for the first set amount (e.g., $7,000) in expenses for each member in a contract year. After those expenses have been paid, the MCP will reimburse the provider/group/IPA for verified expenses that exceed the set amount.

If the provider's contract has a stop-loss clause, it is important that the medical biller be aware of the set amount. The biller will need to file a claim with the MCP for any services that exceed that set amount. The biller also should be familiar with that portion of the provider's contract with the MCP, as there are often limits put on the billing. For example, the MCP may require that claims be submitted within a specified time period, or that preauthorization be obtained before the services are rendered. Some contracts also may stipulate that the year runs from July 1 to June 30. If the biller is unfamiliar with the terms required to achieve stop-loss reimbursement, the provider could stand to lose a substantial sum of money.

Often the MCPs will require that a claim for reimbursement be submitted on specific forms. An example of this form is shown in Figure 7-16 ●.

Incorrect Denials

If a provider/group/IPA arranges, refers, or renders services or equipment not covered under a plan, the provider/group/IPA must inform the member ahead of time that the services or equipment are

FIGURE 7-15

Claims Transmittal Form

Provider Network Services

CLAIMS TRANSMITTAL FORM

Date: _____

To: Claims Services

From: _____, Administrator for _____

The attached claims are the responsibility of [the HMO].

Authorization Number _____

____ Inpatient hospital (IP) charges

____ Outpatient surgery (OPS) facility charges

____ Anesthesia for approved IP or OPS

____ Radiology for approved IP, OPS, or SNF

____ Pathology for approved IP, OPS, or SNF

____ Emergency services that resulted in admission to inpatient status

____ Ambulance

____ Durable medical equipment

____ Dialysis facility charges

____ Radiation therapy

____ Member not on roster for date of service. Include relevant roster page(s).

NOTE: Use a separate form for each type of plan expense. Multiple providers may be grouped if the authorization number is the same.

  [The HMO] will not send denial notices for services that are the responsibility of the Group/IPA.

  Refer to the Medical Services Agreement for questions of coverage and financial responsibility.

Excess Risk Limit Cost Summary

I. Group Name: _____   Enrollee Name: _____   II.

    Address: _____   Enrollee PF #: _____

    _____   Date of Elegibility: _____

    Contact Person: _____   Contract Year: _____

    Phone Number: _____   For HIV/AIDS cases, list qualifying hospital stays:

    Date Submitted: _____

		Type of submission	
__ Original		__ Medicare	
__ Supplemental		__ Commercial	
__ Resubmittal		__ OO Care	
__ AIDS/HIV		__ CCC	

III.

Provider of Service / Provider #	Date of Service	CPT4, RVS, or SMA code	Units	Billed Amount	Amount Paid	For HMO use only
					TOTAL THIS PAGE:	

FIGURE 7-16

Excess Risk (Stop-Loss) Form

not covered by the plan and that the member is liable for coverage. The provider/group/IPA should have a form for the member to sign stating the understanding that such services are not a covered expense. If the member is not informed of the noncoverage and financial liability in advance, the member cannot be held liable for the cost of the services or equipment.

If the MCP has a Medicare HMO plan, it must agree to cover at least the minimum of services that are covered under Medicare. Therefore, it is important that providers and their billers understand what items are covered under Medicare so that these items are not denied.

Many MCPs have a limit on the number of visits or units that a member may utilize during a year (e.g., twenty chiropractic visits). When the member has exhausted the benefits under such an arrangement, it is important to notify the member of having reached the limit and that any additional treatments will not be covered by the plan. Failure to do so could cause the provider/group/IPA to be liable for the services.

It is important that billers note in a patient's file if he or she is recovered under an MCP plan. If a member receives services that should have been preauthorized, and the provider is a contracted member with a plan, the provider forfeits the fee for those services.

PRACTICE **PITFALLS**

Example: Sarah James is seen by Dr. Dorman. She indicates that she is covered by Medicare when she is actually covered by a Medicare HMO. Dr. Mark Dorman is contracted with the Medicare HMO to which Ms. James belongs. Thinking that Ms. James is covered by Medicare, he renders services that need preauthorization by the HMO. Because the provider did not inform Ms. James in advance that the services were not preauthorized or were not covered by the HMO, the services will be denied. Because he is a contracted provider with the HMO, Dr. Dorman is not allowed to bill the patient for these services. Therefore, the provider forfeits his fee.

To prevent this from happening, it is important to verify insurance coverage before the first visit, and also to ask each patient on subsequent visits about any changes in insurance coverage since the previous visit.

CHAPTER REVIEW

Summary

- Managed care contracts were created in an attempt to bring health care costs under control by having providers share some of the financial risks of health care with the patient and the insurance carrier.
- There are numerous types of managed care organizations, including HMOs, PPOs, gatekeeper PPOs, EPOs, PHOs, and MSOs.
- HMOs are one of the most common managed care trends. HMOs pay providers a set capitation amount each month for the patients on their eligibility roster, and in return the provider is expected to cover many of the services that member needs. A written contract will dictate those services that the provider will cover and those that the HMO will cover.
- The provider must complete numerous forms to keep the MCP informed of services rendered and the daily operations of the practice.

Review Questions

Directions: Answer the following questions without looking back into the material just covered. Write your answers in the space provided.

1. What is a PPO? _____

_____

_____

2. What should a biller do if a patient requests treatment but is not included on the provider's eligibility roster?

_____

_____

_____

3. What is a TAR, and what is its purpose? _____

_____

_____

4. What is a gatekeeper PPO? _____

_____

_____

5. What are ten reasons for the rising cost of health care in America?

_____

_____

_____

_____

6. Which of the following models represent the original concept of HMO services?

   • Staff model

   • Group model

   • Network model

7. Why is it critical for the provider to check the member's identification card prior to providing treatment?

_____

_____

8. What four reasons would indicate that a second opinion may be necessary?

_____

_____

_____

_____

9. What is a clean claim?

_____

_____

10. What criteria must be met in a denial letter?

_____

_____

_____

_____

   If you are unable to answer any of these questions, refer back to that section in the chapter, and then fill in the answers.

Activity #4: Locating the Key Terms

Directions: Complete the crossword puzzle by filling in a word from the key words that fits each clue.

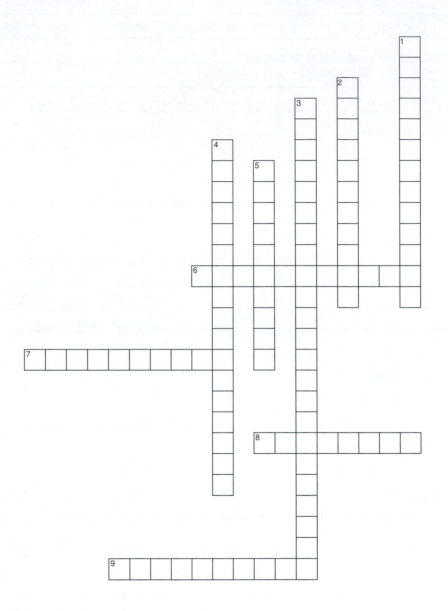

Across

6. An attempt by insurers to control health care costs using a number of different methods

7. A monthly payment made to a provider in exchange for providing the health care needs of a member

8. An attempt to limit payments by an insured person or a group/IPA in the case of a catastrophic illness or injury to a member

9. Verbal expressions of dissatisfaction with a provider or services

Down

1. When a patient transfers care from a provider

2. An insurance policy that protects the company against catastrophic medical costs levied against its plan, either by a single employee or by all employees as a whole

3. Providers who do not agree to provide services at a reduced amount in exchange for the referrals from an insurance carrier within a PPO

4. A process whereby insurance carriers review the treatment of a patient and determine whether or not the costs will be covered

5. Written complaints made by a member regarding dissatisfaction with a provider or services

Activity #5: Matching Key Terms

Directions: Match the following terms with the proper definition by writing the letter of the correct definition in the space next to the term.

1. _____ Independent Practice Associations

2. _____ Health Maintenance Organizations

3. _____ Exclusive Provider Organization

4. _____ Social Health Maintenance Organization

5. _____ Terminated member roster

6. _____ Management Service Organization

7. _____ Primary care provider

8. _____ Provider Hospital Organization

9. _____ Preferred Provider Organization

a. An organization that provides the full range of Medicare benefits offered by standard HMOs plus additional services

b. A plan where the insurance carrier contracts with providers to join their "network." These providers agree to provide services at a reduced amount in exchange for the referrals from the carrier, and the carrier agrees to reimburse network providers at a higher percentage than providers outside the network.

c. The provider a patient has chosen for primary medical care

d. A separate corporation set up to provide management services to a medical group for a fee

e. A plan in which the patient must select a PCP and can use only providers who are part of the network or who are referred by the PCP

f. An organization of providers and hospitals that band together for the purpose of obtaining contracts from payer organizations

g. Lists those members whose coverage has been terminated or who have chosen to terminate this provider as their PCP

h. A group of medical organizations and providers who have banded together to form their own HMO

i. Organizations or companies that provide both the coverage for care and the care itself. Members pay a set amount every month, and the HMO agrees to provide all their care, or to pay for the covered care they cannot provide.

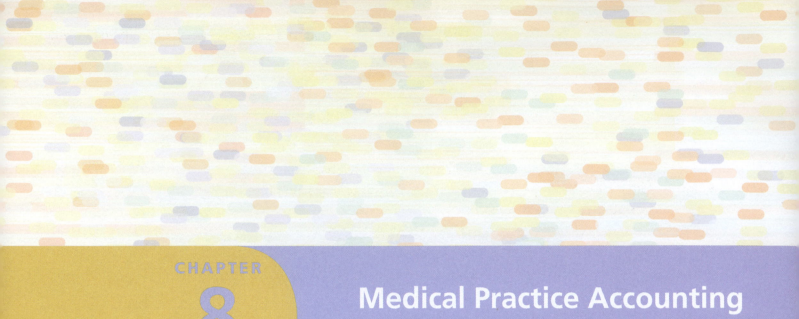

Medical Practice Accounting

Key Words and Concepts you will learn in this chapter:

Accounting control summary

Accounts payable

Accounts receivable

Adjustments

Balance billing

Bankruptcy

Cumulative trial balance

Daily journal

Day sheet

Defendant

Deposit slip

Deposit ticket

Dunning notice

Explanation of Benefits (EOB)

Insurance tracer

Patient aging report

Patient ledger card

Patient receipt

Patient statement

Pended

Petty cash fund

After completion of this chapter you should be able to:

- Explain and use the ledger card and patient statements.

- Describe an electronic practice management system.

- Properly post payments to the patient account.

- Properly create a payment plan.

- Properly handle a collections call.

- Explain and use the daily journal.

- Properly balance petty cash using a petty cash count slip and petty cash receipts.

- List the main reports a medical office may use and their purposes.

Petty cash receipt   Skip

Petty cash count slip   Statement of account

Post   Statute of limitations

Billing is not the only function of the medical biller. Once a bill has been sent
out, it is the biller's responsibility to collect on that bill and to make sure that
the patient's account is properly credited.

   Often the biller begins by submitting a claim to the patient's insurance carrier.
When payment is received from the carrier it is credited against the patient's
account. The patient, or a secondary insurance carrier if there is one, is then
billed for any remaining amount left unpaid on the claim.

   If payment is not received from the insurance carrier in a timely manner, an
insurance tracer is sent on the claim. If payment is not received from the
patient in a timely manner, the medical biller is responsible for handling collections on the account. If necessary, the account may be sent to small claims court
in an effort to collect.

▶ **CRITICAL THINKING QUESTION:** Why is it so important to a provider to receive payments from
insurance carriers in a timely manner?

Accounts Payable/Receivable

The main function and purpose of any bookkeeping system is to provide a way to keep an accurate account of money received and money paid out. Most accounting systems are set up on a
principle of accounts receivable and accounts payable. In simple terms, money owed to the
practice is considered **accounts receivable**, and money the practice owes to others is referred to
as **accounts payable**. In any business, the objective is to have more money coming in than
going out.

   Because the medical office provides a service and also functions as a business, one of the
responsibilities of the medical biller includes the continued updating of financial records. The
biller often is responsible for collecting payments for services from patients. This amounts to
most, if not all, of the accounts receivable a medical practice may have. Therefore, it is important
for the medical biller to ensure all accounts are paid in a timely manner.

   Because of this, billers must keep highly accurate records of patients and the services they
receive, bill for those services promptly, record payments, conduct balance billing in a timely
manner, and institute collections procedures when necessary.

   Often, the practice will have a second person (if not the provider) who is responsible for
handling all accounts payable. However, it is important that the medical biller be aware of any
major purchases that the practice may make and also have a general idea how much the office
expenses are each month. For example, the medical biller who is aware that the practice has
approximately $10,000 in expenses each month will know what needs to be collected to cover
those expenses.

   Several bookkeeping systems may be used in the medical office to keep track of incoming
and outgoing finances manually or electronically. Most computerized billing systems include a
patient accounting function. Thus, they are used not only to generate the claim but also to record
all patient charges and payments. Most medical offices are now using a computerized system,
although some offices still have not made the switch from manual to computerized.

   If a computerized system is used, the accounting system is automatically set up when a
patient's information is entered into a record. When a claim is created, it is automatically posted
to the patient's account. To **post** means to list items such as payments or charges in a log. When
payments are received the information is recorded (posted) on a payment screen, and the amount
paid is automatically deducted from the amount the patient owes.

FIGURE 8-1

Pegboard accounting system
© Michal Heron/Pearson Education

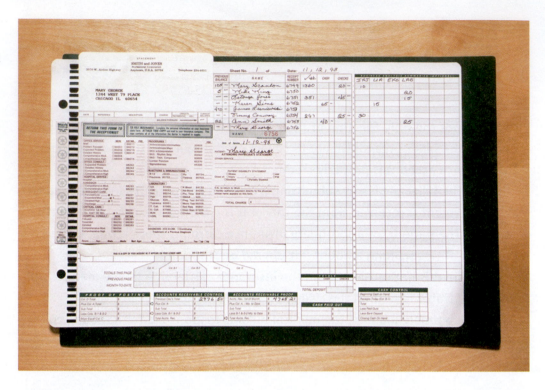

The pegboard system is one of the most frequently used manual systems because it is the simplest to use (Figure 8-1 •). Ledger cards, charge slips, and daily journal sheets all are used in the pegboard system. This system uses no-carbon-required (NCR) material on its forms to allow information written on one form to be recorded on all the rest.

▶ **CRITICAL THINKING QUESTION:** Why might an office choose to not use a computerized book-keeping system? What might the advantages and disadvantages be to the use of a computerized system versus a manual system or vice versa?

Patient Ledger Card/Statement of Account

The patient's account information is often kept on a patient ledger card, also known as a **statement of account** (Figure 8-2 •). The **patient ledger card** is used to indicate a chronological record of all services rendered to a patient and to record all payments and adjustments made on the patient's account.

Each service, payment, or adjustment should have its own line or column on a ledger card. Any services provided are added to the remaining balance (if there is one), and any payments received are subtracted from the remaining balance. **Adjustments** are changes that can either increase or decrease the remaining balance on an account.

Items should be entered in chronological order. Thus, the charges for services performed would be entered before any payments for those services. The remaining balance shown on the last line of the ledger card is the amount that is still owed on the patient's account.

To post items to a ledger card, complete the items as listed below.

- *Responsible Party.* Enter the name of the person ultimately responsible for payment of this bill. This is often the patient, or the parent or guardian of a minor patient.
- *Address.* Enter the address of the person ultimately responsible for payment of this bill.
- *Telephone #.* Enter the telephone number of the person ultimately responsible for payment of this bill.
- *Patient Name.* Enter the name of the patient. Each patient should have a separate ledger card. Never place more than one patient's account information on a card.
- *Account Number.* Enter the patient's account number.
- *Special Notes.* This is where any special circumstances regarding this patient and the account may be good to note.

Paul Provider, M.D.
5858 Peppermint Place
Anytown, USA 12345
(765) 555-6768

Ledger Card/Statement of Account

RESPONSIBLE PARTY: _____

ADDRESS: _____

TELEPHONE #: _____

PATIENT NAME: _____PATIENT ACCOUNT #: _____

SPECIAL NOTES: _____

Date	Description of Service	Charge	Payments	Adjustments	Remaining Balance

FIGURE 8-2

Patient ledger card/statement of account

- *Date.* Enter the date of the transaction. This is the date services were rendered in the case of most charges, or the date a payment was received for services.
- *Description of Service.* Enter a description of the reason this account is being changed. If recording charges, indicate the services that were performed. If recording a payment, indicate that it is a payment and who is making the payment (e.g., Green Insurance Carrier Payment, check #1234). If recording an adjustment, indicate the reason for the adjustment (e.g., adjustment to Medicare-allowed amount).
- *Charge.* Indicate the charge for any services that were performed. If recording a payment, leave this space blank.
- *Payments.* Enter the amount of the payment. If there is no payment, leave this space blank.
- *Adjustments.* Enter the amount of the adjustment. If there is no adjustment, leave this space blank.
- *Remaining Balance.* Add the amount of any charges to the previous amount in this field. Subtract the amount of any payments from the previous amount in this column. Adjustments can be either increases or decreases to the patient's account.

It is important to always keep the patient's ledger card updated. Any changes to the patient's account should be promptly noted. This can prevent numerous problems with the patient's account, including interest charges or late charges being assessed.

Insurance Payments

The insurance carrier is often the first entity to make a payment on a claim. Once the insurance carrier has processed the claim, it will send an Explanation of Benefits with the check (if applicable) to the party designated as the payee. If benefits are assigned, this would be the provider. If benefits are not assigned, this would be the patient. If the patient is designated as the payee, the provider will not receive any contact from the insurance carrier. It is the biller's responsibility to collect the full amount due for services from the patient.

Understanding an Explanation of Benefits

When benefits are assigned to the provider, the insurance carrier creates an **Explanation of Benefits (EOB)** for the claim and sends copies of the EOB to the provider and the patient . The payment is sent directly to the provider. This EOB lists the patient, the date of the service, and the service performed. It also lists the amount that was allowed for the procedure, the percentage covered by insurance, and the amount that the insurance carrier will pay.

If benefits are not assigned to the provider, the EOB is sent to the patient, along with the payment amount. The full amount should be collected from the patient, regardless of what was paid by the insurance carrier (unless Medicare or Medicaid is involved).

It is important to check the EOB carefully against the patient's account. Be sure the codes that were paid were the ones that were billed. Errors can often occur in the inputting of codes, thus causing improper calculation of the benefits.

There are many different EOB styles and formats. EOBs may list one patient or several on the same page. If several are listed together, be sure that payment credits are given to the proper patients. Some providers choose to list each procedure separately on their records and to record the amount received for each service. Others combine all the services provided on the same date and apply the payment to that total.

If the EOB combines payments for several dates of service, be sure to separate the payment amounts according to the proper dates. Some EOBs do not contain information that is detailed enough to do this. In such a case, add together the amounts billed on the claim and apply the total amount against this.

See the sample EOB in Figure 8-3 ●. On this EOB, Abby Addison received a hospital consultation, two hospital visits, and a hospital discharge. All charges were allowed (though not at the billed amount) and were paid at 90 percent. However, the patient had not yet met $100 of her deductible, so this amount was taken from the $126 that otherwise would have been paid by the carrier on the first line item.

On this claim, the billed amount was $450. Because the insurance only paid $193.50, the patient (or any additional insurance if the patient is covered by more than one policy) should be balance billed for the remaining $256.50.

Rover Insurers, Inc.
5931 Rolling Road
Ronson, CO 81369

December 15, CCYY
Claim For: Abby Addison
Claim Number: 478-78-4
Group Policy Number: 41935
Member's ID Number: 001-00-RED

Dear Ms. Addison:

We received a claim for you. The following details the benefits that were paid on this claim. Please save this form for your tax records. If you have any questions, please contact the customer service office.

DATE OF SERVICE	PROCEDURE	BILLED AMOUNT	ALLOWED AMOUNT	% OF PAYMENT	PAYMENT AMOUNT	DENIED AMOUNT	REASON CODE
11/06/CCYY	HOSP CONSULT	$200.00	$140.00	90%	$ 36.00**	$ 60.00	55
11/07-08/CCYY	HOSP VISIT	$150.00	$100.00	90%	$ 90.00	$ 50.00	55
11/09/CCYY	HOSP D/C	$100.00	$ 75.00	90%	$ 67.50	$ 25.00	55
TOTAL		$450.00	$315.00		$193.50	$135.00	

55 Denied amount exceeds the amount covered under your plan.
** $100 applied to deductible.

FIGURE 8-3
Sample Explanation of Benefits

ACTIVITY #1

Understanding the Explanation of Benefits Form

Directions: Using the Explanation of Benefits in Figure 8-3, please answer the following questions.

1. What is the name of the patient? _____
2. What is the total amount billed on the claim? _____
3. What is the total amount allowed on the claim? _____
4. What is the total claim payment? _____
5. What is the total amount denied? _____
6. What is the reason for the denied amount? _____
7. How much was applied to the deductible? _____
8. What is the EOB date? _____
9. What is the name of the insurance company? _____
10. What was the percentage at which the allowed amount was covered? _____

Patient Payments

When visiting the provider, the patient may wish to make a payment for the amount owed on account or the estimated amount owing after insurance benefits are paid. A receipt should be given to the patient at the time the patient makes a payment. A **patient receipt** (Figure 8-4 ●) is a written acknowledgment that a specific sum of money has been received. A patient walk-out receipt outlines the total activity pertaining to the patient's visit that day. This type of receipt is usually generated from a computerized medical billing system (Figure 8-5 ●).

PAUL PROVIDER, M.D. 5858 Peppermint Place Anytown, USA 12345	RECEIPT			Date _____ CC _____ No.

RECEIPT   Date _____ CC _____ No. ____

Received From _____

Address _____

_____ Dollars $ _____

For _____

ACCOUNT			HOW PAID			
AMT OF ACCOUNT			CASH			
AMT PAID			CHECK			By _____
BALANCE DUE			MONEY ORDER			

FIGURE 8-4

Patient receipt

Posting Payments

When payment on a claim is received, it is important to post the payment to the patient's account. This can be done via a computerized or manual system.

Be sure to record all the pertinent information regarding a payment. This should include not only the name of the person or entity making the payment but also the type of payment (e.g., cash, check, money order) and the number of the check or money order.

Post each of the appropriate amounts from the EOB onto the patient's account. In the case of a Medicare Summary Notice (MSN) or Medicaid Remittance Advice, be sure to write off any amounts that were not allowed. Next, determine the amount that is still owed on the claim.

Balance Billing

If any remaining amounts are owed, one will need to balance bill. **Balance billing** consists of sending an additional bill to another party for payment of any remaining amounts on a claim. If the patient has more than one insurance carrier, a second copy of the claim should be sent to the secondary carrier to coordinate benefits between the two carriers. Be sure to attach a copy of the primary carrier's EOB so that the secondary payer may see how much was paid by the primary payer. Do not alter any of the information on the form. An exact copy of the form should be sent to the secondary insurance carrier. CMS-1500 forms can be ordered to print on carbon copy for this purpose. However, with electronic submission of the CMS-1500, there will be less of a need for printing the form.

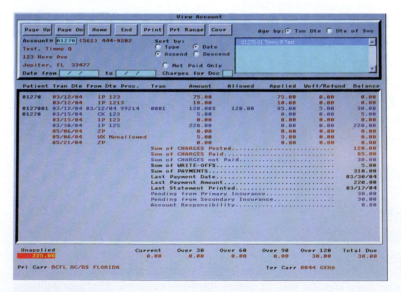

FIGURE 8-5

Example of a computer billing software program

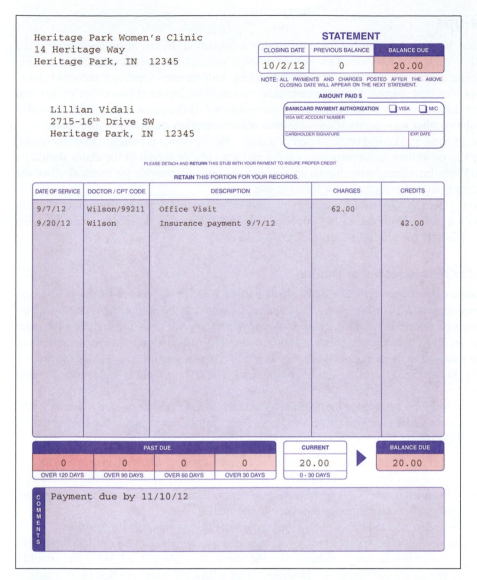

FIGURE 8-6

Sample computerized patient billing statement

If there is no secondary insurance carrier, the patient should be balance billed for any remaining amounts. Patients are usually billed using a patient statement. Most insurance carriers will send a copy of the EOB to the patient at the same time one is sent to the provider. However, some providers prefer to include a copy of the EOB to allow the patient to view how the payment was credited to the account.

Patient Statements

A **patient statement** is an individual summary (organized either by patient or by family) that lists all the services, charges, payments, adjustments, and balances due that occurred during the month. This statement is sent to the patient or family every month. It acts as both a statement of the account and as a bill.

Often patient statements contain a **dunning notice**, which is a statement, or sentence included on the statement, reminding the recipient to make a payment on the account (Figure 8-6 ●). Certain days are more appropriate for sending out patient statements. These dates are usually between the 8th and the 12th of the month and between the 20th and the 27th of the month. Sending out patient statements on these dates receives a higher response because many people receive their paychecks on the 15th and the 30th or 31st of the month.

Follow-ups

A claim may be denied or **pended** (held for further information) by the insurance carrier if the form contains omissions or errors. The most common reasons claims are denied include missing or incomplete diagnoses, diagnoses not corresponding with services rendered, incorrect dates, charges not itemized, incorrect patient insurance information, incorrect procedure codes, and insufficient documentation to substantiate services rendered. If the claim was denied or pended for these or any other reasons, complete or correct the information and resubmit the claim.

If the payment was denied on all or part of a claim and the denial is believed to be incorrect, a letter should be written to the insurance carrier and a review or appeal of the claim should be requested. Every insurance carrier has an appeals process and will provide the medical office the required directions and information or forms to use.

A good system should be established in the medical office that provides a reminder when to follow up on a claim. If the carrier has not been heard from in six weeks after a claim has been filed, it is definitely time to follow up.

When a Claim Is Rejected or Denied

An insurance carrier may reject or deny all or part of a claim. Be aware of the distinction between *rejection* of a claim and *denial* of a claim. A claim may be accepted as filed by Medicare but may be rejected or denied. Denials are subject to appeal, since a denial is a payment determination. Rejections may be corrected and resubmitted. Submissions that are incomplete or invalid are returned to the provider (RTP) with a notation explaining the error. Once the error is resolved by the provider, the claim can be resubmitted. The claim should be resubmitted within sixty days.

Before billing the patient for the remaining balance, it is important to determine why the claim was rejected. Many claims are rejected because of minor errors that can be fixed easily, such as the following:

1. The patient is not listed as covered under the mentioned policy. Many insurance carriers (and their computer systems) track patients according to policy numbers, group numbers, or Social Security numbers. If any of these numbers is incorrect, the claim may be rejected because the patient and the policy numbers do not match.
2. Office visits are rejected because they fall within the follow-up days for a surgical procedure. If the office visit was for a reason (diagnosis) other than as a follow-up to the surgery, be sure this is clearly indicated on the claim. Box 24e of the CMS-1500 should reference the additional diagnosis. Modifiers used with CPT codes are helpful to explain further the purpose of the office visit. For instance, modifier-24 can be used to indicate unrelated evaluation and management (E/M) services by the provider during a postoperative period. The use of modifier-25 shows the payer that a significant E/M service and a procedure were performed on the same day. Some providers (including Medicare) may require additional documentation proving that the visit was unrelated to the surgical procedure.
3. The claim (or some service) is denied as not being medically necessary. If procedures seem unrelated to the listed diagnoses, those procedures may be denied. Be sure that each procedure has an appropriate diagnosis listed for it. If additional room is needed for more diagnoses, procedures can be listed on two separate CMS-1500s, according to their related diagnoses.
4. Item 12, release of information, was not completed. After ensuring that the signature is on file, type "Signature on File" in the box. Some insurance carriers require that the patient's name or the name of the person who signed the release appear in this field, and will reject claims noting only "Signature on File."
5. The patient was not covered at the time the treatment was begun. If special conditions exist that negate the preexisting condition provisions, be sure to attach this information. These special conditions can be the meeting of certain requirements, such as the patient being treatment free for a specified period of time, or the patient's medical insurance was transferred when the patient moved from one job to another.
6. The claim is rejected because the facility or provider is incorrect for the type of procedure being performed. For example, if ear surgery is being performed by an obstetrician, it

FIGURE 8-7

Sample appeal letter dealing with denial because of medical necessity

---

Allied Medical Center
1933 E. Frankford Rd #110
Carrollton, TX 12345

Dear Mr. Hess,

We have received the explanation of benefits for a patient, Mr. Robert Crawford. However, we believe the charges totaling $480.00 for February 25, 2011, through March 14, 2011, have been considered incorrectly.

The EOB states that the March 15th charge of $80.00 is not a medical necessity. When I spoke to you at the claims center earlier this week, your explanation of the denial was because the patient is not homebound and the insurance company believes the visit was for patient convenience and not medically necessary.

In reviewing the nurse's notes for each skilled nursing visit, medical necessity appears to have been established. The March 15th visit should not have been denied. A new infusion therapy was started on that date and the patient required instruction on drug administration.

Skilled nursing visits are a medical necessity to follow up on how well the patient is learning and, indeed, errors in the patient's technique were discovered. Throughout the therapy the patient was fatigued, weak, and felt sick. The patient also felt overwhelmed with the therapies, requiring further instruction and reinforcement. The results of not having skilled nursing visits could lead to further complications, such as not following the drug schedule or performing inaccurate drug administration.

It appears that a review of the nurse's notes would support the medical necessity of the nursing charges. Please reconsider the denied portion of the charges and issue a payment to Value Home Care in the amount of $80.00

Sincerely,

Bill Ingram
Collections Manager, Value Home Care

---

would be rejected. Be sure that the procedure codes listed are correct for those procedures that were performed.

7. The claim is rejected because the patient's gender or age is incorrect for the type of procedure being performed. For example, a male is not treated for gynecological procedures. If the gender is listed incorrectly on the patient's form, the claim could be resubmitted.

Carriers are required to provide the reason why the claim or procedure was rejected or denied. If the wording of why the claim was rejected or denied is not understood, contact the person (or department) listed on the EOB to inquire.

If the error is a minor one, fix the error and resubmit the claim. If more documentation is needed (e.g., an operative report) to justify services performed, include the additional information and resubmit the claim.

If everything on the claim is correct and there is a disagreement with the claims examiner's judgment on the claim, contact the claims examiner and discuss the situation. If no agreement can be reached on the claim, ask what the appeals process is for such a situation. All companies have an appeals or claim review process (Figure 8-7 ●).

Insurance Tracer

If a payment has not been received from an insurance carrier within six weeks of sending in the claim, you should submit an insurance tracer. An **insurance tracer** is a form or letter sent

Paul Provider, M.D.
5858 Peppermint Place
Anytown, USA 12345
(765) 555-6768

INSURANCE TRACER

Date: _____

Dear Insurance Carrier:

We sent a claim to you over six weeks ago and have not heard back from you.
Patient:
Insured:
Address:
SSN/Birth Date:
Group Number:
Claim Amount:
Date Billed:
Date of Services:
Date of Illness or Injury:
Diagnosis:
Employer:
Address:

Please supply the following information on the above named claim within ten days. Payment on this claim is overdue and we would like to avoid involving the patient and the state insurance commissioner in a reimbursement complaint.

Claim pending because:_____

Payment in progress. Check will be mailed on:_____

Payment previously made. Date: _____

To whom:_____

Check #: _____ Payment Amount: _____

Claim denied. Reason: _____

Patient notified: Yes   No

Remarks: _____

Thank you for your assistance.

Completed by: _____

FIGURE 8-8

Insurance tracer

to the insurance carrier to inquire about the status of a previously submitted claim. Be sure to include the patient's name, Social Security number or insurance number, policy name and number, and the patient's address. Also include the date of services, the diagnosis, and information regarding the patient's employer.

Many medical offices have a form letter for this purpose (Figure 8-8 ●). Payments from insurance carriers should normally be received within four to six weeks. When the payment is received, the amount of payment should be compared with the actual claim originally sent. The payment should then be posted to the patient's account.

ACTIVITY #2

Completing an Insurance Tracer

Directions: Using the following information, complete an insurance tracer form for each patient. The tracer forms can be found in Appendix A. The information required for the tracer forms are provided below in addition to the information provided either in the patient chart or in the Patient Data Table and Provider Data Table in Appendix A.

	Patient	Date Billed	Date of Service	Date of Illness	Diagnosis	Amount Billed
1.	Abby Addison	02/01/CCYY	01/16/CCYY	01/16/CCYY	401.9	$210.00
2.	Bobby Brumble	02/01/CCYY	01/16/CCYY	05/04/CCYY	250.0X	$103.00
3.	Cathy Crenshaw	02/01/CCYY	01/16/CCYY	01/16/CCYY	491.9	$160.00
4.	Daisy Doolittle	02/08/CCYY	01/16/CCYY	01/16/CCYY	243	$120.00
5.	Edward Edmunds	02/08/CCYY	01/16/CCYY	05/07/CCYY	414.00	$165.00

Collections

The patient is always financially responsible for payment of services rendered, regardless of whether he or she is covered by insurance (Figure 8-9 ●). The following are two exceptions: (1) if the patient is a minor, in which case the financial responsibility lies with the parent(s) or legal guardian or (2) if the patient was injured on the job and the services rendered are related to this injury, in which case the company's workers' compensation carrier would be responsible for payment.

After the claim is paid by the insurance carrier and posted to the patient's account, any remaining balance is billed to the patient. This is typically done by mailing out a copy of the patient's ledger card and/or EOB to the patient with a letter explaining how much the patient owes the practice. If no payment has been received within thirty days, a follow-up reminder should be sent to the patient or individual (such as a parent) who is the individual responsible for payment of the bill.

If payment is not received within fifteen days of the second notice, send a courtesy collection notice reminding the patient that payment is now seriously delinquent, followed by a courtesy call ten days later. Keep accurate records of when each contact was made and the outcome of that contact. Also record the date follow-up should be performed if a payment is not received. The longer an account ages, the less likely you will be able to recover the money due.

Providers often are wary of becoming "bill collectors" because the image is not consistent with that of a healer. However, if revenues are not collected in a timely manner, it can be difficult for the provider to meet the cost of the practice's overhead and other obligations. Therefore, a balance must be achieved that allows for the collection of revenues without tarnishing the provider's image. The best way to achieve this is to set reasonable credit limits and to stress to patients that they are responsible for payment of the bill. Create a credit agreement, and then ask each patient to sign and date it. Also make sure that patients understand that by signing the credit agreement, they are agreeing to abide by its terms.

Office staff should be wary of making their credit policy too stringent. You do not want to lose patients because they cannot afford your terms. If you need to put a little pressure on clients without alienating them, try using a third party (e.g. your accountant).

When collections are being sought by telephone, there are laws to be followed under the Fair Debt Collection Practices Act. Harassing, frightening, or abusive calls are a violation of this act, as are calling during odd hours or calling the patient's friends or neighbors (Figure 8-10 ●).

FIGURE 8-9

Collecting payment from a patient
© Michal Heron/Pearson Education

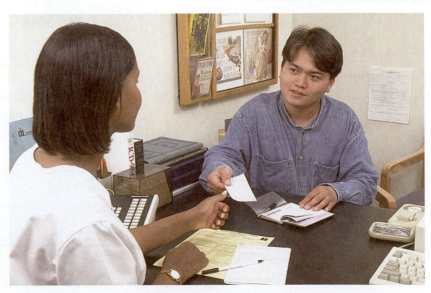

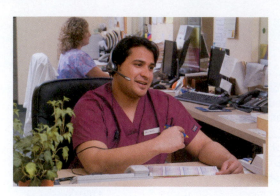

FIGURE 8-10

Making collection calls

A **statute of limitations** is the maximum time that a debt can be collected from the time the debt was incurred or became due. The statute of limitations varies from state to state, so check with your state legislature.

When all other methods of collection are exhausted, a collection agency may be retained to collect delinquent accounts. Most collection agencies charge a percentage of the account once the debt is collected. Therefore, usually only large amounts are sent to a collection agency. Many companies use a standard collection letter (Figure 8-11 ●). If the standard collection notice does not gain a response within thirty days, a delinquent notice should be sent (Figure 8-12 ●).

▶ **CRITICAL THINKING QUESTION:** Why does HIPAA advocate an electronic submission of bills? To research this question, visit the Internet and find the answer.

Collections Procedures

The medical biller often needs to work as a bill collector in order to obtain reimbursement for amounts not covered by insurance or other sources. Usually, these amounts need to be collected from the patient. Occasionally, as a result of an error on a previous claim payment, it may become necessary for a medical biller to recover monies that were paid in error. For these reasons, we will cover the basic laws and regulations regarding collections.

Although the specific laws and regulations vary from state to state, you should become familiar with several general guidelines, including these:

1. You are never allowed to make frightening or abusive calls. This includes making any threats to the person, calling names, or making derogatory statements. Racial or ethnic statements should never be made.
2. It is illegal to call people at odd times of the day. In most states, this means any time between 8:00 p.m. and 8:00 a.m. In some states, it is also illegal to contact people at their place of employment.
3. It is illegal to request collection through another party, including friends or neighbors. This means that you are not allowed to leave a message with anyone other than the debtor concerning details of the collection attempt. This includes, but is not limited to, the amount you are trying to collect, any payment amounts or details that may have been worked out, and the nature of the bill. If you call the debtor and reach a family member or roommate, you are allowed to leave a message giving your name, company, and phone number and requesting that the person you are trying to contact return your call.

Paul Provider, M.D.
5858 Peppermint Place
Anytown, USA 12345
(765) 555-6768

Dear Sir/Madam:

   We are currently showing a past due amount on your account. According to our records your payment of $____ was due on/by _____. As of this date, payment has not been received.

   Please remit payment as soon as possible. If you have recently sent payment, please disregard this notice.

Sincerely,

Collections Representative

FIGURE 8-11

Sample collection letter

Paul Provider, M.D.
5858 Peppermint Place
Anytown, USA 12345
(765) 555-6768

Dear Sir/Madam:

   Your account is seriously delinquent. According to our records we have not yet received your payment of $_____. This payment was due by _____ and reflects services that were rendered on _____.

   If payment is not received by _____ we may be forced to send your bill to collections. Doing so may damage your credit rating.

   If you are unable to pay the full amount, please contact our office immediately to set up a payment plan.

Sincerely,

Collections Representative

FIGURE 8-12

Delinquent notice

4. You are not allowed to harass the person from whom you are trying to collect. The legal definition of harassment varies from state to state; however, it is illegal to do things such as call and speak to the debtor several times a day or even several times a week. For this reason, it is important to provide a reminder of the debt and then ask when you can expect to receive a payment. If the patient is unable to pay in full and your company allows payment plans, try to work out a payment plan for the amount owed. Make detailed notes of the conversation in the patient file. You should not contact the person again until after the date payment is expected.

Payment Plans

If the patient cannot pay the entire bill when contacted and the office allows it, payment arrangements should be made. If a payment plan is worked out, whether over the phone or in person, it is advisable to write down the terms of the agreement and have it signed by both parties (the debtor and a representative of the company to which the money is owed).

   If the payment requires more than four installments, the federal Truth in Lending Act will apply. Regulation Z of the Truth in Lending Act requires that a written disclosure be made. When the installment plan is being discussed, the following important points should be covered:

- The amount of the debt
- The amount of the down payment
- The estimated date of final payment
- The amount of each installment
- The date each payment is due (Figure 8-13 ●)

   As previously explained, a statute of limitations is the maximum time a debt can be collected from the time it was incurred or became due. Remember that the statute of limitations varies from state to state, so check with your state legislature. You should always be aware of the statute of limitations within your state, as the entire debt must be paid off before this time or the provider will forfeit any amounts remaining unpaid.

Truth in Lending Form

Many providers utilize a preprinted form for payment plans. This ensures that they comply with all requirements of the Truth in Lending Act. The form provided in Figure 8-13 meets all requirements

Paul Provider, M.D.
5858 Peppermint Place
Anytown, USA 12345
(765) 555-6768

Date:
Provider:
Patient's Name:
Patient's Address:

Cash price (total fee):
Less cash down payment:
Unpaid balance of cash price:
Amount financed:
FINANCE CHARGE:
ANNUAL PERCENTAGE RATE:
Total of payments:
Deferred payment price:

Patient hereby agrees to pay to (provider's name) at the address shown above, the total payments shown above in _____ monthly installments of $____, first installment being payable _____20 ____, and all such installments on the same day of each consecutive month until paid in full.

Signature _____   Date_____

FIGURE 8-13

Payment plan letter

of this act if it is printed on the provider's letterhead. Please note that the words FINANCE CHARGE and ANNUAL PERCENTAGE RATE must appear in capital letters.

● **ONLINE INFORMATION:** To read more about the Truth in Lending Act, visit the following Web site: truthinlendingact.uslegal.com/credit-truth-in-lending/truth-in-lending-act.

Payment Schedule Form

A payment schedule form is designed to track the payment history of a patient making payments through an installment plan. Some providers prefer to use a payment schedule that may be placed on half of an 8.5 × 11-inch sheet of paper (with the Truth in Lending Form contained on the right-hand side of the paper), or with a payment schedule attached to or printed on the back of the Truth in Lending document.

A payment schedule lists the due date of each installment, the paid amount of the installment, the date the payment was received, and any follow-up notes (usually notes of a phone call if the payment was not received on time). Some practices will use the follow-up area to include the check number of the payment. This helps to track the payment if there are any questions.

Using a form such as this allows the biller to easily see how many payments have been received and if the patient is behind or ahead in payments. It also helps to determine if a patient has missed a payment. Occasionally, a payment will be missed, and the patient will then pay subsequent payments on the due date. Patients may believe they are up to date on their payments when in fact they are a month behind. By using a payment schedule form, you can quickly access this information.

Tracing a Skip

A **skip** is a person who has received services without payment and has moved and left no forwarding address. Skips are usually identified by mail being returned to the medical office by the post office and postmarked "Return to Sender" or "Address Unknown." In attempting to trace a skip, use the information on the patient information sheet. The person shown in the "Person to Contact in Case of Emergency" space should be contacted. Another source is the local Department of Motor Vehicles. If the patient owns a car, it must be registered. The motor vehicle department may be able to provide information regarding the patient's whereabouts. Under no circumstances should information regarding the patient's medical condition be given to the third party.

Tracing a skip is a very tedious and challenging task, and it requires tact as well as patience. If the methods mentioned here prove to be futile, the account may be written off or turned over to a collection agency.

Bankruptcy

Bankruptcy laws allow protection for a debtor. By filing for **bankruptcy**, a debtor announces the inability to pay creditors and requests relief for debts from the bankruptcy court. A provider who is owed money by a patient is considered to be a creditor for that patient.

If the patient includes the outstanding provider's fees as part of a bankruptcy filing, the fees owed may be discharged by the court. This means that the debtor does not have to pay the debt.

A claim should be filed on all bankruptcy proceedings, regardless of whether one is requested. This protects the provider in case he or she does not receive notice that a claim is required. If a claim is not filed within a specified period of time (usually ninety days) the creditor relinquishes any claim on the debtor. The proper claim forms can be obtained from the bankruptcy court, and standard forms are available in many stationery stores.

As soon as an office is informed that a patient has filed bankruptcy, the provider is no longer allowed to attempt collection on that account. This often includes accounts not only of the patient but also accounts of all members of the patient's family. If the account was turned over to a collection agency, immediately notify the collection agency that the patient has filed bankruptcy. Many providers will write off the patient's debt when they are notified of the bankruptcy filing. This prevents statements from continuing to be sent out.

A letter should be sent by certified mail to the patient if the provider wishes to discontinue treatment for the patient. Even if the patient refuses to sign and return the letter, the provider is allowed to discontinue treatment of the patient, without being charged with patient abandonment, thirty days after receipt of the letter. See Figure 8-14 ● for a sample letter for discontinuance of treatment as a result of a bankruptcy filing letter.

Paul Provider, M.D.
5858 Peppermint Place
Anytown, USA 12345
(765) 555-6768

Dear _____:

We are sorry to hear about your recent financial difficulties. Unfortunately, due to your situation, Dr. --- will no longer be able to treat you and your family. We will continue treatment for the next 30 days to allow you to find a new provider; however, during this period payment must be made in cash prior to services rendered. We will be happy to inform you of an estimate of the cost of services prior to an appointment to allow you to bring in the required funds.

When you have chosen a new provider, and upon your written request, we will be happy to provide copies of any medical reports or information on your treatment to the new provider.

Please sign and date one copy of this letter to acknowledge understanding, and return it to our offices in the enclosed envelope. Thank you very much.

Sincerely,

Paul Provider, M.D.

FIGURE 8-14

Letter for discontinuance of treatment as a result of bankruptcy filing

Small Claims Court

At times, a patient who is able to pay his account will refuse to pay. In such cases, it may be necessary to take the patient to small claims court and ask for a judgment against the person.

Attorneys are not allowed in small claims court, so each party represents itself. Each side tells its side of the story and the judge renders a decision. The maximum limit is $5,000 per case in most areas. Your claim should ask for all money that the defendant owes you, plus any collection costs, court costs, and any other costs incurred in attempting to collect the debt.

Before filing a claim, you must show that you have attempted to recover the money and that your efforts have not been successful. This means that you have billed the patient at least three times and sent collection letters demanding payment. If the patient makes no attempt to pay the bill, contact the municipal courthouse in your area and request a plaintiff claim form.

Complete the plaintiff claim form and send it to the court with any required filing fees. The **defendant** (the person you are suing) will be notified of the lawsuit and you will be given a court date.

On the scheduled date, show up in court and bring any and all available documentation to support your case. You should include copies of the pertinent portion of the medical record showing the services performed, the billing for those services, and any letters or copies of statements that show collection attempts.

The judge will take all the evidence into consideration and render a verdict. Often the verdict will come several weeks after the court date. If the decision is in your favor, the defendant will be ordered to pay you the money. If not, you are unable to collect the money requested.

Many states have a provision for the defendant to pay "through the court." In such a case, the court collects the money and reimburses you. There is usually a charge for this service, often based on the amount of money being collected. However, this charge can be much less than trying to collect from someone who still refuses to pay, even though the court has ruled against the defendant. If you choose this option, be sure to discuss it with the clerk of the court before trial.

Practice Accounting

As a medical biller, you are often responsible for keeping a petty cash drawer to use for small cash expenses, such as postage, office supplies, and so on, as well as for reconciling the amount in petty cash. At the beginning of each day, you should have a beginning balance in your petty cash drawer. A petty cash receipt should be filled out and placed in the drawer for all cash removed from petty cash. At the end of the day, reconcile petty cash by making sure that the cash on hand plus petty cash receipts for that day's expenses equals the beginning amount of petty cash on that day.

Medical billers are also responsible for maintaining a *cash* account to be used when collecting payments from patients. At the end of each day, prepare a bank deposit slip, listing all payments received from patients on that day.

When a patient makes a payment, place the check or cash in the petty cash drawer. If change is needed, remove the proper change from the petty cash drawer and replace it with a petty cash receipt.

Petty Cash

Most offices have a **petty cash fund** to start the business day. This fund is used to make change for patients who are making cash payments and for purchasing miscellaneous small office supplies. Keeping track of this fund on a daily basis is essential.

PETTY CASH COUNT SLIPS. Most offices use a **petty cash count slip** (Figure 8-15 ●) to keep track of the amount of money kept in petty cash. The petty cash count slip has space to write the date and time at the top. The remainder of the slip shows various denominations of currency and coins.

To use the petty cash count slip, count the number of each denomination available. Put the number of items on the first line, then multiply the denomination by the number of items. This is the amount of money you have for that denomination.

Once you have counted all the money in the drawer, total the amount on the petty cash count slip. Most offices also will require the person making the count to sign the slip with his or her name or initials.

FIGURE 8-15

Petty cash count slip

PETTY CASH COUNT

DATE _____

TIME _____

	QUANTITY	AMOUNT
CURRENCY		
$100	_____	_____
$50	_____	_____
$20	_____	_____
$10	_____	_____
$5	_____	_____
$1	_____	_____
TOTAL		_____
COINS		
$1	_____	_____
Half $	_____	_____
Quarters	_____	_____
Dimes	_____	_____
Nickels	_____	_____
Pennies	_____	_____
TOTAL		_____
RECEIPTS TOTAL +		_____
GRAND TOTAL		_____

This count is often performed at the beginning of the day, before any money is taken from or added to petty cash, and at the close of the day. The morning's petty cash count slip is usually kept in the petty cash box for the day (Figure 8-16 ●).

PETTY CASH RECEIPTS. At times, the money in petty cash will be needed to pay for small office supplies or other items for the office. This can range from purchasing a few pens to ordering a cake to celebrate an employee's birthday.

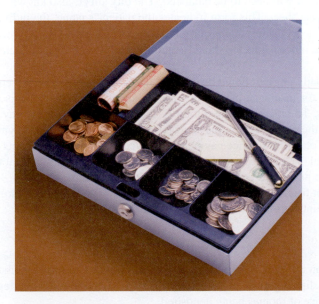

FIGURE 8-16

Petty cash drawer
© Getty Images, Inc.—Photodisc

```
┌─────────────────────────────────────────────────────────┐
│          RECEIVED OF PETTY CASH              01278        │
│                                                           │
│   NUMBER _____ DATE _____   │
│   AMOUNT _____    │
│   FOR _____    │
│   _____      │
│   _____      │
│   CHARGE TO ACCOUNT _____      │
│   _____   _____      │
│   APPROVED BY                 RECEIVED BY                 │
└─────────────────────────────────────────────────────────┘
```

FIGURE 8-17

Petty cash receipt

Usually only a few people are allowed to take money from petty cash. Each time cash is removed, the medical biller should get the permission of a supervisor. This is usually documented using a **petty cash receipt** (Figure 8-17 ●). Each person who takes money from petty cash should sign a petty cash receipt showing the date the money was taken, the amount, and for what it is to be used.

Petty cash receipts should be kept in the petty cash box until a purchase receipt and change are obtained. This allows all reimbursements and outgoing monies to be monitored and approved by a supervisor.

After purchases are made, the receipt and any change should be returned to the petty cash drawer. Be sure that the amount of the receipt and the change equal the amount that was originally taken from petty cash. Indicate on the petty cash receipt the amount of change returned. Then staple the purchase receipt to the petty cash receipt.

At times, someone may purchase an office supply with, and need to be reimbursed with, petty cash funds for the out-of-pocket expense. A petty cash receipt also should be completed for these types of purchases. The exact amount should be returned to the person and the purchase receipt stapled to the petty cash receipt.

Petty cash receipts should be kept in the petty cash drawer. When reconciling funds at the end of the day, petty cash vouchers should be counted as cash. This will help you to determine if your amounts have balanced.

All petty cash receipts should be consecutively numbered and treated as amounts paid out.

The Day Sheet/Daily Journal

At the end of the day, the day sheet will need to be balanced. The **day sheet**, also known as the **daily journal**, is used as a balance sheet. This form indicates the patient's name, the individual fee charged for the day, any payments made, and the current balance (Figure 8-18 ●). All receipts for the day and any insurance or other payments should equal the cash/check total collected on the daily journal.

The beginning line on the daily journal should be the petty cash total for the day. All entries should be made on the journal for insurance payments, cash payments, or any other miscellaneous payments or adjustments. To balance, make a total of the cash receipts for the day, any petty cash disbursements, and the petty cash on hand. Make another receipt for all payments made in the office or by mail. Total all insurance payments received. Combine the receipts total and the insurance payments total. Total the payments column on the daily journal. This total is equal to the combined insurance payments, cash receipts, and petty cash totals.

If the daily journal does not balance, go back through the charge slips and ledger cards for the day. By comparing the amounts written, you should be able to find your error.

Deposit Slips

All checks should be stamped on the back with a bank deposit stamp, then information about it should be entered on a deposit slip (Figure 8-19 ●). A **deposit slip** (also referred to as **deposit ticket**) is an overview and balance of monies being deposited.

Paul Provider, M.D.
5858 Peppermint Place
Anytown, USA 12345
(765) 555-6768

Day Sheet/Daily Journal

Date	Name	Description of Service	Charge	Payments	Adjustments	Remaining Balance

FIGURE 8-18

Day sheet/daily journal

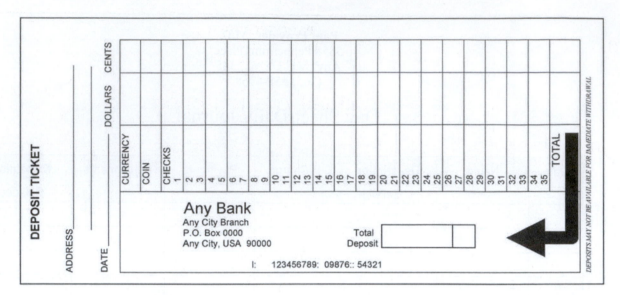

FIGURE 8-19

Deposit slip/Deposit ticket

Be sure to fill out the deposit slip with the correct account number since several companies maintain more than one bank account. The deposit slip has space for coin, cash, and check deposits. Add up the amount of money you have in currency and enter it in the first box. Next, add up the amount of coins you have and list it in the second box.

Checks are listed individually. Fill in the bank number of the check. This is a four- to six-digit number with a hyphen in the middle (e.g., 66-123). This number refers to the bank and the branch of the bank that the check is drawn on. Next to this number and below the previous amounts, list the amount of the check. If you run out of space for all of your checks, there is usually additional space on the back of the deposit slip.

When all amounts have been entered, total them and put the amount at the bottom. This will give you the total amount of your deposit.

Office Reports

Numerous reports are designed to help the medical office run smoothly and to keep track of the cash flow. These include the daily journal (see above), patient statements (see above), the accounting control summary, cumulative trial balance, and patient aging report.

Accounting Control Summary

The **accounting control summary** is a weekly or monthly report form that shows each day's charges, payments, and adjustments for the period indicated. The medical biller uses this form to double-check the figures against his or her records. This ensures that all information that is to be recorded reaches the computer properly and has been entered correctly. It also lists items that were not entered.

Items may not be entered or "held in suspense" for a variety of reasons, including wrong account numbers, incorrect spellings, missing code numbers, and no master record for the family.

Cumulative Trial Balance

The **cumulative trial balance** lists each patient alphabetically and shows any charges, payments, or adjustments to the patient's account. This allows the medical office to keep track of all accounts and the amounts that are owed and have been paid.

Patient Aging Report

A **patient aging report** (Figure 8-20 ●) allows the medical biller to categorize a patient account's outstanding balance by the length of time the charges have been due.

PAUL PROVIDER
5858 Peppermint Place
Anytown, USA 12345
(765) 555-6768

Patient Aging Report

Patient	Current	31 – 60 Days	61 – 90 Days	91+ Days	Total

FIGURE 8-20

Patient aging report

CHAPTER REVIEW

Summary

- Keeping accurate patient accounts is one of the most important jobs of a medical biller. Patients must not only be billed for the services they receive, but insurance carriers must be billed, payments must be posted to accounts, and patients must be balance billed for any remaining amounts on claims.
- If payment is not received from an insurance carrier in a timely manner, an insurance tracer must be completed.
- Collections also are an important aspect of the biller's job. Some patients will refuse to pay their bill, and so collection attempts must be made. At times, this involves tracing a skipped patient or filing a claim in small claims court. If the patient files bankruptcy, all collections on the account must stop and the patient must be properly informed if the provider refuses to continue to treat the patient.
- It is important to keep a daily journal of the office transactions, an accounting control summary, a cumulative trial balance, and patient aging reports. It is the medical biller's responsibility to reconcile petty cash and prepare a deposit slip of the day's receipts.

Review Questions

Directions: Answer the following questions without looking back into the material just covered. Write your answers in the space provided.

1. What information is listed on a patient statement? _____
_____
_____

2. Under the Truth in Lending Act, what items must be included in a payment plan? _____
_____
_____

3. What is the purpose of the ledger card? _____
_____

4. If you are attempting to collect on a bill, is it legal to call the person names or to make derogatory comments regarding the person's sex, race, or ethnic background? _____
_____
_____

5. What information are you allowed to give if you call a debtor and speak with a roommate or other family member? _____
_____

6. What is the purpose of the petty cash count slip, and how do you use it? _____
_____
_____

7. What is the purpose of the daily journal? _____
_____

8. What is included on a daily journal? _____
_____
_____

9. What is the purpose of the petty cash receipt? _____

    _____

10. What are some of the most common accounting reports used in a medical office, and what
    is their purpose?

    _____

    _____

    _____

If you are unable to answer any of these questions, refer back to that section in the chapter, and
then fill in the answers.

Activity #3: Word Search

Directions: Find and circle the terms listed below. Words can appear horizontally, vertically,
diagonally, forward, or backward.

1. Accounting control summary
2. Adjustments
3. Cumulative trial balance
4. Defendant
5. Explanation of Benefits
6. Patient aging report
7. Pended
8. Post
9. Statute of limitations

```
Y T P Z N B W G Y Y V T U I E B J X Q I V E E J X I F R Y N
D R V A D I W N P K F Y S C T B B F L X S C U G V S B X R S
M P A Z T X S S Q L V G N O M B W W A T T N W W L P P L T X
E I N M P I H L V Y M K P W P I K A I H G A J J Z I B Z K K
V P Y R M L E V L B B W S G S Q S F V R X L O P N X C K A C
Q S P D T U C N T D O I B G H G E E J U O A E D Q W A H E I
P C F Z R E S M T W D M S D U N N V H Z Z B J A V L G Z L I
Q Z O H E F I L R A M G K E E X O J B F V L C I D J X C P Q
F S M J G H P I O L G M X B D H P W N K P A H N X Y D L W A
X H K Q V K K Q W R K I F F B M H W J U U I G Z F B W Y B P
K C L H G F N W E P T O N O Q U W Y Z Q D R C Z M G A U U M
E X U Q O P P Z Q J N N K G K X X A C L B T S W T F B N B X
J R O P C O C R D O Q K O D R B L R T K C E Z E E Y X G T X
H P O J M L V E I N N F H C X E I E J B U V E L S K Y M W Q
L S K J J Y F T X M G S P Z G N P W N C U I O G S Q C O E K
M J D M U E A E U M D K K Z U N H O X N G T T X O F V X A B
E Q T B N N Q Z R T N S Q M Q V I C R D A A Y L K N Y E Y W
E X B D A B H R L S Z V K X Q R Z T D T C L S S T E B I G V
Z Y A L D A A I A Q T L S R P J W R N E G U V M G T H E Y P
B N P F D K D A Y Q S N U E E H L Q H U M M O M A S P A U Y
T X D E D N E P Z E T A V R J B J D Z R O U K N D O T X H A
E S T A T U T E O F L I M I T A T I O N S C K Y J G T I C H
L H R R D U N F R H Z D D H B U S Z X B X V C M U H Q T O M
Y K Y Q X O V L N X N D D E O Q B I R Z I Z K A S V V K S P
P F B I K A K H O P X O A V J T T T L L H R P J T K U V C M
A A Z P W H D F S Y D Z K W H V C M V H Y N W Z M V H V Q K
B E A H U F H R F F P Z W X X B P Z D E G E H X E T D H J C
C R W A H P Q L B H S T U R K R J Z P A X A R D N N M O A O
K U M Y E F P U J R J J I A S D P M S H V Z A H T S D L R N
A F L M Q V E T L S X M W Y V Z Q C P O T L N C S I M L I Z
```

Activity #4: Matching Key Terms

Directions: Match the following terms with the proper definition by writing the letter of the correct definition in the space next to the term.

1. _____ Accounts payable

2. _____ Statement of account

3. _____ Balance billing

4. _____ Petty cash receipt

5. _____ Daily journal

6. _____ Patient statement

7. _____ Dunning notice

8. _____ Insurance tracer

a. A daily balance sheet that shows the patient's name, the individual fee charged for the day, any payments made, and the current balance

b. A form or letter sent to the insurance carrier to inquire about the disposition of a previously submitted claim

c. A statement or sentence reminding the recipient to make a payment on their account

d. An individual summary (either by patient or by family) that lists all the services, charges, payments, adjustments, and balance due that occurred during the month

e. Money paid out, usually for goods or services

f. Sending an additional bill to another party for payment of any remaining amounts on a claim

g. A form that is used whenever money is removed from the petty cash fund indicating how much money was removed and who received it

h. A card used to indicate a chronological record of all services rendered to a patient

Activity #5: Completing an Encounter Form and Patient Receipt

Directions: Based on the following scenarios and using Dr. Paul Provider's information, complete an encounter form and patient receipt. Then post the payment to the patient ledger card. Next, balance the day sheet/daily journal. Finally, create a bank deposit slip for the payments made. Refer to the Patient Data Table and Provider Data Table in Appendix A for additional information, along with the forms needed to complete this activity.

1. The following services were billed for: Abby Addison   Date of Service: 01/16/CCYY

   Diagnosis: Hypertension

   99205–Comprehensive High-Complexity Exam ($160)

   8100–Urinalysis ($30)

   36415–Venipuncture ($20)

   Patient made a cash payment of $60 on this visit.

2. The following services were billed for: Bobby Brumble   Date of Service: 01/16/CCYY

   Diagnosis: Diabetes

   99211–Minimal Exam ($35)

81000–Urinalysis ($30)

82948–Glucose Fingerstick ($18)

36415–Venipuncture ($20)

Patient made a payment by check of $75 on this visit.

3. The following services were billed for: Cathy Crenshaw   Date of Service: 01/16/CCYY

   Diagnosis: Chronic Bronchitis

   99204–Comprehensive Moderate Complexity Exam ($140)

   36415–Venipuncture ($20)

   Patient made a payment by check of $110 on this visit.

4. The following services were billed for: Daisy Doolittle   Date of Service: 01/16/CCYY

   Diagnosis: Congenital Hypothyroidism

   99203–Detailed Low-Complexity Exam ($100)

   36415–Venipuncture ($20)

   Patient made a cash payment of $15 on this visit.

5. The following services were billed for: Edward Edmunds   Date of Service: 01/16/CCYY

   Diagnosis: Coronary Artery Disease

   99214–Detailed Moderate-Complexity Exam ($60)

   93000–EKG ($55)

   81000–Urinalysis ($30)

   36415–Venipuncture ($20)

   Patient did not make a payment.

SECTION

MEDICAL CODING

4

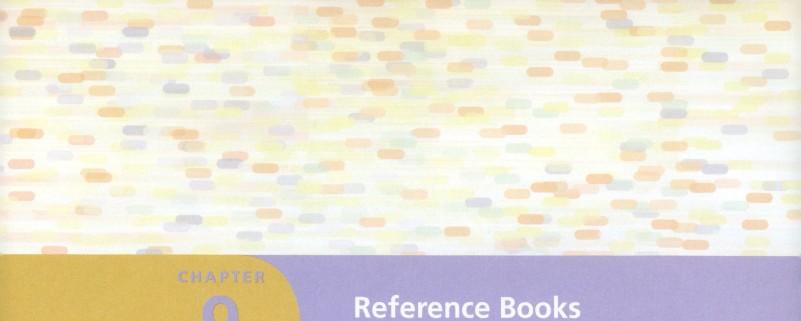

Reference Books

Key Words and Concepts you will learn in this chapter:

Air ambulance

Base call charge

Controlled drugs

Enteral therapy

Generic drugs

Health Care Common Procedure Coding System (HCPCS)

International Classification of Diseases—9th Revision, Clinical Modification (ICD-9-CM)

Legend drugs

Medically oriented equipment

Medical dictionary

Medications

Nonlegend drugs

Orthotics

Over-the-counter drugs (OTCs)

Parenteral therapy

Pharmaceuticals

Physicians' Desk Reference (PDR)

Prescription legend

After completion of this chapter you should be able to:

Recognize *The Merck Manual, Physicians' Desk Reference* (PDR), a medical dictionary, *Current Procedural Terminology* (CPT), and *ICD-9-CM*, and explain their use.

Determine if a pharmaceutical is a prescription or a nonprescription drug.

List the sections of the PDR and the information each section contains.

Properly use the PDR.

Explain the purpose and use of the *Health Care Common Procedure Coding System* (HCPCS).

Describe the two levels used in HCPCS coding.

Properly code procedures or items using HCPCS.

A **reference book** is a source of information to which a reader is referred. In health claims billing, coding, and examining, a number of books are used as reference books. These include *International Classification of Diseases—9th Revision, Clinical Modification* (ICD-9-CM); *Provider's Current Procedure Terminology* (CPT); *Relative Value Study* (RVS); *Health Care Common Procedure Coding System* (HCPCS); *Physicians' Desk Reference* (PDR); medical dictionaries; and *The Merck Manual*. Each of these books is discussed briefly in this chapter. The ICD-9-CM, ICD-10-CM, and CPT are presented individually and in further detail in Chapters 10, 11, and 12.

▶ **CRITICAL THINKING QUESTION:** Why is it important in your field of study to know how to use the various types of reference books available to prepare health claims?

Medical Dictionaries

A **medical dictionary** lists medical terms and their definitions, synonyms, illustrations, and supplemental information. Numerous medical dictionaries are available. As a rule, this reference should be used primarily for verifying a diagnosis or affected body area, or for checking definitions and spelling. As with most dictionaries, entries are arranged alphabetically.

When using a medical dictionary, it is important that you first read through the foreword and any instructions or general guidelines contained in the front of the book. Because each publisher uses different symbols and information, you must read these instructions to understand the symbols and terms and their meanings. In addition to basic definitions, many medical dictionaries include other information regarding words and terms.

When using the medical dictionary it is imperative that the medical biller read through the entire entry. If terms are used in the definition that the medical biller does not understand, the unknown word also should be looked up, either in the medical dictionary (if it is a medical term) or in a standard dictionary (if it is not).

Numerous diseases, conditions, or terms are very similar to each other in spelling or pronunciation but vastly different in meaning. It is important to use the proper term and its proper spelling when billing and coding a claim.

The Merck Manual

The Merck Manual is used to assist in identifying the symptomatology, prognosis, treatment protocols, etiology, and other miscellaneous information regarding diagnoses.

The Merck Manual has two main sections: a listing of diseases and an index. The index is arranged alphabetically by disease. To find a particular disease, simply locate the disease and its corresponding page number in the index. The information provided includes the diagnosis, symptoms, prognosis, and treatment.

Physicians' Desk Reference (PDR)

Medications are drugs (often called **pharmaceuticals**) used to treat diseases, symptoms, or discomforts (e.g., pain medications). The ***Physicians' Desk Reference*** (**PDR**) is a medical reference book that provides comprehensive information about the particular use of a drug; how the drug works in the body; possible side effects; and warnings against use for the elderly, pregnant women, and for people with other health complications (Figure 9-1 ●). The PDR is published annually with supplements published as necessary during the year.

Two types of drugs are listed in the PDR: legend and nonlegend. **Legend drugs** are drugs that can only be obtained with a prescription. The

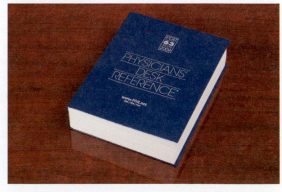

FIGURE 9-1

Physicians' Desk Reference

© Michal Heron/Pearson Education

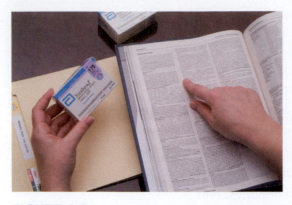

FIGURE 9-2

The PDR is used for reviewing information related to a drug.
© Michal Heron/Pearson Education

prescription legend appears on the label and is the pharmaceutical manufacturer's warning. The product label must include the statement "Caution: Federal law prohibits dispensing without a prescription." Legend drugs are indicated with the symbol Rx. **Nonlegend drugs** are drugs that can be obtained without a prescription. Nonlegend drugs also are known as **over-the-counter drugs (OTCs)**. Some drugs are closely monitored or controlled, and consequently they are called controlled drugs. **Controlled drugs** are drugs that are tightly controlled by federal mandates because of their addictive, experimental, toxic, or other highly volatile properties (Figure 9-2 ●).

The PDR is divided into six sections:

1. *Manufacturer's Index (white).* Arranged alphabetically by manufacturer, then by drug name. The name and address of the manufacturer are included. This section includes prescription and nonprescription drugs.
2. *Product Name Index (pink).* Arranged alphabetically by drug name. Prescription and non-prescription drugs are included. This section is usually used first to locate the manufacturer's name and the page number for further information.
3. *Product Category Index (blue).* Arranged alphabetically by drug action category—that is, according to the most common use of the drug. If the drug is an antidepressant, it is listed under the antidepressant category; if it is an antacid, it is listed under the antacid category.
4. *Product Identification Section (gray).* Arranged alphabetically by manufacturer, then by brand name. This section contains the actual size and full-color reproductions. Only the reproductions submitted by the manufacturer are included.
5. *Product Information Section (white).* Arranged alphabetically by manufacturer, then by brand name. Most pharmaceuticals are described by indications and usage, dosage, administration, description, clinical pharmacology, supply warnings, contraindications, adverse reactions, overdosage precautions, and other miscellaneous information.
6. *Diagnostic Product Information (green).* Arranged alphabetically by manufacturer, then by product. This section provides a description of diagnostic products only.

Generic Versus Brand Name Drugs

A pharmaceutical manufacturer bears the cost of all research, development, and testing of a new drug. When a pharmaceutical company develops a drug, it can file for and may receive patent protection for that particular drug. **Proprietary drugs** are pharmaceuticals that are patented or controlled by a manufacturer. The manufacturer copyrights the trade or brand name. This allows the company the right to manufacture the drug exclusively under a brand name for a period of time. After the patent has expired, any company may manufacture the drug. Other companies that begin manufacturing the drug after the patent period expires do not incur the research and development costs. Therefore, they can produce an equivalent drug for a lot less money. The drugs produced by other manufacturers are generic drugs. **Generic drugs** are nonproprietary drugs not protected by trademark, and their name is usually descriptive of the drug's chemical structure.

When making a generic drug, the manufacturer must provide appropriate safety data to the U.S. Food and Drug Administration (FDA). These data include sufficient proof that the generic product has the identical active ingredient(s) and is as effective as the brand name drug in all respects. When the generic drug meets these requirements, it is considered "therapeutically equivalent."

Most manufacturers of generic drugs also make brand name drugs. In fact, 70 percent to 80 percent of all generic drugs are made by the same manufacturers that make the brand name drugs. The profit made on the generic drugs helps to offset some of the research and development costs of other brand name drugs.

Prescription Plans

Prescription medications are usually covered under benefit plans in one of two ways: (1) under a separate, free-standing plan for outpatient, prescription medicines only or (2) under Major Medical as any other eligible expense, subject to all applicable deductibles, copayments, limitations, and exclusions.

Separate prescription service plans establish networks of participating pharmacies and then assume responsibility for the claims processing. Such plans usually include some if not all of the following components:

1. The claimant is not required to pay for his or her prescription with a large cash outlay. Instead, a small specified copayment amount, chosen by the group, is paid by the claimant for each prescription (copayments usually range from $8 to $30).
2. The pharmacy accepts an identification card as evidence that payment will be made by the plan; it then bills the plan for the unpaid balance.
3. A claim form is not required from the cardholder. The pharmacy bills the payer directly.
4. The member is required to go to a participating pharmacy to fill prescriptions. Otherwise, either the claimant will be responsible for full payment for the medication or a reduced percentage may be paid.
5. Each prescription filled will provide a supply for a specified number of days—thirty-, sixty-, or ninety-day maximum.

Prescription service plans typically exclude the following types of expenses:

1. Devices or medical/surgical supplies of any type, such as bandages, gauze, and so on (Hypodermic needles and syringes may be covered for diabetics.)
2. Drugs dispensed while the member is confined in a facility, including those given on the day of discharge
3. Immunization agents, biological sera, blood, plasma, or other blood agents
4. Investigational or experimental drugs
5. Health foods, food supplements, vitamins, and appetite suppressants

As with most other plan provisions, the covered and excluded charges vary from plan to plan. Therefore, the benefits should be verified.

ACTIVITY #1

Demonstrating the Use of the PDR

Directions: Look up the following medications in the PDR. Indicate in the space provided whether or not the drug is prescription by writing in the status symbol. Also, indicate the trade name if the generic name is given; indicate the generic name if the trade name is given. The manufacturer's name is indicated in parentheses.

	Name	Symbol
1. Fluorouracil Cream (Roche)	_____	_____
2. Proventil (Schering)	_____	_____
3. Spectazole (Ortho-McNeil)	_____	_____
4. Fenfluramine Hydrochloride (Robins)	_____	_____
5. Valium Injectable (Roche)	_____	_____
6. Klonpin (Roche)	_____	_____
7. Psyllium Husk Fiber (Proctor & Gamble)	_____	_____
8. Metaproterenol Sulfate (Boehringer Ingelheim)	_____	_____
9. Pentazocine Hydrochloride and Acetaminophen (Winthrop)	_____	_____
10. Flonase (Glaxo-Smith-Kline)	_____	_____
11. Dilantin Injection Parenteral (Parke-Davis)	_____	_____
12. Sotradecol Injection (Elkins-Sinn)	_____	_____
13. Aldomet Tablets (Merck)	_____	_____
14. Mandol (Lilly)	_____	_____
15. Viagra (Pfizer)	_____	_____

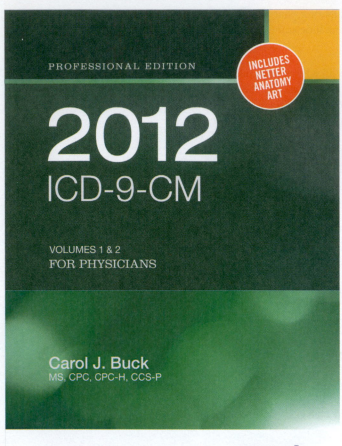

FIGURE 9-3
ICD-9-CM code book

Reprinted by permission of the American Medical Association.

ICD-9-CM and ICD-10-CM

The *International Classification of Diseases—9th Revision, Clinical Modification* (**ICD-9-CM**) is an indexing of diseases and conditions (Figure 9-3). The ICD-9-CM serves a dual purpose for health benefits personnel: First, it enables the medical biller and the claims examiner to convert English language descriptions of an illness, injury, or other condition into a numerical code; second, it allows for the classification of diseases for statistical purposes. Symptoms, diseases, injuries, and routine services are identified with either a three-, four-, or five-digit code, which may be entirely numerical or may be alphanumeric.

The ICD-9-CM consists of three volumes:

- *Volume I.* A tabular listing of diseases.
- *Volume II.* An alphabetical index of diseases by English language description.
- *Volume III.* A numerical and alphabetical listing of hospital inpatient procedures, also referred to as ICD-9-PCS (Procedure Coding System).

Volumes I and II are used by all medical providers. Volume III is used only by hospitals for inpatient procedures.

The *International Classification of Diseases—10th Revision, Clinical Modification* (ICD-10-CM) is an update to ICD-9-CM that will go into effect on October 1, 2013. At that time, ICD-9-CM will no longer be used. As with ICD-9-CM, ICD-10-CM serves a dual purpose for health benefits personnel: First, it enables the medical biller and the claims examiner to convert English-language descriptions of an illness, injury, or other condition into a numerical code; second, it allows for the classification of diseases for statistical purposes. Symptoms, diseases, injuries, and routine services are identified with three-, four-, five-, six-, or seven-digit codes, all of which will be alphanumeric. ICD-10-CM codes are more specific than ICD-9-CM codes and provide more consistent data regarding patients' medical conditions. ICD-9-CM is thirty years old, uses outdated terms, and is inconsistent with current medical practice. Also, the structure of ICD-9-CM limits the number of new codes that can be created, and many ICD-9 categories are full. The change to more specific codes in ICD-10 increases the number of diagnosis codes from 14,000 ICD-9-CM codes to over 68,000 ICD-10-CM codes. ICD-10-CM consists of two volumes:

- *Volume I.* A tabular listing of diseases.
- *Volume II.* An alphabetical index of diseases by English-language description.

In addition, ICD-10-PCS will be a separate volume that replaces ICD-9-CM, Volume 3. ICD-10-PCS is a numerical and alphabetical listing of hospital inpatient procedures. The code structure has significant changes, and the number of codes is increased from 3,800 to over 72,000. ICD-10-PCS will also be adopted on October 1, 2013.

ICD-9-CM is discussed in further detail in Chapter 10. ICD-10-CM and ICD-10-PCS are discussed in detail in Chapters 11 and 12.

Provider's Current Procedure Terminology (CPT)

The *Provider's Current Procedure Terminology* (**CPT**) is a systematic listing for coding the procedures or services performed by a provider (Figure 9-4 •). (Within this text, the word *provider* is used generically to apply to any provider of services other than a hospital or other facility.) Each procedure is identified with a five-digit numerical code. The purpose of the CPT is to provide a uniform method of accurately describing medical, surgical, and diagnostic services, which facilitates an effective means of communication among providers, patients, and claim administrators.

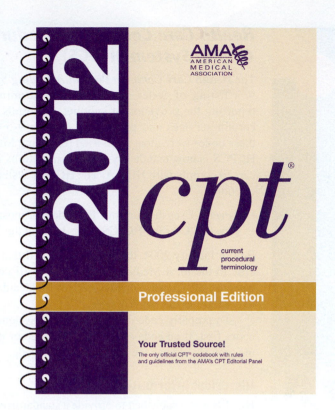

FIGURE 9-4
CPT coding book
Reprinted by permission of the
American Medical Association.

The CPT has six major sections:

1. *Evaluation and Management*—99201–99499
2. *Medicine*—90281-99607
3. *Surgery*—10021-69990
4. *Anesthesia*—00100–01999
5. *Radiology/Nuclear Medicine*—70010–79999
6. *Pathology & Laboratory Tests*—80047–89398

The CPT and its use are discussed in detail in Chapter 12.

ACTIVITY #2

Selecting the Correct Reference Book—Part 1

Directions: Determine the correct reference book needed to answer the following questions, then use that reference to find the answer. Do not be concerned if you do not understand all the words in the description or answer.

1. What is a synonym (word with the same meaning) for the common cold? _____
   _____

2. How long is a person contagious with the common cold? _____
   _____

3. Name two symptoms of a cold. _____
   _____
   _____

4. What causes the common cold? _____
   _____
   _____

5. What is the incubation period for this disease? _____
   _____
   _____

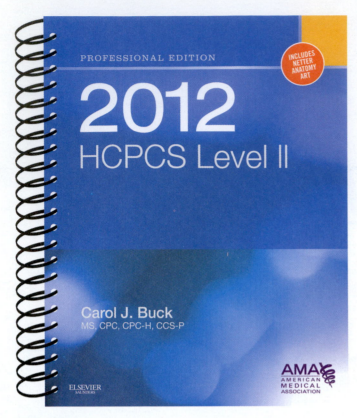

FIGURE 9-5

HCPCS Level II coding book

Reprinted by permission of the American Medical Association.

Health Care Common Procedure Coding System (HCPCS)

The *Health Care Common Procedure Coding System* (**HCPCS**) is a listing of codes and descriptive terminology used for reporting the provision of supplies, materials, injections, and certain services and procedures (Figure 9-5 ●). In the past, these codes were most often used for billing Medicare services. HCPCS is now mandatory for all transactions involving health care to comply with HIPAA. The HCPCS system has two levels of coding:

- *Level I.* Uses the current CPT codes for most procedures.
- *Level II.* Uses the HCPCS codes listed in the HCPCS manual.

Before January 2004, there was a Level III that used codes specific to the local Medicare carrier. Level III codes were eliminated by the Centers for Medicare & Medicaid Services (CMS) to conform to the HIPAA laws.

To properly code using the HCPCS system, check Level II codes first. If no code exists for the service or item you are billing, you should use the appropriate CPT code.

Historical Information

HCPCS was established to provide a standardized system to code items and services provided in the delivery of medical care. This system is necessary to ensure that insurance claims processed by Medicare, Medicaid, and other health insurance programs are processed in a consistent manner. HCPCS is based on the American Medical Association (AMA) Current Procedure Terminology (CPT) with additional codes and modifiers developed by the Health Care Financing Administration (HCFA). HCPCS is made up of two coding levels (HCPCS Level I (CPT) was initially developed in 1966; HCPCS Level II was established in 1983):

- *Level 1.* The first level contains only the CPT codes and modifiers. Maintenance of these codes is the responsibility of the AMA, and updates are done on a yearly basis. There are over 7,000 CPT codes; however, the CPT is limited in its selections for materials, supplies, and injection codes. For example, the code 99070 is used for all supplies.
- *Level 2.* The second level includes the CMS designated codes. These are nonprovider services, such as Durable Medical Equipment, Prostheses and Orthotics. A few providers' services that were not found in the CPT codes were assigned HCPCS codes, such as J codes for injections. HCPCS codes are alphanumeric, beginning with A0000 and continuing through V5999. More than 2,400 HCPCS codes are updated yearly.

Although the acronym HCPCS is technically used to denote both levels of the coding system, it is commonly used to denote just Level 2, which differs from the more commonly used CPT codes.

Because numerous changes are made every year to the CPT and HCPCS codes, it is imperative that the biller use the most current edition of the CPT and HCPCS manuals. The use of the most current edition is a requirement of HIPAA.

Coding Using the HCPCS Manual

Procedure coding is a way for providers to report to an insurance carrier the exact service(s) performed for their patients. The CPT covers many provider services. However, it is not all-encompassing, and Medicare carriers need more detailed information on certain types of services, including medical equipment, supplies, and the injection of drugs.

With the advent of the HCPCS J codes, the biller can now enter a code to indicate which drug is being given to the patient.

Most versions of the HCPCS manual contain an index. This index lists most of the procedures or items that are included in the manual. However, not all items are included. For example, some HCPCS indexes do not list all the drugs included in the J code section. Still, most of the drugs are listed in alphabetical order, making it easy to locate the correct code.

To locate an HCPCS code for an item or service, use the index. The index will provide the specific HCPCS code for that item or service. If there is more than one applicable code, the index will list all codes or may list a range of codes. However, just looking in the index is not enough. After identifying the code, locate the code in the lettered section and read the information provided. There may be additional information regarding the code, or there may be references to other codes that may be more appropriate.

For example, use your HCPCS manual to locate code L3806. The correct description for this code would be "Wrist-hand-finger-orthoses (WHFO); long opponens, no attachment, custom fabricated."

Sections of the HCPCS Manual

The HCPCS manual is categorized into numerous sections (Table 9-1 ●). Each section begins with a letter, and each code within that section begins with the same letter.

ACTIVITY #3

Determining the Correct HCPCS Code for Injections

Directions: Determine the correct HCPCS codes for the following procedures/items.

1. Injection of thiamine HCl, 100 mg   1. _____
2. Injection of azithromycin, 500 mg   2. _____
3. Injection of testosterone suspension, up to 50 mg   3. _____
4. Injection of lorazepam (Ativan), 2 mg   4. _____
5. Injection of iron dextran 50 mg   5. _____

TABLE 9-1 Categorization of HCPCS Manual (2011)

Category	Code
Transportation Services	A0021–A0999
Medical and Surgical Supplies	A4000–A7527
Administrative Miscellaneous and Investigational	A9000–A9999
Enteral and Parenteral Therapy	B4000–B9999
CMS Hospital Outpatient Payment System	C1000–C9999
Durable Medical Equipment	E0100–E9999
Temporary Procedures and Professional Services	G0000–G9999
Behavioral Health and Substance Abuse Treatment Services	H0001–H9999
Drugs Other than Chemotherapy	J0100–J9999
Temporary Codes Assigned to DME Regional Carriers	K0000–K9999
Orthotic	L0100–L4999
Prosthetic	L5000–L9999
Other Medical Services	M0000–M0301
Laboratory Services	P0000–P9999
Temporary Codes Assigned by CMS	Q0000–Q9999
Diagnostic Radiology Services	R0000–R9999
Temporary National Codes Established by Private Payors	S0000–S9999
Temporary National Codes Established by Medicaid	T1000–T9999
Vision Services	V0000–V2999
Hearing Services	V5000–V5999

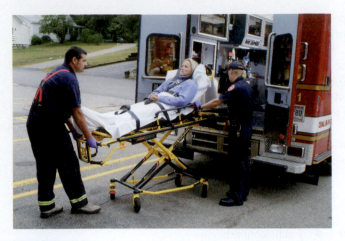

FIGURE 9-6

Transporting a patient by ambulance

© Pearson Education

TRANSPORTATION SERVICES. These codes are used to report transportation services, including ambulance and air ambulance services.

Ambulance Service. Ambulance expenses are incurred in the transfer of an injured or sick person to a medical facility (Figure 9-6 ●). These expenses are not considered professional or hospital services. The ambulance service bills the patient for this service, separate from any hospital or physician services.

An ambulance expense is covered under the following conditions:

1. The ambulance must be medically necessary and not for the patient's convenience.
2. Transportation is provided by a professional ambulance/paramedic service.
3. Transportation is to the nearest facility capable of treating the patient.
4. Transportation is provided from one facility to another when the necessary treatment cannot be obtained from the first hospital.
5. Transportation to home from a facility is provided if the patient is unable to travel in an upright position. Exceptions such as this vary by plan, so refer to the plan provisions before processing.
6. Charges for ambulance services are covered when either emergency room or inpatient hospital charges also are billed. An exception would be in the case of an insured who is dead on arrival at the hospital.
7. Transportation to a facility is covered if the claimant is dead on arrival, even though no treatment or charges are incurred at the facility.

Expenses commonly billed by an ambulance service include these:

• *Base call charge.* This is the amount automatically charged for the ambulance to respond to a call even if the patient is not subsequently transported.
• *Oxygen.* Includes oxygen supplies.
• *Mileage.*
• *Linens.*
• *Emergency response charge.* This is an extra expense in addition to the base charge, which may be added if the patient's condition is severe enough that resuscitation efforts or other types of stabilization measures are required.
• *Paramedic response charge.* If paramedics rather than emergency medical technicians (EMTs) are used, an extra expense may be added.

Air Ambulance. An **air ambulance** is a helicopter or other flight vehicle used to transport a severely injured or ill person to a hospital. Air medical transport may be covered if:

1. The facility in the area where the patient is injured cannot manage the patient's condition and it is medically necessary to transfer the patient by air to another facility more equipped to treat the patient.

ACTIVITY #4

Determining the Correct HCPCS Code for Ambulance Service and Life Support

Directions: Determine the correct HCPCS codes for the following procedures/items.

1. Ambulance service, basic life support emergency transport   1. _____
2. Ambulance service, advanced life support emergency transport   2. _____
3. BLS routine disposable supplies   3. _____
4. Ambulance oxygen and oxygen supplies, life-sustaining situation   4. _____
5. Advanced life support, level 2   5. _____

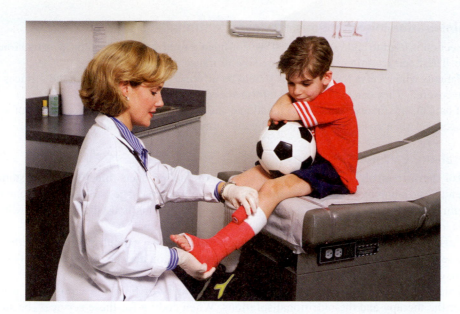

FIGURE 9-7
Medical supplies are needed for many services.
© Michal Heron/Pearson Education

2. Ground transport time would be prolonged and, thus, compromise the patient's medical status.

Coverage is limited to the regular air ambulance charge for transportation to the nearest facility that can handle the case.

Medical and Surgical Supplies

Perishable medical and surgical supplies may be covered under the insurance plan if the items can be used only by the patient and are medically necessary in the treatment of the illness or injury. Medical and surgical supplies (Figure 9-7 ●) include the following:

1. Disposable, nondurable supplies and accessories required to operate medical equipment or prosthetic devices
2. Necessary drugs and biological items put directly into equipment (such as nonprescription nutrients)
3. Initial and replacement accessories essential for operating medical equipment
4. Supplies furnished and charged by a hospital, surgical center, or provider as part of active therapy, such as elastic bandage, cast, and cervical collar

Examples of medical supply items include diabetes testing strips, catheters, syringes, ostomy pouches, and so on. Do not include items or supplies that could be used by the patient or a member of the patient's family for purposes other than medical care.

ACTIVITY #5

Determining the Correct HCPCS Code for Medical and Surgical Supplies

Directions: Determine the correct HCPCS codes for the following items.

1. Ostomy pouch, drainable; for use on barrier with locking flange (two-piece system)   1. _____
2. Tracheostomy care kit for new tracheostomy   2. _____
3. Paraffin, per pound   3. _____
4. Surgical trays   4. _____
5. Vabra aspirator   5. _____

Administrative Miscellaneous and Investigational

This section is used to code services that are considered to be experimental or investigational in nature. These services often are not covered by insurance carriers.

Patients who receive these services should be informed ahead of time that the services may not be covered. They can then make an informed decision regarding their care.

If patients are involved in an investigational study (e.g., to study the effectiveness of a drug or procedure), their costs may be covered by the entity that is monitoring the study.

Enteral and Parenteral Therapy

Enteral therapy involves the administration of nutritional products directly into the stomach, duodenum, or jejunum. A tube is inserted through the nasal passage, stomach, duodenum, or jejunum depending on the viability of surrounding organs. This is used for patients who are unable to chew, swallow, or tolerate food in the digestive system.

Parenteral therapy involves administering substances to a patient via a tube inserted into a vein (e.g., medications or nutritional supplements). Nutrition may be given to patients whose digestive system cannot tolerate food.

This section of the HCPCS manual includes codes for both the equipment used to deliver the therapy and the nutritional solutions. When coding for these services, be sure to include all codes that apply to the given situation.

CMS Hospital Outpatient Payment System

The codes in this section are used to bill for services that are covered under the Outpatient Prospective Payment System (OPPS). This system uses the Ambulatory Payment Classifications (APCs) to bill for outpatient hospital services. This payment classification system will be discussed in detail in Chapter 15.

Durable Medical Equipment

Durable medical equipment (DME) is an item that can be used for an extended time without significant deterioration (i.e., it can stand repeated use). Therefore, an item that can be rented and returned for reuse would meet the requirement for durability. Medical supplies of a disposable nature, such as incontinent pads and surgical stockings, would not qualify as durable.

Medically oriented equipment is primarily and customarily used for medical purposes (i.e., it is designed to fulfill a medical need). Therefore, it is generally not useful in the absence of an illness or injury. For example, an air conditioner may be used in the case of a heart patient to lower room temperature and reduce fluid loss. However, because the primary and customary use is nonmedical in nature, an air conditioner cannot be considered medical equipment. If the item could be used in a regular manner in the absence of a diagnosis, it is probably nonmedical in nature.

DME BILLING PROCEDURES. Most plans allow for the purchase or temporary rental of equipment and supplies when prescribed by a provider. However, certain requirements must be satisfied.

Basically, three tests must be applied to items billed as DME in determining whether or not the items may be covered under a plan:

1. Does the item satisfy the definition of DME?
2. Is the item reasonable and necessary for the treatment of an illness or injury or for improvement of the functioning of a malformed body part?
3. Is the item prescribed for use in the patient's home?

Only when all three conditions are met will the item be covered by the plan.

An item may meet the definition of DME and yet not be covered by the plan. Two things should be considered:

1. *Reasonableness.* This evaluates the soundness and practicality of the DME approach to therapy, including factors such as:
   a. Is the need for the unit based on failures of other less costly approaches?
   b. Have more conservative means been attempted?

c. What benefits will be derived from the unit?

d. Do the benefits justify the expense?

2. *Necessity.* Equipment is necessary when it is expected to make a meaningful contribution to the treatment of the patient's illness or injury or to the improvement of the functioning of a malformed body part.

Many plans cover the use of oxygen under DME benefits. Even though the oxygen itself is not durable, the canister in which the oxygen is contained and transported is durable (Figure 9-8 ●), and it therefore falls under the category of DME. Charges for delivery of the DME and oxygen are usually covered.

RENTAL VERSUS PURCHASING DETERMINATIONS. If the rental fee for DME is greater than the purchase price, rental is allowed up to but not exceeding the purchase price. Purchase of the item is not required. However, the member should be notified that an expense that is higher than the purchase price may not be allowed.

For DME to be purchased or rented temporarily, the equipment must be prescribed for use in the home. Therefore, any facility that meets at least the minimum requirements of the definition of a hospital or skilled nursing facility is usually excluded from consideration. A patient's home can be considered, but is not limited to, the following:

- His or her own home, apartment, or dwelling
- A relative's home
- A home for the elderly

REPAIRS, REPLACEMENT, AND DELIVERY OF DME. Repairs are covered when necessary to make the equipment functional. If the expense for repairs exceeds the estimated cost of purchasing or renting new equipment for the remaining period of medical need, payment is limited to the lower amount.

Replacements are usually covered in cases of irreparable damage or wear, or when the patient's physical condition has changed. Replacements as a result of wear or changes in the patient's physical condition must be supported by a current provider's order. Replacements as a result of loss may or may not be covered, depending on the circumstances. Usually, replacement is not covered when disrepair or loss results from a patient's carelessness.

DME BILLING REQUIREMENTS. All claims for DME should be documented with the following information:

1. *A description of the equipment prescribed by the provider.* If the item is a commonly used item, a detailed description may not be necessary. However, with new equipment, it is important to try to obtain a marketing or manufacturer's brochure that indicates how the item is constructed and how it functions.

2. *A statement of the medical necessity of the equipment.* This should be in the form of a prescription showing the imprinted name, address, and telephone number of the prescribing provider. The related diagnosis should also be indicated.

3. *An indication as to whether the item is to be rented or purchased, and the rental or purchase price.*

4. *The estimated length of time that the equipment will be needed.* This information will aid in the analysis of whether a rental or a purchase is more economical.

5. *An indication as to where and for how long the equipment will be used.*

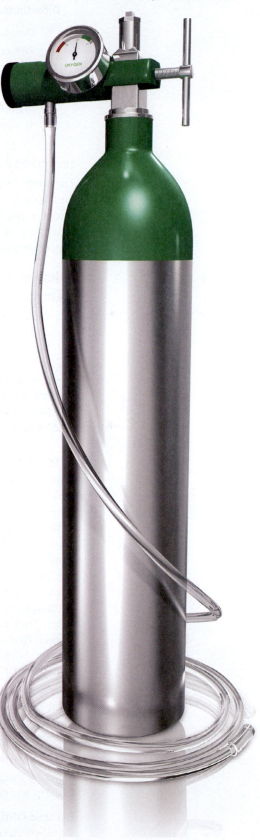

FIGURE 9-8

Canisters in which oxygen is contained and transported are durable.

© dream designs/Shutterstock.com

ACTIVITY #6.

Determining the Correct HCPCS Code for Durable Medical Equipment

Directions: Determine the correct HCPCS codes for the following items.

1. Over-bed table   1. _____
2. Walker, folding, wheeled, adjustable or fixed height   2. _____
3. Raised toiled seat   3. _____
4. Hospital bed, fixed height, with any type side rails with mattress   4. _____
5. Dry pressure mattress   5. _____

Temporary Procedures and Professional Services

The codes listed in this section are often temporary codes set up to identify professional services for which no corresponding CPT code exists. These often are services that are covered by Medicare but may or may not be covered by other insurance carriers.

Many of these codes are deleted when a corresponding CPT code is created. Thus, it is important to use the HCPCS manual for the current year when coding these services.

Behavioral Health and Substance Abuse Treatment Services

The codes in this section identify rehabilitative services, such as alcohol or drug abuse treatment. These services are often covered under the mental health portion of a health plan.

Many insurance carriers are recognizing the role that drug and alcohol abuse plays in affecting the health of the patient. For that reason, many carriers will reimburse for rehabilitative services. In addition, many companies will cover the costs for these services if they think it will help them to retain a good employee.

Many of these codes are specific to a certain type of facility. It is important to determine the type of facility providing the treatment before using the codes in this section.

Drugs Other Than Chemotherapy

This is one of the most frequently used sections when coding administration of medications. J codes indicate the name of the drug, the dosage, and the method of administration. When coding drug usage, it is important to verify the dosage amount and method of administration contained in the code description. The amount is often a standard dosage amount, or portion of a dosage amount. Most medications are administered IM, IV, or SC rather than orally. There are a limited number of oral medications included.

Each method of administration can have a different code. In order to code properly, you must take into account the drug used, the amount given, and the administration method used. Although the drugs in this section are somewhat alphabetical, many drugs will appear out of order. They may be in order of their brand name, as that is the name that was applied to the drug when it first came out (and when the HCPCS code was first assigned).

Temporary Codes Assigned to DME Regional Carriers

This section contains codes that were temporarily assigned for use by Durable Medical Equipment Regional Carriers (DMERCs). All Medicare DME claims should be submitted to one of the four regional carriers. The proper regional carrier for the claim is dependent on the residence of the beneficiary, not the point where the DME item was purchased.

● **ONLINE INFORMATION:** For a list of the DMERCs and the areas they serve, you can go to the Medicare Web site at www.cms.gov/DMEPOSFeeSched/Downloads/DMEPOS_Jurisidiction_List.zip and download the .zip file.

Because DME claims are sent to and processed by different carriers than are medical and professional services, it is important not to mix DME and services on the same claim.

These codes often will further define a piece of durable medical equipment that was ordered for a patient. For example, this section will list several additional types of wheelchairs and wheelchair attachments. The codes in this section are often deleted when no longer needed. This can be a result of an additional code being created in the regular DME codes (E codes), or from the equipment no longer being considered valid treatment for a given condition or situation. These codes should only be used when you are instructed to do so by the DMERC in your area. Otherwise, the closest regular DME codes should be used.

Because these codes are temporary, numerous changes are made to this listing every year. For that reason, it is important to always use a current HCPCS manual when coding in this section.

Orthotics

Orthotics are devices used to correct a deformity or disability. They also are used to correct misalignment of the joints, especially the joints used for walking. Orthotics can be as small as a lift placed inside the shoe or as large as a brace to correct curvature of the spine.

When billing for an orthotic device, you will need to include a copy of the prescription with the complete diagnosis. Some carriers may even require pictures to be taken to document the need for the device. Other carriers may request literature from the manufacturer of the device explaining how the device is used and the benefits to the patient.

Before billing for these items, it is best to contact the insurance carrier and ask what its guidelines are. The carrier can inform you of any documentation you will need to submit with the claim. Submitting the documentation at the same time as you submit the claim can prevent a delay in processing.

Prosthetics

Prosthetic devices are designed to replace a missing body part or to restore some function to a paralyzed body part. Prosthetic devices include the making and application of an artificial part medically necessary to replace a lost or impaired body part or function, such as an artificial arm or leg.

Prosthetics are intended to replace body parts that are permanently damaged. Many carriers will accept the provider's decision that the body part needs to be replaced. If the judgment of the attending provider is that the condition is of long or indefinite duration, the test of permanence is met.

Covered expenses associated with prosthetics include the following:

- Shipping and handling as part of the purchase price
- Temporary postoperative prostheses
- Replacement charges when replacement is a result of a change in the patient's physical condition, and not for wear and tear (Children often need replacement prostheses every six to 12 months, depending on their growth rate and other factors).

Other Medical Services

This section contains very few codes. The reason this section is so small is that most procedures that would be listed here are already listed in the CPT. Thus, the CPT would be the main coding manual for these medical services. Often, the codes that are included in this section are considered new or experimental.

The modifiers included in this section will often designate the type of provider involved. This can include psychologists, clinical social workers, and so on.

Laboratory Services

The codes in this section are for pathology and laboratory tests. Many of these codes are not listed in the CPT.

Some of the codes in this section are for the testing of blood or blood parts (e.g., plasma, platelets) to ensure that they are free of disease before being transfused into a patient. There also are codes for the separation of blood into the various specific components that a patient might need.

A few of the tests in this section (e.g., Pap smears) can be split into the technical component (the person or facility taking the test or drawing the blood) and the professional component (the person interpreting the test results). If the provider performs the test, but does not interpret the results, it is important to use the modifier -TC to indicate that the charge is for the technical component.

Temporary Codes Assigned by CMS

This section is used for creating temporary codes. This list will contain codes that are current, as well as codes that have been superseded by a permanent HCPCS code. Some codes will be superseded by a CPT code that has been added to the CPT.

This section includes many types of procedures and services. Many of these codes pertain to new drugs that have been added to the market. As with the other temporary code sections, the items in this section will be changed frequently, so it is important to use the current HCPCS manual when coding.

Diagnostic Radiology Services

This short section is for recording transportation of x-ray or EKG equipment to a nursing home or other facility. In situations in which more than one patient is to be seen, or where the patient is too fragile to be moved, it is easier to transport the equipment to the patient.

Vision Services

The codes in this section are used to report services performed on or pertaining to the eyes, including eyeglasses, contacts, prosthetic eyes, lenses, or other items pertaining to the care and use of the eyes or vision correction.

The codes in this section can be very specific regarding the type of lenses used and other factors. Because of this, special training may be needed to code these services properly. Any devices ordered in this section must have a prescription written by an authorized provider. A copy of this prescription should be submitted with the claim.

Hearing Services

The codes in this section are used for reporting services in regard to hearing. This includes hearing testing, as well as devices used to assist those who are hearing impaired (e.g., hearing aids). Other assistive living devices (e.g., telephone amplifier, television caption decoder) are also included in this section. There also are codes for speech-language services such as speech screening.

A prescription written by an authorized provider must be provided for any devices ordered in this section. A copy of this prescription should be submitted with the claim.

Modifiers

Each section of the HCPCS manual has modifiers that are unique to that section. It is important that medical billers check the modifiers for each section before billing a claim. Without the proper modifiers, claim payment may be delayed or denied. This is especially true in the case of Medicare claims. Not including the appropriate modifier also can cause incorrect reimbursement.

Modifiers in the HCPCS manual are usually two-digit letter codes. In some cases, two separate one-digit letter codes will be combined to make up a single two-digit letter code. For example, in the transportation services section, the first letter indicates where the patient was picked up and the second letter indicates where the patient was delivered.

CHAPTER REVIEW

Summary

- The ICD-9-CM is used to code diagnoses and conditions.
- The CPT is used to code procedures and services rendered by providers.
- The PDR assists in determining whether a drug is prescription or nonprescription, and lists some of the properties (e.g., manufacturer, chemical makeup, side effects, appearance) of a specific drug.

- Medical dictionaries list medical terms and their meanings.
- *The Merck Manual* can assist in determining whether a service or procedure is appropriate for a given diagnosis or condition.
- There are two levels of HCPCS coding.

    Level 1. Contains only the CPT codes and modifiers.
    Level 2. Includes the codes found in sections A through V of the HCPCS manual.

Review Questions

Directions: Answer the following questions without looking back into the material just covered. Write your answers in the space provided.

1. Which manuals are used for coding diagnoses? _____

    _____

2. The full name of the PDR is _____

3. If you needed to verify a diagnosis, affected body area, or spelling of terms and definitions, you would probably refer to the _____

    _____

4. What are medications? _____

    _____

5. Explain the difference between a legend and a nonlegend drug. _____

    _____

6. Name the six sections of the PDR.

    a. _____

    b. _____

    c. _____

    d. _____

    e. _____

    f. _____

7. (True or False?) Controlled drugs can be purchased over the counter. _____

8. What is the HCPCS manual used for? _____

    _____

9. What are the two coding levels of HCPCS?

    a. _____

    _____

    b. _____

    _____

10. What are the three tests that are applied to DME items to determine if they will be covered under a plan?

    a. _____

    _____

b. _____

_____

c. _____

_____

If you are unable to answer any of these questions, refer back to that section in the chapter, and then fill in the answers.

Activity #7: Selecting the Correct Reference Book—Part 2

Directions: Determine the correct reference book needed to answer the following questions, and then use that reference to find the answer. Do not be concerned if you do not understand all the words in the description or answer.

1. What do the initials AIDS and HIV stand for? _____

_____

2. Which of the following is the correct diagnosis code for AIDS? 079.53, V01.7, 042, or 795.71?

_____

_____

_____

3. Describe AIDS. _____

_____

_____

4. How is AIDS transmitted among adults? _____

_____

_____

5. How is AIDS transmitted to infants? _____

_____

6. What is the description of the code 43842, and is it an appropriate treatment for an AIDS patient? _____

_____

_____

7. What are the descriptions of the codes 86701, 86702, and 86703, and are any of them an appropriate procedure for a suspected AIDS patient? _____

_____

_____

_____

8. If the patient is a Medicare patient and receives an injection of interferon, would you use the code J9213 or 90772, and why? _____

_____

_____

_____

9. What precautions should medical personnel take when treating someone with AIDS?_____

_____

_____

_____

10. What book would tell you if a specific drug was considered effective against the given condition?

_____

_____

_____

Activity #8: Selecting the Correct Reference Book—Part 3

Directions: Determine the correct reference book needed to answer the following questions, and then use that reference to find the answer. Do not be concerned if you do not understand all the words in the description or answer.

1. What is the English-language description for the diagnosis code 696.1? _____

_____

2. Describe the disease from question 1. _____

_____

_____

3. What are erythematous papules? _____

_____

_____

4. What is the cause of the disease in question 1? _____

_____

5. Name two symptoms or signs of this disease.

    a. _____

    b. _____

6. Name two possible treatments for this disease.

    a. _____

    b. _____

7. What is the English-language description for the procedure code 97028? _____

_____

8. Is procedure code 97028 a valid treatment for diagnosis code 696.1? _____

9. Should a patient with this disease expose themselves to sunlight? _____

10. Does smoking affect this condition? If so, in what way? _____

_____

Activity #9: Determining the Correct HCPCS Code—Part 1

Directions: Determine the correct HCPCS codes for the following procedures/items.

1. Moisture exchanger, disposable, for use with invasive mechanical ventilation   1. _____
2. Detailed and extensive oral evaluation—problem focused   2. _____
3. Application of desensitizing medicaments   3. _____
4. Injection of calcium gluconate, per 10 ml   4. _____
5. Air pressure mat   5. _____
6. Cellular therapy   6. _____
7. Stomach tube (Levin type)   7. _____
8. Sitz bath chair   8. _____
9. Jaw motion rehabilitation system   9. _____
10. Dialysis equipment, unspecified   10. _____
11. Replace quadrilateral socket brim; molded to patient model   11. _____
12. Cardiokymography   12. _____
13. Lenticular, nonaspheric, per lens, bifocal   13. _____
14. Speech screening   14. _____
15. Assessment for hearing aid   15. _____
16. Oral thermometer, reusable   16. _____
17. Collagen skin test kit   17. _____
18. Injection, tetracycline, 200 mg   18. _____
19. Ambulatory surgical boot   19. _____
20. Prosthetic implant   20. _____
21. Potassium hydroxide (KOH) preparation   21. _____
22. Transportation of portable EKG to nursing home   22. _____
23. Infusion of normal saline solution, 250 cc   23. _____
24. Botulinum toxin type A, 2 units   24. _____
25. Orthodontic treatment (non-contract fee)   25. _____
26. House call   26. _____
27. Rollabout chair, 6-inch casters   27. _____
28. Dialysis blood leak detector   28. _____
29. Splint   29. _____
30. Men's orthopedic oxford shoes   30. _____

Activity #10: Determining the Correct HCPCS Code—Part 2

Directions: Determine the correct HCPCS codes for the following procedures/items.

1. Synthetic vascular graft material implant   1. _____
2. Artificial larynx, BV type   2. _____
3. Thoracic low-profile extension, lateral   3. _____
4. Azithromycin dihydrate capsules, 1 gm   4. _____

5. Infusion chemo treatment   5. _____

6. Triam A injection, 10 mg   6. _____

7. Sterile syringe, 30 cc   7. _____

8. Amalgam, 2 surfaces, primary   8. _____

9. Tigan injection, 100 mg   9. _____

10. Raised toilet seat   10. _____

11. Apnea monitor, with recording feature   11. _____

12. Dexasone LA injection   12. _____

13. Assessment for hearing aid   13. _____

14. Epoetin alpha injection, 1,500 units (non ESRD)   14. _____

15. Hot water bottle   15. _____

16. Bed board   16. _____

17. Cervical collar molded to patient   17. _____

18. Celestone Soluspan, 3 mg   18. _____

19. Nonelastic binder for extremity   19. _____

20. Canal preparation and fitting   20. _____

21. Pediatric speech aid   21. _____

22. Fresh, frozen plasma   22. _____

23. Preparation of vaginal wet mount   23. _____

24. Gas impermeable contact lens   24. _____

25. Reverse osmosis water purifier   25. _____

26. Reimplantation of tooth   26. _____

27. Tylenol, nonprescription   27. _____

28. Duoval-Pa   28. _____

29. Hemodialysis machine   29. _____

30. Insulin injection, 100 units   30. _____

Activity #11: Match the Following Terms

Directions: Match the following terms with the proper definition by writing the letter of the correct definition in the space next to the term.

1. _____ Reference book

a. An index used for billing injections, medication, supplies, and durable medical equipment

2. _____ Durable medical equipment

b. Equipment that is primarily and customarily used for medical purposes

3. _____ Provider's Current Procedure Terminology

c. A drug that may be purchased without a prescription; also known as a nonlegend drug

4. _____ Durable Medical Equipment Regional Carriers

d. An indexing of diseases and conditions

5. _____ *International Classification of Diseases—9th Revision, Clinical Modification*

e. Source of information to which a reader is referred

6. _____ Medically oriented equipment

7. _____ *Health Care Common Procedure Coding System*

8. _____ Over-the-counter drug

f. One of four regional Medicare carriers responsible for the processing of durable medical equipment claims

g. A systematic listing for coding the procedures or services performed by a provider

h. Equipment that can withstand repeated use, is primarily and customarily used to serve a medical purpose, is generally not useful to a person in the absence of an illness or injury, and is appropriate for use in the home

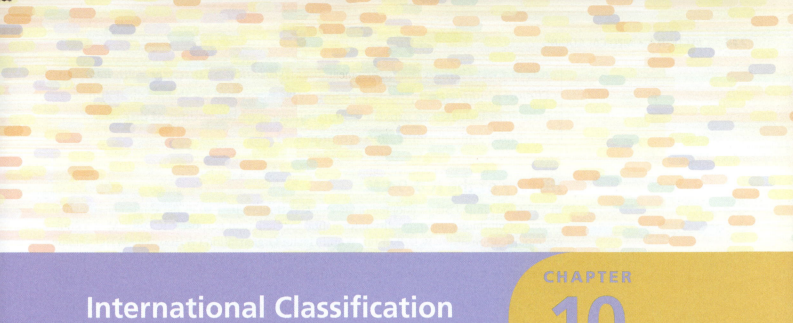

International Classification of Diseases (ICD-9-CM) Coding

After completion of this chapter you should be able to:

Discuss the history of the ICD-9-CM and why it was created.

Describe the contents of each volume of the ICD-9-CM.

Describe how each volume of the ICD-9-CM is arranged.

State the guidelines concerning ICD-9-CM coding.

Describe main terms and how they are used.

Identify and describe the common signs and symbols used in the ICD-9-CM.

List the important factors to be aware of when using ICD-9-CM codes for billing.

Describe how to handle downgrading of codes and concurrent care situations.

Convert the English-language description of an illness or injury into a numeric ICD-9-CM code.

Key Words and Concepts you will learn in this chapter:

Benign
Concurrent care
E code listing
Eponyms
ICD-9-CM
Main terms
Malignant
Malignant CA in situ
Malignant primary
Malignant secondary
Neoplasm
Subterms
V code listing

ICD-9-CM refers to the *International Classification of Diseases—9th Revision, Clinical Modification.* This is a coding system devised by the medical and insurance industry to provide standardization of the coding of diseases, conditions, impairments, and symptoms.

History of the ICD-9-CM

In 1979, the United States adopted the ICD-9-CM (Figure 10-1 ●) as the single classification system of morbidity and mortality information for statistical purposes. ICD-9-CM is a clinical modification of the ICD-9 of the World Health Organization (WHO). The WHO version has been in existence since the early 1900s. The WHO originally created the ICD as a means of compiling data on morbidity and mortality and allowing hospitals and clinics to restore and retrieve diagnostic data.

In 1956, the American Hospital Association and the American Association of Medical Record Librarians (now known as the American Health Information Management Association, or AHIMA) undertook a study of the efficacies of coding systems for diagnostic indexing. That study concluded that the ICD provided a good framework for hospital indexing.

In 1977, the National Center for Health Statistics convened a steering committee to provide advice and counsel on revisions that should be made to the ICD-9-CM. This created the ICD-9-CM, which is a clinical modification of WHO's ICD-9-CM.

Each year the ICD-9-CM is updated. On release of the revised information by the U.S. Department of Health and Human Services, numerous publishing companies print their own version of the information contained in the ICD-9-CM. All these publications contain the same basic information; however, publishers add various options—such as color coding, section tabs, helpful symbols, and various instructions and aids— to make theirs the most preferred version. The decision of which publisher's version of the ICD-9-CM to use is simply a matter of individual or company choice.

▶ **CRITICAL THINKING QUESTION:** How does the use of standardized codes, such as ICD-9-CM codes, help communication between the medical office and insurance carriers?

Contents of the ICD-9-CM

The ICD-9-CM comprises three volumes.

Volume I. The tabular or numerical listings of diagnoses are structured numerically according to body system. The body systems are arranged as follows:

1. Infectious and Parasitic Diseases
2. Neoplasms
3. Endocrine, Nutritional, and Metabolic Diseases, and Immunity Disorders
4. Diseases of the Blood and Blood-Forming Organs
5. Mental Disorders
6. Diseases of the Nervous System and Sense Organs
7. Diseases of the Circulatory System
8. Diseases of the Respiratory System
9. Diseases of the Digestive System
10. Diseases of the Genitourinary System
11. Complications of Pregnancy, Childbirth, and the Puerperium
12. Diseases of the Skin and Subcutaneous Tissue
13. Diseases of the Musculoskeletal System and Connective Tissue

FIGURE 10-1

ICD-9-CM code book

Reprinted by permission of the American Medical Association.

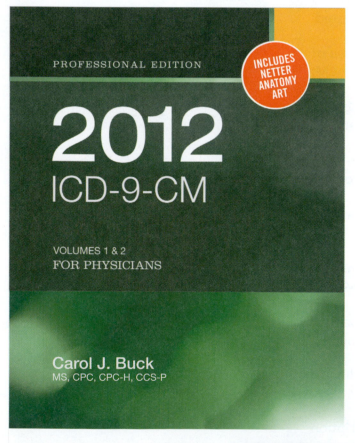

14. Congenital Anomalies
15. Certain Conditions Originating in the Perinatal Period
16. Symptoms, Signs, and Ill-Defined Conditions
17. Injury and Poisoning

Volume I also contains a section that provides a listing of factors affecting the health status of an individual (V codes).

Volume I is used when:

- An ICD-9-CM code is provided, but there is no language description of the diagnosis, or
- A language diagnosis is included, but an ICD-9-CM code is not indicated and the terms used by the provider cannot be found in Volume II. If you can identify the body system, you may be able to locate an appropriate ICD-9-CM code.

A number in parentheses after a code is the page number in Volume II that can be checked to verify the code. Table 10-1 ● shows the codes for Volume I.

Volume II. Volume II is divided into four sections:

- An alphabetical index of diseases and injuries
- A table of drugs and chemicals
- An alphabetical index of external causes of injuries and poisonings (accidents) (E codes)
- A summary of additions and revisions to Volume I

Volume III. A numeric listing of surgical procedure codes are found here. Volume III contains both a tabular listing and index. The tabular listing has procedures arranged according to body sections. The body sections are arranged as follows:

1. Operations on the Nervous System
2. Operations on the Endocrine System
3. Operations on the Eye
4. Operations on the Ear
5. Operations on the Nose, Mouth, and Pharynx
6. Operations on the Respiratory System
7. Operations on the Cardiovascular System
8. Operations on the Hemic and Lymphatic System
9. Operations on the Digestive System
10. Operations on the Urinary System
11. Operations on the Male Genital Organs
12. Operations on the Female Genital Organs
13. Obstetrical Procedures
14. Operations on the Musculoskeletal System
15. Operations on the Integumentary System
16. Miscellaneous Diagnostic and Therapeutic Procedures

The index lists procedures in alphabetical order. The medical biller should confirm any choice of code by looking in the tabular listing and checking all referrals, exclusions, and notes included.

How to Use the ICD-9-CM

The ICD-9-CM is structured to move from a general diagnosis to a more specific diagnosis by adding on digits. It uses three-, four-, or five-digit codes. Three-digit codes are the most general. By adding additional digits, a more precise diagnosis is identified.

A variety of different types of medical insurance processing systems are available. No matter the system, very precise coding is required.

When performing ICD-9-CM coding, the medical biller should always code to the highest number of digits possible: the highest degree of specificity. This includes four- and five-digit subclassifications wherever they occur. **Subterms** are secondary classifications under a main term.

TABLE 10-1 ICD-9-CM: Organization of Volume I

Number	Body System/Classification
001–139	Infectious and Parasitic Diseases
140–239	Neoplasms
240–279	Endocrine, Nutritional, and Metabolic Diseases, and Immunity Disorders
280–289	Diseases of the Blood and Blood-Forming Organs
290–319	Mental Disorders
320–389	Diseases of the Nervous System and Sense Organs
390–459	Diseases of the Circulatory System
460–519	Diseases of the Respiratory System
520–579	Diseases of the Digestive System
580–629	Diseases of the Genitourinary System
630–679	Complications of Pregnancy, Childbirth, and the Puerperium
680–709	Diseases of the Skin and Subcutaneous Tissue
710–739	Diseases of the Musculoskeletal System and Connective Tissue
740–759	Congenital Anomalies
760–779	Certain Conditions Originating in the Perinatal Period
780–799	Symptoms, Signs, and Ill-Defined Conditions
800–999	Injury and Poisoning
V01–V91	Supplementary Classification of Factors Influencing Health Status and Contact with Health Services
E000–E999	Supplementary Classification of External Causes of Injury and Poisoning

General Guidelines for ICD-9-CM

The following basic guidelines should be kept in mind when locating and using the proper ICD-9-CM code:

1. Read through the introduction of the ICD-9-CM to ensure your understanding of any color coding, symbols, abbreviations, and terms that the book uses. Be aware that different publishers may use different symbols and colors.

2. Always use both the Alphabetic Index Listing (Volume II) and the Numeric Tabular Listing (Volume I). Volume II alone will not give you any exclusions, referrals, or instructions for the codes, including the need for four- or five-digit subclassifications.

3. When performing inpatient coding, always code the principal diagnosis. The official Uniform Hospital Discharge Data Set (UHDDS) definition of the principal diagnosis is "the condition established after study to be chiefly responsible for occasioning the admission of the patient to the hospital for care."

   a. For outpatient coding, do not code symptoms or the suspected condition if a final diagnosis is indicated. Symptoms and suspected conditions are usually accompanied by terms such as *probable, suspected, questionable,* or *Rule out (R/O).*

   b. It is understood that some conditions will not be fully diagnosed until test results have provided further understanding of the condition; in such cases, code conditions to the highest degree of certainty for the encounter. For example, many codes contain a fourth or fifth digit, which is for "unspecified" conditions or types. Often this will be indicated by the abbreviation NOS for "Not Otherwise Specified." These codes are acceptable if this is the highest level of certainty documented by the provider at this encounter.

4. Code the diagnosis to the highest number of digits possible. For example, do not use only three digits to describe a condition when four- and five-digit subclassifications exist for that category.

5. Code only the diagnosis determined by the provider and any complications. Do not list any codes for previous conditions that were previously treated and that no longer exist.

6. The main diagnosis, condition, or reason for the encounter should be listed first. All other conditions that coexist at the time of treatment and that affect the treatment are to be coded following the main diagnosis. If several conditions equally resulted in the encounter, the

provider may choose which to list first, unless instructed otherwise by the ICD-9-CM Official Guidelines or instructional notes.

7. When a patient is seen for ancillary diagnostic services only, the appropriate V code (see "V Codes") should be listed first, and the diagnosis or condition that is the underlying reason for the tests should be listed second. If a second code is not listed, delays in claim processing or denial of benefits may result.

    For example, if a chest X-ray is taken (coded V72.5) and no second code is listed, the claim may be denied if there are no benefits for routine chest X-rays.

8. When a patient is seen for ancillary therapeutic services only, the appropriate V code should be listed first, and the diagnosis or condition that is the underlying reason for the services should be listed second.

9. Diagnosis codes for chronic diseases or conditions may be coded as often as needed when the patient has repeated encounters for the chronic disease or condition.

10. Diagnoses that relate to earlier episodes of care or are chronic and have no bearing on the current treatment are to be excluded.

11. When billing for surgical procedures, use the correct code to indicate the diagnosis or reason for the surgery. If a postoperative diagnosis is different from the preoperative diagnosis, and the postoperative diagnosis is known at the time the claim is submitted, you should code the postoperative diagnosis.

12. Adjectives (acute, chronic, and the like) may appear as subterms. For example, the diagnosis of acute pelvic inflammatory disease may be located in the following manner:

    a. Look up the condition—disease.
    b. Under disease, refer to the subheading (site) of pelvis, pelvic.
    c. Locate the specific condition—inflammatory (female) (PID).
    d. Finally, locate manifestation, acute—614.3.

13. Cross-reference to synonyms, closely related terms, and code categories beginning with "See" and "See also"—for example, "Pelvic-peritonitis (See also peritonitis, pelvic, female)."

14. Carefully read any and all notes under the main term. These can include exclusions, referrals, and examples of diagnoses or conditions.

15. Carefully note any modifiers associated with the main term. Compare these with any qualifying terms used in the diagnosis statement.

16. Watch for subterms listed under a main term. Subterms become more specific the further down they go.

These guidelines should be memorized and used whenever you are attempting to assign an ICD-9-CM code. They will ensure a higher degree of accuracy and a higher rate of correct benefit payment on claims.

Main Terms

The alphabetic index is arranged by condition, disease, or syndrome. These identifying names are called the main terms and are the keys by which this volume is structured. The **main terms** usually identify disease conditions rather than locations. For instance, when coding a gastric ulcer, the main term would be ulcer and the anatomic site would be gastric. The main terms may be listed as proper medical terms or ill-defined terms or as eponyms. **Eponyms** are illnesses or conditions named after a person (e.g., Gerhardt's Disease). Certain conditions may be listed under more than one term. For example, Streptococcal tonsillitis (Figure 10-2 ●) can be located in two ways:

- Under *tonsillitis* (subheading: *streptococcal*)
- Under *infection* (subheading: *streptococcal, site—sore throat*)

Streptococcal is not a condition; it is the type of organism involved in an infection.

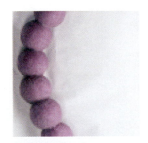

FIGURE 10-2

A chain of streptococci

© Denis Finnin and Jackie Beckett/Pearson Education

PRACTICE **PITFALLS**

Carefully read through the beginning sections of your ICD-9-CM manual. This will give you a lot of additional information on properly using the manual. This is one of your best sources for learning how to use the ICD-9-CM.

Some other examples of conditions that may be listed under more than one term include the following:

- Dislocated shoulder
- Pulmonary edema
- Pelvic abscess
- Prolapsed uterus
- Fractured radius
- Sick sinus syndrome
- Chronic hepatitis
- External hemorrhoids

It is important to note that a diagnosis may be described as an acute or chronic condition. Acute conditions are usually severe and sudden in onset, whereas a chronic condition develops and worsens over a period of time.

ACTIVITY #1

Identifying the Main Term

Directions: Identify the main term and write it in the space provided.

Acute bronchitis	_____
Heart palpitations	_____
Rectal leukoplakia	_____
Pernicious anemia	_____
Bacterial meningitis	_____
Ulcerative colitis	_____
Rosacea acne	_____
Recurrent urethritis	_____
Diabetes mellitus	_____
Internal hemorrhoids	_____

Exceptions

In some instances, the ICD-9-CM is organized differently so that the main terms do not identify disease conditions. These exceptions include the following:

1. Obstetric conditions, which are found under "Delivery," "Pregnancy," or "Puerperal" (*Puerperal* refers to the period immediately following delivery.)
2. Complications of medical and surgical conditions, which are located under "Complications" (However, they can also be found under the condition. For example, "evisceration" of an operative wound can be found under *evisceration* and *complication*. It is recommended that you look under the condition.)
3. Late effects of diseases and injuries, which are under the main term "late effects"
4. In some situations, a claim or bill may provide a "diagnosis" that is not a sickness or injury per se. For example, *exposure to, history of, problem with,* or *vaccination* are not diagnoses but may be considered appropriate main terms.

Appropriate sites or modifiers are listed in alphabetical sequence under the main terms with further subterm listings as required. For example, the diagnosis of open tibia/fibula fracture may be located as follows:

See Fracture heading

Locate tibia as a subheading

Site—with fibula

Description—open = 823.92

PRACTICE **PITFALLS**

The medical biller is limited to the available number of spaces on the billing form. List only the main conditions up to the number of spaces provided.

Once you have identified the code in the indexed listing (Volume II), cross-reference your selection with the tabular listing in Volume I. This will ensure that you have selected the proper code. It also will allow you to code to the highest degree of specificity.

Be sure to research any exclusions, referrals ("See also"), and examples to ensure that your code is correct. Also be sure to refer to the three- and four-digit classification headings. These headings often have further information or list the fourth and fifth digits that apply to all following codes in that classification.

For example, let's use the dislocated shoulder mentioned previously. The index lists the three-digit classification for a dislocated shoulder as 831. However, a four-digit classification will tell whether the injury is open or closed, and a five-digit classification will pinpoint the diagnosis as to the more precise location of the injury. Also, note that a chronic or recurrent shoulder dislocation has an entirely different three-digit classification of 718.

Now turn to classification 831 in the tabular listing. You will see that the five-digit sub-classifications are listed directly below the three-digit classification heading. This is followed by the three-digit classifications and the four-digit classifications.

The reason for this order can be better understood when you look at the codes 800–804. Each of these codes is for a fracture of the skull. The five-digit codes that immediately follow the classification heading can be used with any of the three- or four-digit classifications that begin with the numbers 800, 801, 803, or 804. The classifications for 804 appear several pages later. This is why it is important to always look back to the four- and three-digit classification headings when coding.

NEOPLASMS. A **neoplasm** is a growth (tumor) that results from abnormal cell activity (Figure 10-3 ●). Selecting an ICD-9-CM code for a neoplasm involves identifying the following factors:

- The pathologic status of the growth—benign or malignant
- The site of the growth—breast, lung, bladder
- The cell type (e.g., oat cell)

This information is not always provided on medical reports, claims, or bills. Therefore, as with any other diagnosis, the code selected will be based on the available information. The more information provided, the more specific the code.

For coding growths or tumors, you need to become familiar with the ICD-9-CM Neoplasm Table (NT) located in Volume II. This table is organized alphabetically by site (location). Because the site is not always known, there is an entry for "unknown site or unspecified."

On the right side of the Neoplasm Table are six columns from which to select an ICD-9-CM code based on the given diagnosis. The first three columns relate to malignant neoplasms. Malignant means that the cancer or growth is growing. Malignant growths will spread throughout the body until they kill the patient. The first three columns are defined as follows:

Malignant primary. *Primary* means that the site of the tumor is the point of origin of the neoplasm.

Malignant secondary. *Secondary* means that the site of the tumor in question is not where the disease originated. It has spread to this location from the primary site.

Malignant CA in situ. *In situ* means that the malignant growth is still localized in one area and has not spread within the organ of origin.

The last three columns in the neoplasm table include codes related to the following neoplasms:

Benign. This term describes a localized growth that does not spread (metastasize) and is not usually terminal.

FIGURE 10-3

Lichen planus, a type of neoplasm that can appear in the oral cavity

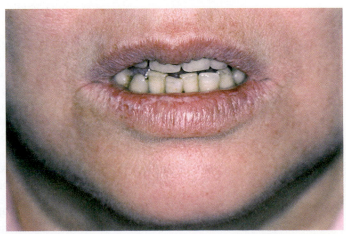

Uncertain behavior. In this situation we have determined that the growth is malignant or benign but the behavior of the growth is yet to be determined. In cases in which the information does not establish which type of manifestation is present and the growth could be either, this coding may be used. As a rule, this column should be used only when the neoplasm's behavior is stated to be uncertain by a pathologist or provider or is listed as such in the alphabetic index.

Unspecified. A growth is unspecified when it is not identified as benign or malignant; the type of growth is always one or the other.

The first step in coding growths is to determine whether the growth is benign or malignant. If the status is indicated, go directly to the table under either the malignant or benign column, according to the site of the growth. Choose the malignant column based on the specifics of the diagnosis—primary, secondary, or in situ.

For example:

Diagnosis: Benign Neoplasm of Breast

ACTION: **1.** Find neoplasm first in Volume II
                 2. Under neoplasm look up breast
                 3. Then look in the column for benign
                 4. Code is 217

Diagnosis: CA in Situ—Uterus

ACTION: **1.** Find neoplasm first in Volume II
                 2. Under neoplasm look up uterus
                 3. Then look for malignant
                 4. The code is 233.2

Diagnosis: Brain Tumor

ACTION: **1.** Find neoplasm first in Volume II
                 2. Under neoplasm look up brain
                 3. Then look for unspecified
                 4. The code is 239.6

If a growth is identified as malignant but is not further identified as primary, secondary, or CA in situ, code it is as primary.

The terms *CA, cancer, carcinoma,* and *sarcoma* always indicate a malignancy. Other terms, such as *fibroma* and *adenoma,* require you to check the alphabetical listing (not the Neoplasm Table) of Volume II to determine whether the condition is benign or malignant. Subsequently, the proper column in the Neoplasm Table can be referenced.

For example:

If the diagnosis is:	Look under the main term:
Pelvic fibroma	Fibroma
Adenoma	Adenoma
Adenosarcoma	Adenosarcoma
Papilloma, eyelid	Papilloma
Osteosarcoma	Osteosarcoma

In most cases, looking under the appropriate main term will direct you to the correct column in the Neoplasm Table. In some circumstances, however, you will be given a valid ICD-9-CM code by the provider and you will not need to reference the Neoplasm Table at all.

As you can see, the reference under the main term identifies whether the neoplasm is benign or malignant. In the case of adenosarcoma, a valid ICD-9-CM code (189.0) is given and the Neoplasm Table did not have to be checked. Remember that M codes are disregarded. Also note that the "See also" reference, which is usually optional, must be followed in the case of neoplasms. Over time, you may learn which neoplasms are benign or malignant and may be able to go directly to the Neoplasm Table.

LESIONS. Although lesions are similar to neoplasms, they are treated differently by the ICD-9-CM. Lesions should be handled as indicated in the following statements:

> ### ACTIVITY #2
>
> ## Determining the Correct ICD-9-CM Code
>
> **Directions:**   Locate the appropriate ICD-9-CM code and write it in the space provided.
>
> 1. Benign breast tumor   _____
>
> 2. CA in situ, uterus   _____
>
> 3. Lung tumor   _____
>
> 4. Secondary CA, pancreas   _____
>
> 5. Primary CA, pylorus   _____
>
> 6. Carcinoma in situ, trachea   _____
>
> 7. Malignant tumor duodenum   _____
>
> 8. Cancer, rectum   _____
>
> 9. Sarcoma, skin   _____
>
> 10. Brain tumor   _____

If the diagnosis simply states "lesion," look under the main term lesion alphabetically in Volume II.

If the diagnosis is "benign lesion," look under the main term *lesion.*

If the diagnosis is "malignant lesion," look under one of the malignant columns in the Neoplasm Table in Volume II.

SPRAINS/STRAINS. Sprains and strains are coded according to the site of injury. Strains of the musculoskeletal system are included under the main term *Sprain.* There is a separate main term reference for strains that are not related to the musculoskeletal system (such as eyestrain). If the location of a musculoskeletal strain or sprain is unknown, use code 848.9 (musculoskeletal system). Normally, 848.9 is used as a temporary code while additional information is requested from the provider.

DISLOCATIONS. As with strains and sprains, dislocations are coded according to the site of injury. For a unspecified open dislocation code 839.8 should be used. (See previous paragraph.) For an unspecified closed dislocation 839.8 would be used.

A closed dislocation may be simple, complete, partial, uncomplicated, or unspecified (type). Open dislocations include infected, compound, and dislocation with a foreign body.

Chronic, habitual, old, or *recurrent* dislocations may be coded as "dislocation, recurrent, and pathologic."

FRACTURES. As with strains, sprains, and dislocations, fractures are coded according to the site of injury. Various types of fractures are shown in Figure 10-4 ●.

Closed fractures include the following descriptions, with or without delayed healing: comminuted, linear, depressed, march, elevated, simple, fissured, slipped epiphysis, greenstick, spiral, impacted, and unspecified.

Open fractures include compound, infected, missile, puncture with or without a foreign body, with or without delayed healing.

Assume that the fracture is closed unless wording indicates otherwise.

When multiple fractures are involved, it is easier to look under the names of the bones involved than to look under "Fracture, multiple."

V Codes

The **V code listing** is a supplementary listing of factors that affect the health status of the patient. Often there are reasons for an encounter that relate to a disease or condition but do not constitute a diagnosis. There are three main types of occurrences:

1. ***When a person who is not ill has an encounter with a health care provider for a specific purpose that is not in and of itself a disease or condition.*** These encounters can include a visit from a person who is getting a vaccination or a checkup, who is acting as an organ or tissue donor to another person, or who wants to discuss a problem that is not considered a disease or condition (e.g., fertility problems, genetic counseling).

FIGURE 10-4

Various types of fractures

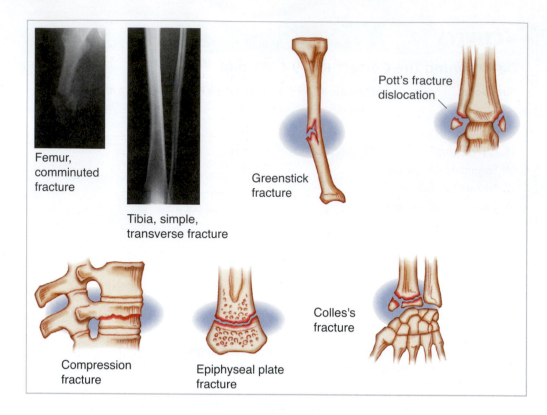

2. *When a patient with a chronic or recurring condition visits a health care provider for service associated with treatment of that condition.* This can include a cast change, dialysis for renal disease, monitoring of pacemaker, and other similar situations.
3. *When a situation arises that influences the person's health but is not a disease or condition.* Such situations include exposure to potential health hazards (e.g., tuberculosis, polio), animal bites that require rabies vaccination, and the fact that a person's physiology or family history suggests a factor that should be borne in mind when treatment is received (e.g., carrier of suspected infectious diseases, history of cancer or other diseases, allergies to medicines).

When performing diagnosis coding in circumstances 2 and 3 above, the V code should be used as a supplementary code (not the primary diagnosis code). The diagnosis or condition that underlies the reason for the treatment (circumstance 2) or that caused the patient to seek medical attention (circumstance 3) should be coded as the primary diagnosis. V codes are arranged according to the following headings:

V01–V06 Persons with potential health hazards related to communicable diseases

V07–V09 Persons with need for isolation, other potential health hazards and prophylactic measures

V10–V19 Persons with potential health hazards related to personal and family history

V20–V29 Persons encountering health services in circumstances related to reproduction and development

V30–V39 Liveborn infants according to type of birth

V40–V49 Persons with a condition influencing their health status

V50–V59 Persons encountering health services for specific procedures and aftercare

V60–V68 Persons encountering health services in other circumstances

V70–V82 Persons without reported diagnosis encountered during examination and investigation of individuals and populations

As a medical biller, you should examine the V codes and familiarize yourself with the situations they define.

E Codes

The **E code listing** is a supplementary classification of external causes of injury and poisoning. E codes are used to indicate the cause of the injury, not the injury itself. Therefore, an E code should always be an additional code, not a primary diagnosis code. For example, a patient was a pedestrian struck by a car and suffered a fractured femur. The diagnosis would be fractured femur (code 821.00), and the cause would be pedestrian struck by automobile (E814.7).

> ### PRACTICE **PITFALLS**
>
> The diagnosis coded must support the services rendered. On the claim form, the diagnosis that relates to each procedure performed is placed next to the procedure code. Therefore, each procedure performed should have a diagnosis that substantiates the need for that procedure.

To correctly code E codes, consult the index located in section 3 of Volume II (behind the table of drugs and chemicals). This index is used the same way the index to diseases and conditions is used. First, locate the cause in the index, then turn to the tabular listing to confirm your choice and to ensure correct four- and five-digit subclassifications.

The beginning of the E code section contains definitions of the terms involved in describing causes. Medical billers should familiarize themselves with these definitions because they are vital to proper coding. When coding transport accidents, the following headings are used:

- Railway (E800–E807)
- Motor Vehicle (E810–E819)
- Motor vehicle nontraffic accidents (E820–E825)
- Other Road Vehicles (E826–E829)
- Water Transport (E830–E838)
- Air and Space (E840–E845)

If you are coding an accident that involves more than one type of vehicle, the order listed here should be followed. For example, let's code an accident between a car and a streetcar. Since a streetcar is considered a railway vehicle, the car would take precedence. Therefore, you would look under the motor vehicle section to find motor vehicle accident involving collision with train (E810). The four-digit subclassification would then be added to this number to describe the activity of the patient at the time of the accident (motor vehicle accident section heading).

If you are coding machinery accidents (nontransport vehicles), you should use category E919.x. This allows for a broad description of the type of machinery and activity that made up the cause of the injury. If you wish to provide a more detailed description, the International Labour Organization has created a Classification of Industrial Accidents According to Agency. However, this classification should be used in addition to the appropriate E code, not in place of it. Some versions of the ICD-9-CM reproduce this classification listing.

On October 1, 2010, two new E code sections went into effect: E000, External Cause Status, and E001–E030, Activity. These sections bring ICD-9-CM E codes closer to ICD-10-CM external cause codes. The E001–E030 section identifies the activity an individual is engaged in when a health condition or injury is incurred; the E000 section differentiates between an individual's civilian or military status. Activity and status codes should be used in addition to external cause codes for the cause, intent, and place of occurrence of the condition or injury. As with the new ICD-9-CM codes, multiple external cause codes may be coded to identify all components of the patient's condition. The external cause status section contains four new codes within one new category:

- E000.0 Civilian activity done for income or pay
- E000.1 Military activity
- E000.2 Volunteer activity
- E000.8 Other external cause status
- E000.9 Unspecified external cause status

The following are examples of broad categories found in the activity section:

- E001 Activities involving walking and running
- E002 Activities involving water and water craft

- E003 Activities involving ice and snow
- E012 Activities involving arts and handcrafts
- E013 Activities involving personal hygiene and household maintenance
- E014 Activities involving person providing caregiving
- E019 Activities involving animal care
- E029 Other activity
- E030 Unspecified activity

Signs and Symbols Used in the ICD-9-CM

Most coding books use signs and symbols to alert you to specific situations with codes. However, different versions of the coding books may have different signs and symbols or none at all.

Listed below are some of the common signs and symbols used in the ICD-9-CM and their meaning:

- • This code is new to this edition of the ICD-9-CM. It has just been added to the list of ICD-9-CM codes.
- ▲ This code has been changed from last year's edition of the ICD-9-CM.
- 4 A fourth digit is required to properly use this code.
- 5 A fifth digit is required to properly use this code.

Many ICD-9-CM codes also have signs or symbols for nonspecific codes or unspecified codes. These codes should only be used as a last resort when no other code is appropriate.

Some ICD-9-CMs also will use colors to signify the fourth- or fifth-digit requirement. For example, a pink box may appear behind the code number.

It is important to understand the meanings of these signs and symbols as they are used in your version of the ICD-9-CM. Without understanding them, your chances of improperly coding a claim can increase greatly.

The details of the signs and symbols used in your version of the ICD-9-CM should appear in the beginning of the book. You should read this section carefully before beginning coding.

Concurrent Care

Often, reimbursement problems arrive when two providers are seeing a patient at the same time for two unrelated medical conditions. This is known as **concurrent care**. Claims were frequently denied as duplication of services when the patient was seen by two providers on the same day, when no duplication actually occurred.

Before 1992, a CPT modifier (75) denoted concurrent care. This modifier has since been dropped. Now there are two ways to ensure the possibility of payment from the payer:

1. Submit two separate claim forms, one for each provider, which list two completely separate diagnoses and the related services that were provided.
2. If the separate providers were members of the same medical group and payment is to be made to the medical group, then all services should be submitted on the same claim form. However, two separate diagnoses should be listed, and the procedures performed for each should be substantiated by the referencing of the separate diagnoses next to the procedure.

ICD-9-CM Volume 3

Volume 3 (Procedure Index and Procedure Table) of ICD-9-CM contains procedure codes, whereas Volumes 1 and 2 contain diagnostic codes. Procedure codes are numbers used to identify specific health interventions taken by medical professionals. The format for Volume 3 is the same as for Volume 1, except the codes consist of two digits before the decimal point and one or two digits following the decimal point. Most conventions for Volume 3 are the same as those for Volume 2 except that some subterms appear immediately below the main term rather than following alphabetizing rules.

▶ **CRITICAL THINKING QUESTION:** How would an incorrect selection of an ICD-9-CM code impact a patient?

ICD-10-CM

Every year the ICD-9-CM is updated, incorporating new diagnoses and revising or eliminating old ones. However, since these are limited revisions, the book continues to be called the ICD-9-CM. Each time there is a major revision of the ICD, it is assigned a new version number. The ICD-9-CM is for the ninth such revision.

ICD-10-CM is the tenth such revision and is effective October 1, 2013. The next two chapters in this text discuss the transition to and use of ICD-10-CM.

CHAPTER REVIEW

Summary

- The ICD-9-CM is the primary book used when coding diagnoses on health claims. It is made up of three volumes. Volume I is the tabular listing of diagnoses and conditions. Volume II is the indexed or alphabetic listing of diagnoses and conditions. Volume III is the tabular and alphabetic listing of procedures.
- To accurately code a diagnosis, locate the main term for the condition under the indexed listing in Volume II. The numeric code located should be checked against the information provided in Volume I, and all referrals, exclusions, and additional digit subclassifications should be consulted to ensure that the right code has been chosen.
- When coding procedures in Volume III, first consult the index, then cross-reference the code with the information provided in the tabular listing.
- Diagnoses that do not substantiate services rendered, match the proper location of services, or otherwise conflict with additional information on the claim form will result in delays and denials of benefit payments.

Review Questions

Directions: Answer the following questions without looking back into the material just covered. Write your answers in the space provided.

1. Volume _____ is the tabular listing of diagnoses in ICD-9-CM.

2. If only a language description of the condition is provided, Volume _____ should be used to locate the numerical listing.

3. Main terms are used to identify the _____

   _____

4. (True or False?) Benign lesions are listed in the Neoplasm Table. _____

5. (True or False?) Always assume fractures are "open" unless otherwise indicated. _____

6. (True or False?) The more digits in the code, the more general the diagnosis. _____

7. (True or False?) Obstetrical-related conditions are handled differently from other main terms. _____

8. (True or False?) "Rule out" is a definitive diagnosis. _____

9. Volume II is used in some instances to determine whether a neoplasm is _____ or _____.

10. The ICD-9-CM is comprised of _____ volumes.

If you are unable to answer any of these questions, refer back to that section in the chapter, and then fill in the answers.

Activity #3: Finding the Main Term and Determining the Correct ICD-9-CM Code—Part 1

Directions: Based on the condition, look up the appropriate ICD-9-CM code and write it in the space provided. Also underline the main term.

Condition	Code
1. Tuberculous pleurisy	1. _____
2. Nontoxic nodular goiter	2. _____
3. Pernicious anemia	3. _____
4. Bacterial meningitis	4. _____
5. Tricuspid valve disease	5. _____
6. Upper respiratory infection (acute)	6. _____
7. Bronchitis	7. _____
8. Acute bronchitis	8. _____
9. Diabetes mellitus without mention of complication	9. _____
10. Normal delivery	10. _____
11. Metacarpus osteoarthrosis	11. _____
12. Other dyspnea and respiratory abnormality	12. _____
13. Exposure to hepatitis	13. _____
14. Gallbladder disease	14. _____
15. Acne	15. _____
16. Murine (endemic) typhus	16. _____
17. Ulcerative colitis	17. _____
18. Malignant neoplasm of orbit	18. _____
19. Urticaria pigmentosa	19. _____
20. Malignant neoplasm of cerebrum	20. _____
21. Degenerative skin disorders	21. _____
22. Rosacea acne	22. _____
23. Artificial insemination	23. _____
24. DTP inoculation	24. _____
25. Generalized hyperhidrosis	25. _____
26. Swimmer's ear (acute)	26. _____
27. Heart palpitations	27. _____
28. Paramacular lesion of the retina	28. _____
29. Rectal leukoplakia	29. _____
30. Plasma cell leukemia not in remission	30. _____

Activity #4: ICD-9-CM Crossword Puzzle—Part 1

Directions: Based on the diagnosis description, look up the appropriate ICD-9-CM code and write it in the crossword puzzle space provided.

Crossword Game 1

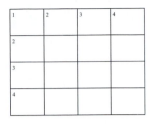

Across

1. Atrophic skin spots

2. Open wound of pharynx

3. Relapsing fever

4. Malignant neoplasm of parotid gland

Down

1. Hallucinations

2. Foot and mouth disease

3. Malignant neoplasm of nasopharynx lateral wall

4. Headache due to lumbar puncture

Crossword Game 2

Across

1. Acute appendicitis with peritoneal abscess

2. Blister on heel

3. Femoral artery aneurysm

4. Big spleen syndrome

Down

1. Urethral calculus

2. Chronic coronary insufficiency

3. Mumps

4. Fish tapeworm infection

Activity #5: Finding the Main Term and Determining the Correct ICD-9-CM Code—Part 2

Directions: Based on the condition, look up the appropriate ICD-9-CM code and write it in the space provided. Also underline the main term.

Condition	Code
1. Proximal fibular open dislocation	1. _____
2. Gangrene of the tunica vaginalis	2. _____
3. Obstructed gangrenous hernia	3. _____
4. Hypercholesterolemia	4. _____
5. Other ovarian dysfunction	5. _____
6. Sudden infant death syndrome (SIDS)	6. _____
7. Glomerulohyalinosis diabetic syndrome	7. _____
8. Gonococcal salpingo-oophoritis (chronic)	8. _____
9. Bladder neck stricture	9. _____

10. Popliteal thrombophlebitis   10. _____

11. Ulcerative colitis   11. _____

12. Superior mesenteric artery syndrome   12. _____

13. Renal artery thrombosis   13. _____

14. Recurrent urethritis   14. _____

15. Enuresis   15. _____

16. Diabetes mellitus   16. _____

17. Endogenous obesity   17. _____

18. Essential hypertension   18. _____

19. Inguinal hernia   19. _____

20. Tendon sheath ganglion   20. _____

21. Borderline glaucoma   21. _____

22. Glioblastoma of the forearm   22. _____

23. Ulcerative gastroenteritis   23. _____

24. Hallux valgus   24. _____

25. Heart disease   25. _____

26. Heat prostration   26. _____

27. Epidural hematoma of the brain   27. _____

28. Internal hemorrhoids   28. _____

29. Familial hypercholesterolemia   29. _____

30. Endocrine imbalance   30. _____

Activity 6: ICD-9-CM Never-Ending Circle Challenge

Directions: Starting with the marked line, look up the ICD-9-CM codes and enter one digit on each
line. Use the last number of the previous code as the first number of the following code
(e.g., ICD-9-CM codes 001.3, 384.5, and 500.23 would be written 0 0 1 3 8 4 5 0 0 2 3).

Never-Ending Circle
Game 1

1. Complicated open wound of ear

2. Deprivation of water

3. Stuttering

4. Chicken pox

5. Overdose of appetite suppressants

6. Blackwater fever

7. Patella fracture

8. Quartan malaria

9. Hemophilia C

10. Other nonthrombocytopenic purpuras

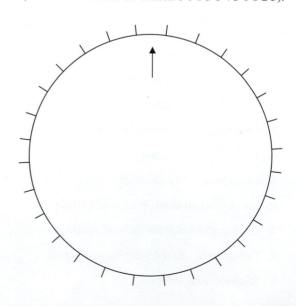

Never-Ending Circle
Game 2

1. Abscess on the chin

2. Tuberculosis of the eye

3. Culture shock

4. Insect bit on the lip

5. Hemorrhoids without complication

6. Vaginal infertility

7. Acute bronchitis

8. Tetanus

9. Diaphoresis

10. Eye penetrated with foreign body

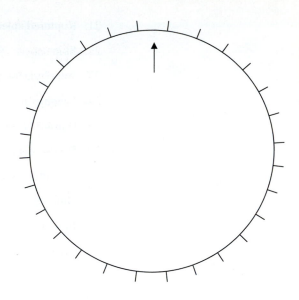

Activity #7: Finding the Main Term and Determining the Correct ICD-9-CM Code—Part 3

Directions: Based on the condition, look up the appropriate ICD-9-CM code and write it in the space provided. Also underline the main term.

Condition	Code
1. Hypothyroidism	1. _____
2. Fetal alcohol intoxication	2. _____
3. Diabetic iritis	3. _____
4. Loss of appetite	4. _____
5. Embryonal liposarcoma	5. _____
6. Atrophic spots of skin	6. _____
7. Necrosis of the liver	7. _____
8. Ameloblastic sarcoma	8. _____
9. Septicemia salmonella	9. _____
10. Squamous cell carcinoma of the skin, in situ	10. _____
11. Open cuboid infected fracture	11. _____
12. Recurrent elbow dislocation	12. _____
13. Weight gain failure	13. _____
14. Anemia in end-stage renal disease	14. _____
15. Thyroid disease	15. _____
16. Degenerative nephritis	16. _____
17. Neurofibromatosis	17. _____
18. Cardiovascular observation	18. _____
19. Tibial osteosarcoma	19. _____
20. Stirrup otosclerosis	20. _____

21. Ruptured spleen   21. _____

22. Skin sepsis   22. _____

23. Anaphylactic shock   23. _____

24. Diaphysitis   24. _____

25. Carotid artery stenosis   25. _____

26. Post status asthmaticus   26. _____

27. Capsulitis of the knee   27. _____

28. Glue ear syndrome   28. _____

29. Epilepsy   29. _____

30. Trichinosis   30. _____

Activity #8: ICD-9-CM Crossword Puzzle—Part 2

Directions: Based on the diagnosis description, look up the appropriate ICD-9-CM code and write it in the crossword puzzle space provided.

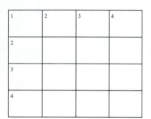

Crossword Game 1

Across

1. Cheek abscess

2. Arteriosclerotic vascular

3. Sebaceous cyst, breast

4. Secondary malignant neoplasm of the skin of the breast

Down

1. Maternal obesity syndrome

2. Elbow strain

3. Malignant lymphoma

4. Chronic gonorrhea

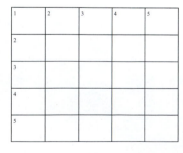

Crossword Game 2

Across

1. Accident involving two cars colliding, driver injured

2. Temporal bone fracture, open

3. Generalized osteoarthrosis, lower back

4. Dysgammaglobulinemia

5. Salmonella osteomyelitis

Down

1. Failure of sterile precautions during a surgical operation

2. Sphenoid bone fracture, open with subdural and extradural hemorrhage

3. Histoplasmosis pericarditis

4. Diabetes mellitus without complication

5. Small round virus

Activity #9: Finding the Main Term and Determining the Correct ICD-9-CM Code—Part 4

Directions: Based on the condition, look up the appropriate ICD-9-CM code and write it in the space provided. Also underline the main term.

Condition	Code
1. Abnormal movements	1. _____
2. Hurthle cell, benign	2. _____
3. Pregnant with twins	3. _____
4. Twisted umbilical cord (during delivery)	4. _____
5. Metastasis to the pancreas	5. _____
6. Semilunar cartilage cyst	6. _____
7. Endometrioid cystadenocarcinoma of middle lobe of lung	7. _____
8. Premature heart contractions	8. _____
9. Severe sunburn of the back	9. _____
10. Chemical burn of gums	10. _____
11. Struck by a falling object	11. _____
12. Deaf mute	12. _____
13. Cruveilhier's disease	13. _____
14. Cholecystic chlamydial disease	14. _____
15. Alzheimer's disease	15. _____
16. Fractured mandible, open	16. _____
17. Fractured larynx	17. _____
18. Fractured femur, subtrochanteric	18. _____
19. Fractured tibia and fibula	19. _____
20. Compound Fx, trochanter	20. _____
21. Fx skull with concussion	21. _____
22. Fx ribs (six), open	22. _____
23. Sprained ankle	23. _____
24. Strain, knee	24. _____
25. Sprain, elbow	25. _____
26. Sprained foot	26. _____
27. Eye strain	27. _____
28. Dislocated joint (infected), open	28. _____
29. Dislocated jaw, recurrent	29. _____
30. Dislocated collar bone, open	30. _____
31. Giant cell carcinoma	31. _____
32. Dermatofibroma protuberans	32. _____

33. Leydig cell tumor (male)   33. _____

34. Glomangioma   34. _____

35. Intramuscular lipoma   35. _____

36. Sebaceous cyst   36. _____

37. Leukemia   37. _____

38. Oat cell lung carcinoma   38. _____

39. Papillary hydradenoma   39. _____

40. Mucoid adenoma of the auricle   40. _____

41. Juxtaglomerular tumor   41. _____

42. Malignant insulinoma   42. _____

43. Basophil adenoma of the nose   43. _____

44. Malignant renal intraductal papilloma   44. _____

45. Abdominal fibromatosis   45. _____

46. Aldosteronoma   46. _____

47. Epithelial neoblastoma   47. _____

48. Nabothian gland neoplasm (secondary)   48. _____

49. Myxochondrosarcoma   49. _____

50. Plasmacytoma, esophagus   50. _____

51. Bowen's disease   51. _____

52. Papillary intraductal carcinoma, salivary duct   52. _____

53. Carcinomatous cyst of the breast   53. _____

54. Ciliary epithelium diktyoma   54. _____

55. Wrist dysgerminoma   55. _____

56. Ependymoblastoma, spinal cord   56. _____

57. Femur osteofibroma   57. _____

58. Jadassohn's blue nevus   58. _____

59. Hutchinson's melanotic freckle   59. _____

60. Myxofibroma, connective tissue   60. _____

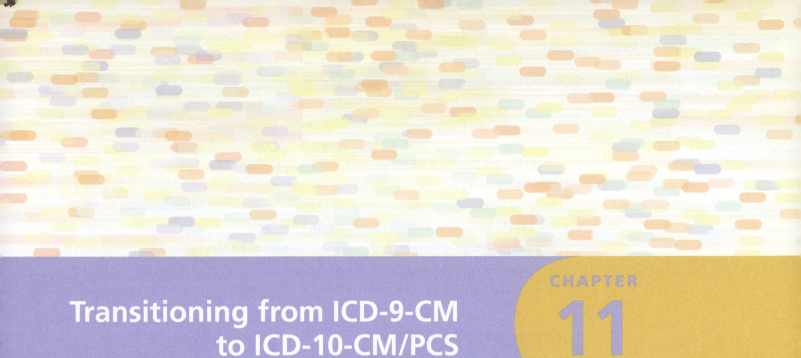

Transitioning from ICD-9-CM to ICD-10-CM/PCS

After completion of this chapter you should be able to:

Discuss the history of ICD-10-CM.

List the benefits of ICD-10-CM.

Describe the overall similarities and differences between ICD-9-CM and ICD-10-CM.

Discuss the overall process for the transition.

Summarize the impact of ICD-10-CM on information systems.

Explain the impact of ICD-10-CM on providers.

Describe the impact of ICD-10-CM on coding professionals.

Discuss the use of data mapping.

Key Words and Concepts you will learn in this chapter:

Accredited Standards Committee (ASC) X12N Version 4010

Backward mapping

Crosswalks

Electronic transactions

Etiology

Forward mapping

General Equivalence Mappings (GEMs)

Glasgow Coma Scale (GCS)

Granularity

ICD-10-PCS (Procedure Coding System)

International Classification of Diseases, 10th Revision, Clinical Modification (ICD-10-CM/PCS)

Laterality

Many-to-one

Morbidity

Mortality

National Center for Health Statistics (NCHS)

National Council for Prescription Drug Programs (NCPDP)

**Official Guidelines for Coding
and Reporting (OGCR)**

One-to-many

Version 4010

Version 5010

> In 2013, the health care industry faces a great challenge: transitioning to a new coding system, ICD-10-CM/PCS. This change not only requires coders to learn how to use the new system on a daily basis; it also mandates updates to all computer systems used by providers, payers, and regulators for billing and coding purposes. In addition, providers will need to change how documentation is done in the medical record along with the type of information that is written in the record (Figure 11-1 ●).

History of ICD-10-CM

The International Classification of Diseases, 10th Revision (ICD-10) is a worldwide reporting system developed by the World Health Organization (WHO) for classifying epidemiological (study of diseases in large populations) and mortality (causes of death) data. ICD-10 was first fully released in 1994, after which time it was gradually adopted internationally by over 130 countries. Countries such as Canada and Australia have already successfully implemented ICD-10 for hospitals, but it is not used in outpatient settings in those countries. The United States, under the direction of the **National Center for Health Statistics (NCHS)**, has adapted and expanded ICD-10 for tracking and billing of both inpatient and outpatient encounters, using terminology and detail consistent with medical practice in the United States. This modification is called **International Classification of Diseases, 10th Revision, Clinical Modification (ICD-10-CM)**.

ICD-10-CM is an updated version of ICD-9-CM. ICD-9-CM has been in use in the United States since 1979 for diagnosis (patient's condition or reason for health services) reporting. ICD-10-CM was developed by the Centers for Disease Control and Prevention (CDC) for all business organizations covered by the Health Insurance Portability and Accountability Act (HIPAA), which are also referred to as covered entities. This expanded version was needed to capture the level of detail regarding **morbidity** (the rate of incidence of disease) and **mortality** data desired by the United States. It also uses terminology consistent with clinical practice in this country. All modifications in ICD-10-CM must conform to WHO conventions for ICD-10. The U.S. version of the ICD-10 diagnosis codes (ICD-10-CM) is much more detailed than it is in other nations. There are about 70,000 codes in the U.S. version compared to about 16,000 codes in the Canadian version and about 22,000 in the Australian version.

FIGURE 11-1

Coder working with a computer system

© Michal Heron/Pearson Education

The United States has been using ICD-10-CM for the limited purpose of coding and classification of mortality data from death certificates since January 1, 1999. HIPAA covered entities are required to adopt ICD-10-CM for medical coding and health claims submission beginning October 1, 2013. This implementation date applies to all providers, such as hospitals, physicians, skilled nursing facilities, rehabilitation facilities, home health agencies, and so on; payers, such as private insurance companies and government Medicare and Medicaid programs; and other HIPAA-covered entities, such as software vendors, clearinghouses, and third-party billing services. ICD-10-CM codes will not be accepted for services rendered before October 1, 2013, and ICD-9-CM codes will not be accepted for services provided after that date.

ICD-10-PCS (Procedure Coding System) was developed by the Centers for Medicare and Medicaid Services (CMS) for use in the United States in inpatient hospital settings only (Figure 11-2 ●). ICD-10-PCS will replace ICD-9-CM Volume 3 procedure codes for hospital inpatient coding in the United States. ICD-10-PCS is not used in other countries. The implementation dates are the same for ICD-10-CM and ICD-10-PCS. ICD-10-PCS is significantly different from ICD-9-CM

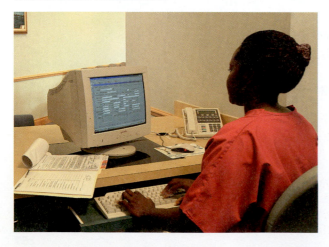

Volume 3 procedure codes and is not discussed in detail in this text. Examples of ICD-10-PCS codes are provided in Chapter 12.

In January 2009, CMS issued two final rules for replacing ICD-9-CM with ICD-10-CM/PCS. The first rule specifies the compliance date for mandatory use of ICD-10-CM/PCS. The second rule updates the HIPAA transaction standards (programming specifications) in order to ensure that computer software programs used by medical facilities can accommodate the use of the ICD-10-CM/PCS codes. The compliance date for the second rule is January 1, 2012.

● **ONLINE INFORMATION:** To read the final rules published in the *Federal Register*, visit
www.cms.gov and search for Federal Register HIPAA standards

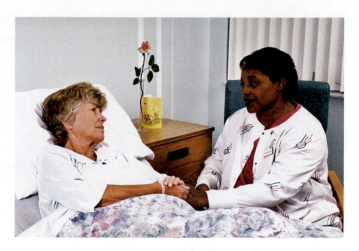

FIGURE 11-2

A patient in a hospital setting

PRACTICE **PITFALLS**

The implementation date of October 1, 2013, applies to the patient's date of service or date of discharge, not the date on which the encounter (patient visit) is coded or billed. There will be a period of time during which medical billers will be working with both the ICD-9-CM for services prior to October 1, 2013, and with the ICD-10-CM for services on or after October 1, 2013. Even when providers have completed billing for all services prior to October 1, 2013, medical billers will still need to work with historical data containing ICD-9-CM codes.

ACTIVITY #1

Determining Which Codes to Use

Directions: Given the situations, indicate if ICD-9-CM or ICD-10-CM codes would be used.

Situation	ICD-9-CM	ICD-10-CM
A patient is in the hospital from January 2, 2013, through January 15, 2013.	❏	❏
On October 1, 2013, you are billing for a patient seen in the office on September 30, 2013.	❏	❏
A patient is in the hospital from October 2, 2013, through October 5, 2013.	❏	❏
A patient arrives at the emergency department at 10:00 p.m. on September 30, 2013, waits for two hours, and the physician enters the exam room at 11:59 p.m.	❏	❏
A patient is admitted to the hospital on September 27, 2013, and discharged on October 1, 2013.	❏	❏
You are working on October 1, 2013, to code for a patient who was admitted to the hospital on September 27, 2013, and discharged September 29, 2013.	❏	❏
A bill that was originally submitted in August 2013 was rejected due to a missing code. On October 5, 2013, you need to update the code and resubmit the bill.	❏	❏
A patient is seen in the office on October 1, 2013, but the clinic's computer system has not yet been updated to ICD-10-CM.	❏	❏

Benefits of ICD-10-CM

ICD-10-CM codes are more specific than ICD-9-CM codes and provide more consistent data regarding patients' medical conditions. ICD-9-CM is thirty years old, uses outdated terms, and is inconsistent with current medical practice. For example, gout is reclassified from ICD-9-CM Chapter 3: Endocrine, Nutritional and Metabolic Diseases, and Immunity Disorders to ICD-10-CM

Chapter 13, Diseases of the Musculoskeletal System and Connective Tissue. This is because gout is now considered to be a disease of the musculoskeletal system rather than a metabolic disorder as it was in 1979. The timeframe for acute myocardial infarction (AMI) is changed from one occurring eight weeks or less after a previous AMI in ICD-9-CM to one occurring four weeks or less in after a previous AMI in ICD-10-CM because this is how cardiologists now define acute myocardial infarction.

The structure of ICD-9-CM limits the number of new codes that can be created, and many ICD-9-CM categories are full. The ICD-10-CM structure allows room to expand the codes to more characters when more specificity is needed. For example, in 2011 a code was added to ICD-9-CM for acquired absence of pancreas. This new code could not be included with other codes for acquired absence of organ because no numbers were left in that section. So, rather than appearing in the most logical place, acquired absence of pancreas was placed in a different section of the tabular listing. Under ICD-10-CM, acquired absence of pancreas is coded in the same section with all other body systems.

The Centers for Medicare and Medicaid Services (CMS) and the American Health Information Management Association (AHIMA) identify numerous benefits that more than likely will result from the use of ICD-10-CM codes. Benefits include the following:

- Patient conditions being more accurately described, reducing the need for attachments to claims
- Higher quality of data made available for tracking quality, safety, and effectiveness of health services
- Reduction of coding errors due to improved consistency across codes and more specific code descriptions
- Improved tracking of domestic and international public health threats, resulting in better response to threats

● **ONLINE INFORMATION:** For further information on the numerous benefits that are expected to result from ICD-10-CM, visit the American Health Information Management Association at www.ahima.org/icd10/replaced.aspx and the CMS Web site at www.cms.gov.

Similarities Between ICD-9-CM and ICD-10-CM

Even though most of the focus on ICD-10-CM is around the differences in the new codes, there are a number of similarities between ICD-9-CM and ICD-10-CM. These similarities will provide a starting point for coders to learn the new systems. This chapter discusses overall similarities between the codes. Chapter 12 addresses the specifics with more examples. Some of the major similarities include the following:

- All codes have three characters before the decimal point, and codes with the same three characters have common traits.
- The alphabetic index is organized in a similar manner with main terms and multiple levels of indented subterms. The process of searching for a code in the index is similar.
- The tabular list is divided into chapters based on body system and **etiology** (causes of disease), and with a few exceptions the chapters appear in the same order. The process of verifying a code in the tabular list is similar.
- Codes have a varying number of digits, and coders must assign codes to the highest degree of specificity.
- Special tables exist for neoplasms and for reactions to drugs and chemicals.
- Instructional notes appear in the tabular list, guiding coders regarding the need for additional codes, included and excluded conditions, and sequencing.
- **Official Guidelines for Coding and Reporting** are required to be followed and are organized into four sections. Many, but not all, of the specific guidelines are the same.
- Many of the conventions (symbols, punctuation, typeface) are the same.

Differences Between ICD-9-CM and ICD-10-CM

There are several types of differences between ICD-10-CM and ICD-9-CM. This chapter discusses overall differences between the codes. Chapter 12 will address the specifics and how they affect assigning codes to patient encounters. Some of the major differences include these:

- The number of codes has increased from 14,000 in ICD-9-CM to more than 68,000 in ICD-10-CM.
- The length of codes has increased from 3 to 5 characters in ICD-9-CM to a length of 3 to 7 characters in ICD-10-CM.
- Code structure has changed from primarily numeric in ICD-9-CM (except for V and E codes) to all codes being alpha-numeric in ICD-10-CM.
- Code formats have been added in ICD-10-CM to include seventh-digit extensions to describe particular circumstances.
- ICD-10-CM terminology and disease classifications have been updated to be consistent with current clinical practice.
- ICD-10-CM codes describe greater levels of clinical detail and specificity than may have been described by a single code in ICD-9-CM.
- ICD-10-CM contains more combination codes that describe multiple related conditions with a single code.

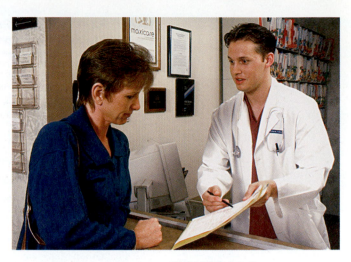

FIGURE 11-3

Both provider and patient can be impacted by the reimbursement process.

© Michal Heron/Pearson Education

Overview of the Transition Process

The transition to convert from ICD-9-CM to ICD-10-CM is one of health care's top priorities and expenditures through the year 2015. Everyone who is part of the health care system or uses its data is impacted, including providers, payers, regulators, vendors, claims clearinghouses, medical billing services, researchers, educational institutions, and support staff in each of these settings (Figure 11-3 ●). All computer systems that collect, transmit, receive, or store diagnostic data need updating due to the expanded length, format, and structure of codes. These changes further impact the budgets of organizations and the productivity of workers.

Fortunately, patients should be minimally directly affected. Patients will be indirectly impacted since it is likely that the overall processing times of claims will be longer, at least during the time when the medical facilities and other entities, such as insurance carriers, get used to the new system and work out all the issues that arise with the implementation of the new system.

Preparing for the Change

When ICD-10 was implemented in countries such as Canada and Australia, the national, provincial, and local governments paid for software upgrades and staff training. In the United States, the costs are incurred individually by each hospital, physician, and health plan. Experience in other countries has demonstrated that the change requires a significant investment of time and money. Health care providers in other countries experienced decreased productivity for many months following the move. Based on the lessons learned from other countries, it is critical that health care organizations in the United States prepare for the transition.

Those who will be directly on the front line of ensuring that the transition occurs as smoothly as possible are found in various positions:

- Health care administrators
- Business owners and managers of hospitals
- Physicians who own their own practice, and the managers of those practices
- Nonphysician providers who practice independently, such as physical therapists, chiropractors, dentists, laboratories, pharmacies, dentists, optometrists, podiatrists, and psychologists

The responsibilities of these individuals include making sure that computer software used in scheduling, finance, performance, intensive care/emergency room, and decision support is up to date to accommodate the expanded size, new structure, and increased number of ICD-10-CM codes. In addition, administrative and clinical staff need to be trained how to use the new codes and software and how the changes in clinical documentation must be achieved. Health care administrators also establish budgets for time and costs related to ICD-10-CM implementation, including expenses for system changes, resource materials, and training. This

TABLE 11-1 A List of Professional Organizations That Provide Guidance for the Transition from ICD-9-CM to ICD-10-CM

Organization Name/Abbreviation	Web Site
American Academy of Professional Coders (AAPC)	aapc.com
American Association of Family Practice (AAFP)	aafp.com
American College of Radiology (ACR)	acr.org
American Health Information Management Association (AHIMA)	ahima.org
American Hospital Association (AHA)	aha.org
American Medical Association (AMA)	ama-assn.org
American Academy of Orthopaedic Surgeons (AAOS)	aaos.org
America's Health Insurance Plans (AHIP)	ahip.com
Health Information Management Systems Society (HIMSS)	himss.org
Medical Group Management Association (MGMA)	mgma.com

includes the costs of any necessary software updates, reprinting of superbills, training, and related expenses.

To ensure that the organization is able to make the transition to ICD-10-CM in a timely manner, health care administrators take the rules and time schedules put forth by regulators and adapt them to their own organization. Guidance for the transition can be obtained through professional organizations. A list of some well-known professional organizations appears in Table 11-1 ●.

Organizations must be ready to bill using ICD-10-CM on October 1, 2013, and certain data processes involving **electronic transactions** (data transmitted via computers) begin sooner. Because the code changes affect nearly every function in an organization, planning begins several years prior to the 2013 implementation date, and monitoring continues for several years after the implementation date. Practices must analyze all systems that submit claims, receive remittances, and exchange claim status or eligibility inquiry and responses to identify software and business process changes. Business processes may need to be changed to capture additional information required by the new HIPAA standards.

Planning for the change also includes planning for staff training. Organizations prepare by identifying who needs to be trained in assigning, using, and working with the new codes; when the training for each is required; and what training methods are to be used. Professional organizations for coders, such as AHIMA and AAPC, recommend that training take place approximately six months prior to the October 1, 2013, compliance date, with training being phased in for different groups of staff.

As part of the transition, organizations should work to identify all information systems and work processes that use ICD-9-CM codes. This could include clinical documentation, encounter forms/superbills, practice management system, electronic health record system, contracts, and public health and quality reporting protocols. By locating the various areas in the organization where ICD-9-CM codes appear, an organization will have a better scope of what will be impacted by the use of ICD-10- CM codes. Wherever ICD-9-CM codes now appear, ICD-10-CM codes will take their place.

In addition, practices need to discuss implementation plans with clearinghouses, billing services, and payers to ensure a smooth transition. The most successful practice takes initiative to contact these business partners and ask about plans for Version 5010 and ICD-10-CM compliance, and when they will finalize systems for both transitions. (The HIPAA-mandated electronic transaction standards for ICD-10-CM codes and related data are referred to as **Version 5010** and replace the previous electronic standards called **Version 4010**.)

The overall process to plan for, implement, and monitor the ICD-10-CM transition requires approximately five years. An example of an ICD-10-CM implementation calendar appears in Table 11-2 ●.

● ONLINE INFORMATION: For further information on AHIMA's preparation checklist, visit www.ahima.org/downloads/pdfs/resources/checklist.pdf

TABLE 11-2 Example ICD-10-CM Implementation Calendar

Year	Tasks	Description
2009	Long-range organization and communication	Brief senior management on the requirements of ICD-10-CM.
		Obtain support and buy-in from senior management and physicians.
		Develop informational material to distribute to managers, staff, and providers.
2010	Research and budgeting	Identify regulatory requirements, educational requirements, and information system requirements.
		Collaborate with information systems vendor to plan changes, costs, timelines, and testing for systems.
		Establish budget for software, hardware, implementation, staff training, testing, and overtime.
		Develop a training plan for each department.
		Begin internal testing of Version 5010 standards for electronic claims.
2011	Implementation planning	Review ICD-10-CM coding guidelines, crosswalks, reimbursement impacts, and new processes that may be required.
		Achieve ability to process Version 5010 transactions for testing and transition with able trading partners.
2012	Preliminary training and business planning	Use Version 5010 standards for all electronic claims.
		Begin preliminary training on the new code set for all affected staff. Begin coder certification in ICD-10-CM.
		Identify what updates are needed for policies and procedures, internal and external reports.
		Evaluate payer and managed care contracts for financial impact.
Early 2013	Education, measurement, and monitoring	Integrate new software into operations and customize code as needed.
		Update forms and paperwork with new codes.
		Finalize testing of all systems with clearinghouses, payers, and electronic transmissions for diagnosis codes and inpatient procedure codes.
		Conduct specialty-specific training of all staff using the code set. Complete coder certification in ICD-10-CM.
		Measure coder productivity; coder knowledge and skill level, and medical record documentation.
10/1/2013	Full implementation	Go live with ICD-10-CM on October 1, 2013.
2014	Monitoring, follow-up, and compliance	Identify and resolve claim errors and denials related to ICD-10-CM.
		Review changes in insurance carrier payment policies.
		Assess and adjust medical records documentation.
		Measure training and productivity outcomes.
		Provide follow-up training as needed.

ACTIVITY #2

Understanding the Impact of ICD-10-CM

Imagine that you are working in a physician office. Your boss has asked you to research how ICD-10-CM will impact your office. Select one of the professional organizations listed in Table 11-1 and research what advice it gives about ICD-10-CM implementation. If there is no link for ICD-10-CM on the Web site's home page, you can search for "ICD-10" within the organization's Web site. Write a one-page memo to your supervisor summarizing your findings.

Impact on Health Care Information Systems

One of the most significant impacts of ICD-10-CM within a health care organization is the impact that the use of these codes has on its health care information systems. Typically an organization has more than one electronic information system that is affected. These may include scheduling, patient registration, medical records, billing, coding, payment posting, quality, and compliance reporting. In large organizations, multiple departments are affected, including laboratory, pharmacy, radiology, medical records, quality assurance, and billing. Reporting to external federal and state regulators is affected. Examples of information reported to regulators are adverse drug events, research, public health, and newborn screenings. Contracts with health plans and payers are also impacted and must be reviewed and modified as necessary to incorporate the new codes.

Electronic transactions are exchanges involving the computerized transfer of health care information between two parties for specific purposes, such as a health care provider submitting medical claims to a health plan for payment. Prior to ICD-10-CM the health care industry used an electronic transaction standard called **Accredited Standards Committee (ASC) X12N Version 4010**. The current version lacks certain functionality required by the health care industry. Therefore, providers must prepare for new standards to continue submitting claims electronically.

In Version 5010, every electronic transaction standard is updated, from claims to eligibility to referral authorizations. Any electronic transaction for which a standard has been adopted should be submitted using Version 5010 on or after January 1, 2012. The implementation of Version 5010 presents substantial changes in the content of the data that providers submit with their claims, as well as the data they receive in response to their electronic inquiries for eligibility or claims status. Unlike the current Version 4010 transaction set, Version 5010 is much more specific in the type of data it collects and transmits.

With the implementation of ICD-10-CM, additional software programming is needed. The new software provides modified field sizes that accommodate longer codes. In addition, the data fields are changed from primarily numeric (with the exception of V and E for the first character) to completely alphanumeric for every character. Other format changes increase the number of diagnosis codes allowed on a claim. Version 5010 has clear rules built in that improve the explanations of claim corrections, reversals, recoupment of payments, and the processing of refunds.

The Version 5010 format does not require the use of ICD-10-CM codes, but it does include a special indicator field that distinguishes whether ICD-9-CM or ICD-10-CM codes are being used in a given transaction. This is necessary because there is a period of time during which providers are processing claims for encounters that occurred both before and after the October 1, 2013, implementation date.

CMS established a three-year timeline for providers to come into compliance with the new electronic standards, as shown in Table 11-3 ●.

Three sets of new health care electronic transaction standards are required for ICD-10-CM, affecting different types of providers. In addition to ASC X12 Version 5010, the **National Council for Prescription Drug Programs (NCPDP)** has established new formats for Medicare Part D

TABLE 11-3 Version 5010 Compliance Timeline

Date	Compliance Step
January 1, 2010	Payers and providers should begin internal testing of Version 5010 standards for electronic claims.
December 31, 2010	Internal testing of Version 5010 must be complete to achieve Level I Version 5010 compliance.
January 1, 2011	Payers and providers should begin external testing of Version 5010 for electronic claims. CMS begins accepting Version 5010 claims. Version 4010 claims continue to be accepted.
December 31, 2011	External testing of Version 5010 for electronic claims must be complete to achieve Level II Version 5010 compliance.
January 1, 2012	All electronic claims must use Version 5010. Version 4010 claims are no longer accepted.
October 1, 2013	Claims for services provided on or after this date must use ICD-10-CM codes for medical diagnosis and inpatient procedures. CPT codes will continue to be used for outpatient services.

pharmacies and suppliers (NCPDP Version D.0) and Medicaid pharmacy plans (NCPDP Version 3.0). Electronic transactions that do not use Version 5010 will not be considered compliant with HIPAA and will be rejected. Table 11-4 ● lists the HIPAA transaction standards and their descriptions. This list helps the medical office specialist understand and appreciate the far-ranging impacts of the change.

● **ONLINE INFORMATION:** For further information on the CMS compliance timeline visit http://www.cms.gov/ICD10/11b15_2012_ICD10PCS.asp#TopOfPage.

TABLE 11-4 **HIPAA Transaction Standards**

HIPAA Standard	Transaction Description
Claims, Encounter, and Payment Information	
ASC X12 837 D	Health care claims—Dental
ASC X12 837 P	Health care claims—Professional
ASC X12 837 I	Health care claims—Institutional
NCPDP D.0	Health care claims—Retail pharmacy drug
ASC X12 837 P NCPDP D.0	Health care claims—Retail pharmacy supplies and professional services
ASC X12 276	Health care claim status inquiry/request
ASC X12 277	Health care claim status response
NCPDP 5.1 NCPDP D.0	Retail pharmacy drug claims (telecommunication and batch standards)
NCPDP 3.0	Medicaid pharmacy subrogation (batch standard) (transmission of a claim from a Medicaid agency to a payer for the purpose of seeking reimbursement for a pharmacy claim the State has paid on behalf of a Medicaid recipient)
ASC X12 835	Health care payment and remittance advice
Coordination of Benefits	
NCPDP D.0	Coordination of Benefits—Retail pharmacy drug
ASC X12 837 D COB	Coordination of Benefits—Dental
ASC X12 837 P COB	Coordination of Benefits—Professional
ASC X12 837 I COB	Coordination of Benefits—Institutional
Eligibility for a Health Plan	
ASC X12 270	Eligibility for a health plan inquiry/request—Dental, Professional, and Institutional
ASC X12 271	Eligibility for a health plan response—Dental, Professional and Institutional
NCPDP D.0	Eligibility for a health plan (request and response)—Retail pharmacy drugs
ASC X12 834	Enrollment and disenrollment in a health plan
ASC X12 820	Health plan premium payment
Referrals	
ASC X12 278	Referral certification and authorization (request and response)
NCPDP D.0	Referral certification and authorization (request and response)—Retail pharmacy drugs
Non-HIPAA-Mandated Formats for Medicare Fee-for-Service (FFS)	
ASC X12 TA1	Transaction acknowledgement
ASC X12 999	Functional acknowledgement
ASC X12 277CA	Claims acknowledgement

ACTIVITY #3

Impact on Information Systems

1. State three ways that ICD-10-CM impacts providers' information systems.

    a. _____

    b. _____

    c. _____

2. State three ways that ICD-10-CM impacts payers' information systems.

    a. _____

    b. _____

    c. _____

Impact on Medical Providers

Providers are impacted by ICD-10-CM in several ways. Physicians who own their own practices experience impacts to operations and budgets (described earlier in this chapter). Providers are also responsible for implementing the needed changes to information systems. They need to make sure the coders they employ receive adequate training. In addition to all these impacts, all providers need to ensure that their own medical documentation provides the additional level of specificity needed under ICD-10-CM. Providers who personally assign some or all diagnostic codes themselves need to learn the coding procedures for ICD-10-CM (Figure 11-4 ●).

Coding changes impact more of the business processes of health care organizations than did the HIPAA transactions or the implementation of the National Provider Identifier (NPI). The impacts of the HIPAA transactions and NPI were generally limited to the transactions with external partners, whereas ICD-10-CM changes impact providers' documentation procedures, record-keeping procedures, fee schedules, medical review edits used by the health plan, and quality measures used in assessing performance.

New Documentation Requirements

FIGURE 11-4

Physician consulting with a medical assistant to ensure the correct code is assigned

© Michal Heron/Pearson Education

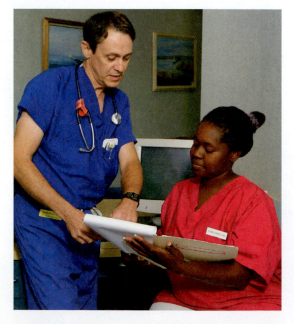

One aspect of ICD-10-CM implementation that directly affects all clinical providers and is of great concern is the potential for increased quantity and detail of documentation. Because ICD-10-CM provides for a greater level of **granularity** and specificity, providers are responsible for ensuring that their documentation provides the required information and that the information is recorded in a way that is easy for coders to abstract. This may result in a reduction in physician and other clinical staff productivity. Effects on productivity continue longer than the expected initial learning curve. The requirement for increased detail never disappears and requires additional time each and every time a provider documents a patient encounter. A 2008 study by Nachimson Advisors entitled "The Impact of Implementing ICD-10 on Physician Practices and Clinical Laboratories: A Report to the ICD-10 Coalition" estimates that physician time spent on documentation increases as much as 15 to 20 percent under ICD-10-CM. The study also estimates that the implementation cost of ICD-10-CM for a three-physician practice could be as much as $83,290, and a 100-physician practice might pay more than $2.7 million.

● **ONLINE INFORMATION:** For further information on the Nachimson study, visit http://nachimsonadvisors.com/Documents/ICD-10%20Impacts%20on%20Providers.pdf

To determine the need for documentation improvement, providers must conduct evaluation studies either internally or with the assistance of external consultants. Random samples of various types of medical records should be evaluated to determine how well the documentation contains the required level of detail mandated by the new coding system. Documentation weaknesses should then be identified, and a priority list of diagnoses and procedures requiring more detail or other changes should be developed.

Even though codes are not actually assigned until the insurance claim is prepared, the impact on providers begins as soon as the patient visit is scheduled. Schedulers often select the reason or purpose for patients' planned visits from a list that is ultimately tied to diagnosis codes. If eligibility needs to be checked, a referral made, or preauthorization is required by the patient's health plan, diagnosis codes are usually necessary. When the patient presents for the visit, the coinsurance, copayment, or deductible payment may be affected by the expected diagnosis or visit type.

The effect on examinations and treatment decisions is a critical and sensitive area for providers. Health plans may update coverage policies to reflect the greater specificity in ICD-10-CM coding. For example, the diagnostic criteria for coverage of a particular treatment could become more specific and, therefore, more limited. Providers may need to document additional details to support a patient's treatment plan. During an office visit, providers may need to alter past treatment protocols or explain to patients why their course of treatment may change due to new insurance company requirements. Again, this impact is not known until health plans review their ICD-10-CM implementation activities and determine what changes need to be made in their policies.

PRACTICE PITFALLS

Although some providers may consider using a code for the "unspecified" version of a diagnosis, rather than taking the time for additional documentation, this can result in payment denials or delays while the health plan requests additional information.

An example of changes in documentation can be seen with comas. ICD-9-CM has one code for coma, with no additional specificity. ICD-10-CM has expanded the codes for coma in traumatic brain injury or sequela of a cerebrovascular accident. The expanded codes reflect the **Glasgow Coma Scale (GCS)**, traditionally used by trauma centers, that rates visual (eye opening), verbal, and motor responses. Three ICD-10-CM codes, one code from each GCS subcategory (visual [eye opening], verbal, and motor), are needed to complete the coding. Therefore, clinicians must document the patient's visual (eye opening), verbal, and motor status in the medical record. They must also document the time when each assessment was conducted in order to assign the appropriate seventh character to the ICD-10-CM code. The options are unspecified time, in the field, at arrival to emergency department, at hospital admission, or twenty-four hours or more after hospital admission. As can be seen in this example, it is critical that the medical staff receive additional training and knowledge regarding ICD-10-CM code requirements. Only with additional training would a staff member understand how to accurately assign and document the coma scale adequately. An example of GCS appears in Table 11-5 ●. Examples of coma coding are discussed in Chapter 12.

TABLE 11-5 Glasgow Coma Scale

Eye Opening Response	Spontaneous—open with blinking at baseline	4 points
	To verbal stimuli, command, speech	3 points
	To pain only (not applied to face)	2 points
	No response	1 point
Verbal Response	Oriented	5 points
	Confused conversation, but able to answer questions	4 points
	Inappropriate words	3 points
	Incomprehensible speech	2 points
	No response	1 point
Motor Response	Obeys commands for movement	6 points
	Purposeful movement to painful stimulus	5 points
	Withdraws in response to pain	4 points
	Flexion in response to pain (decorticate posturing)	3 points
	Extension response in response to pain (decerebrate posturing)	2 points
	No response	1 point

The area of genetic diagnoses also requires documentation and potential treatment changes. For example, ICD-9-CM has one code for Down syndrome. In ICD-10-CM, the codes for Down syndrome require genetic testing to reach the necessary specificity levels that describe the specific type of Down as meiotic nondisjunction, mitotic nondisjunction, or translocation.

In other cases, more patient medical history needs to be obtained. For example, patients being treated for a common condition such as postmenopausal osteoporosis also need documentation of current pathological fractures due to the condition in order to assign the correct code(s).

Impact on Medical Coders

Medical billers and coders are affected by ICD-10-CM on a daily basis. The change date is sudden; there is no easing into it. Any delays or errors in using the new code set directly impact the revenue of the organization. Therefore, coders must be trained and proficient well before the "go live" date so they can be immediately effective. This involves learning the new code set, new coding guidelines, and new or updated software. In this chapter, the general areas of change are discussed. Chapter 12 focuses on the procedures for assigning the actual codes.

Coding Department Changes

The coding department helps identify the current systems and work processes that use ICD-9-CM codes. These may include clinical documentation, encounter forms/superbills, practice management system, electronic health record system, contracts, and public health and quality reporting protocols. The annual changes to both ICD-9-CM and ICD-10-CM place a burden on coding departments to update and maintain all processes that use codes. To make the transition a bit easier, CMS implemented a partial code freeze prior to ICD-10-CM implementation, which has been welcomed by many providers and professional associations because the freeze minimizes the number of code changes during the transition. The process for the partial freeze is described in Table 11-6 ●. The ICD-9-CM Coordination and Maintenance Committee continues to meet twice a year during the freeze. At these meetings the public is allowed to comment on whether or not requests for new diagnosis and procedure codes should be implemented during the freeze, based on the need to capture new technologies or diseases. Any code requests that do not meet the criteria are evaluated for implementation within ICD-10-CM after the partial freeze ends on October 1, 2014.

Because ICD-10-CM requires upgrades to information systems, coders learn new screens and new functions of software for use in coding, medical records, billing, and other functions. Coders also upgrade keyboarding skills from what were primarily numeric data entry skills to full alphanumeric. Coders have always had to use a small combination of alphanumeric keys when using E-codes, V-codes, and HCPCS codes. However, the alphabetic character in ICD-9-CM codes is the first one. In ICD-10-CM, alphabetic characters can occur at almost any position, and nearly all codes have a random sequencing of alphabetic and numeric characters.

▶ **CRITICAL THINKING QUESTION:** Imagine that you are working in a physician practice and your boss has decided to wait until the summer of 2013 to worry about ICD-10-CM. "After all," she says, "CMS always extends its deadlines, and even if it doesn't, most of the rules are the same anyway." Why would you agree or disagree with this statement?

New Terminology

The added detail to ICD-10-CM codes requires additional knowledge of medical terminology, anatomy and physiology, pathophysiology, and pharmacology. Terminology used in ICD-9-CM

TABLE 11-6 Calendar for Partial Code Freeze

October 1, 2011	The last regular annual update to both ICD-9-CMand ICD-10-CM code sets is made.
October 1, 2012	Only limited code updates are made to both ICD-9-CM and ICD-10 code sets to capture new technology and new diseases.
October 1, 2013	No updates are made to ICD-9-CM as the system is no longer a HIPAA standard.
October 1, 2014	Regular updates to ICD-10-CM begin.

TABLE 11-7 Examples of Terminology Differences Between ICD-9-CM and ICD-10-CM

ICD-9-CM Classification	ICD-10-CM Classification
Status asthmaticus	Mild intermittent
	Mild persistent
	Moderate persistent
	Severe persistent
Bleeding/Hemorrhage	*Hemorrhage* used when referring to ulcers
	Bleeding used for diseases such as gastritis, duodenitis, diverticulitis, and diverticulosis
Acute myocardial infarction (AMI)	ST elevation
	Non-ST elevation
Burns	Burns that come from a heat source, electricity, or radiation
	Corrosion used to describe chemical burns

is replaced with more current clinical terminology. Table 11-7 ● shows examples of terminology differences between ICD-9-CM and ICD-10-CM.

New Abstracting Challenges

Just as providers identify areas where ICD-10-CM requires additional documentation details, coders working for those providers learn what details to abstract in order to code the case completely and accurately. In the example given earlier in this chapter regarding provider documentation of coma, coders need to look for the coma scale and time of assessment. Although coders do not assign the coma scale, they need to know it is required and, again, perhaps educate physicians about the need to document it.

In coding for obstetrics in ICD-9-CM, coders are accustomed to assigning a fifth digit for the episode of care: delivered, antepartum, or postpartum, and the presence of a complication. In ICD-10-CM, the episode for care is no longer coded as such, but the trimester of pregnancy is. This should be easily determined from the medical record and does not require additional documentation by physicians, but it does require that coders develop a new methodology.

In coding injuries or conditions to bilateral sites such as eyes, ears, and extremities, ICD-10-CM coders code **laterality** (right or left side). In most cases physicians are accustomed to documenting this information, but coders did not previously assign codes for laterality. Laterality presents an added step in code selection.

Codes for postoperative complications are expanded, and there is a distinction between intraoperative complications and postoperative disorders. Coders must become familiar with the expanded range of code choices and the new terminology.

The codes for external causes of morbidity, known as E-codes in ICD-9-CM, are significantly expanded in ICD-10-CM. Coders learn new main terms in order to locate new codes in the alphabetic index. Codes for legal intervention, war, and military operations are expanded. Most external cause codes in ICD-10-CM also require a seventh-digit extension indicating if the encounter is initial, subsequent, or for sequela. This information should be easily determined from the medical record, but it does represent an additional step in code assignment.

Falls, one of the leading external causes of injury, are described by about 40 codes in ICD-9-CM. ICD-10-CM has approximately 100 types of falls, each requiring one of three extensions for the encounter type as initial, subsequent, or for sequelae, resulting in approximately 300 different codes that can be assigned for falls.

Some external cause codes require information not normally obtained or documented by providers. For example, injuries involving alcohol may require a code for the blood alcohol level of the patient. Such data are often not determined and documented by the provider, but by law enforcement. Place of occurrence codes in ICD-10-CM describe not only the type of location, such as a private dwelling, but the exact location within the residence, such as a kitchen, bedroom, bathroom, or driveway.

New Concepts, Combination Coding, Guidelines

ICD-10-CM contains new coding concepts. For example, blood type is a coding criteria in ICD-10-CM that was nonexistent in ICD-9-CM. Likewise, the concept of injury by underdosing of medication is new in ICD-10-CM. Coders learn what the new concepts are, what they mean, when to use them, and how to assign the correct code.

Some ICD-10-CM codes are less specific than their ICD-9-CM predecessor. For example, ICD-9-CM has approximately thirty-six separate V codes for various types of immunizations, whereas ICD-10-CM has one code for an immunization encounter with the instructional note to use a procedure code to describe the type of immunization given.

Some conditions that require multiple coding in ICD-9-CM are identified with a combination code in ICD-10-CM. For example, diabetes type 2 with diabetic cataract is identified with two codes in ICD-9-CM but with a single combination code in ICD-10-CM that includes both the type of diabetes and the specific complication. Coders learn what situations are combined into a single code and what situations require separate coding.

Many of the "Official Guidelines for Coding and Reporting" are similar between ICD-9-CM and ICD-10-CM, but coders must be alert for those that are different. For example, when coding for anemia in cancer (neoplastic disease), ICD-9-CM directs coders to sequence the codes according to the reason for the encounter. Anemia is sequenced first when it is the primary reason for the encounter. ICD-10-CM guidelines direct coders to always sequence the neoplasm code first.

ICD-9-CM defines acute myocardial infarction (AMI) as one occurring within the past eight weeks, and ICD-10-CM defines AMI as one occurring within the past four weeks or less. Coders learn which guidelines are similar between ICD-9-CM and ICD-10-CM as well as what changes and additions are made.

Coder Training and Certification

Established coders must demonstrate their proficiency in ICD-10-CM to maintain certification. AHIMA and AAPC, the two leading professional organizations for coders, have specific requirements for coders to upgrade their skills to ICD-10-CM. Coders already certified in ICD-9-CM through AHIMA complete a specified amount of ICD-10-CM specific continuing education, based on their specialty and coding credential, beginning in 2011. Coders certified by AAPC take an ICD-10-CM proficiency exam that is available beginning October 2012.

The coding department assesses staff training needs and identifies the specific staff members who code or have a need to know the new codes. The most intensive training regarding the specifics and daily use of ICD-10-CM takes place within six months of the October 1, 2013, implementation date, and some coder education is phased in over a longer time (Figure 11-5 ●). Early training is ideal for managers and lead coders, to acquaint them with an overview of ICD-10-CM changes and preliminary acquaintance with code structure and guidelines. As the implementation date nears, all coders should receive intensive hands-on training on the full set of guidelines and code assignment.

A wide variety of training opportunities and materials are available through professional associations, online courses, webinars, and on-site training. A small practice has the option of teaming up with other local providers. For example, several offices can collaborate to provide training for a staff person from one practice, who can in turn train staff members in other practices. In many communities, physician offices are able to team up with hospitals for training.

The estimated amount of training for coders is 24 to 40 hours, depending on their role, specialty, and type of facility. The most general training is for managers who don't actually use ICD-10-CM codes on a regular basis but need a general awareness of ICD-10-CM code structure, guidelines, and the potential impact to workflow processes. More detailed training is provided for staff who use patient data that contain ICD-10-CM codes but are not responsible for assigning the codes. This would include data analysts who create and use historical data, project future trends, or create management reports. Medical office specialists and coders who assign codes to patient records on a routine basis receive the most intensive training, including a thorough knowledge of the systems, guidelines, and coding methodology. Additional

FIGURE 11-5

Staff training in the use of ICD-10-CM codes is critical to the success of the implementation process.

© Pat Watson/Pearson Education

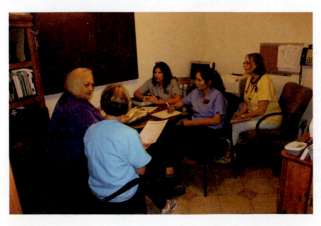

advanced training is needed for coders in individual physician specialties as well as inpatient hospital coders.

● **ONLINE INFORMATION:** For further information on the requirements for certified coders, visit www.aapc.com and www.ahima.org.

ACTIVITY #4

Understanding Certification Requirements

Research the ICD-10-CM requirements for AHIMA, AAPC, or another organization of your choice. Answer the following questions:

1. What are the requirements to maintain certification under ICD-10-CM?
2. Who has to complete the requirements?
3. What is the earliest date proficiency is available?
4. What is the last date by which proficiency must be completed?
5. What is the cost?

Appropriate Use of Data Mapping

General Equivalence Mappings (GEMs), created by jointly CMS and CDC, are the authoritative source for comparing codes between ICD-10-CM and ICD-9-CM. GEMs allow users to map forward and backward between the ICD-9-CM and ICD-10-CM coding systems. GEMs are public domain electronic files designed to give all sectors of the health care industry that use coded data a tool to convert and test systems, link data in long-term clinical studies, develop application-specific mappings, and analyze data collected during the transition period and beyond. This chapter discusses the general purpose and use of GEMs. Details involving translating specific codes are provided in Chapter 12.

GEMs are considered to be maps, not crosswalks. **Crosswalks** imply a one-to-one correlation between codes in two data sets, whereas maps accommodate **one-to-many** (e.g. a single code in ICD-9-CM has several possible equivalents in ICD-10-CM or vice versa) and **many-to-one** relationships (e.g. several codes for instance in ICD-10-CM are combined into a single equivalent code in ICD-9-CM or vice versa). An exact one-to-one matching of the ICD-9-CM and ICD-10-CM codes is not possible due to the changes in structure and concepts in ICD-10. Two **forward mapping** GEM data files list each ICD-9-CM/PCS code respectively and the closest equivalent(s) in ICD-10-CM/PCS. Two **backward mapping** GEM data files list each ICD-10-CM/PCS code, respectively, and the closest equivalent(s) in ICD-9-CM/PCS.

There are four GEM files:

- ICD-9-CM to ICD-10- CM (forward mapping)
- ICD-9- PCS to ICD-10-PCS (forward mapping)
- ICD-10-CM to ICD-9-CM (backward mapping)
- ICD-10-PCS to ICD-9- PCS (backward mapping)

PRACTICE PITFALLS

GEMs are not a substitute for learning how to use ICD-10-CM codes appropriately. GEMs are intended to be used with large volumes of data that need to be compared or analyzed over a time span that includes pre- and post-October 1, 2013, dates. GEMs are not intended to be used by coders to assign codes for specific patient encounters. Doing so would be misuse of data and potentially fraudulent coding practices.

ICD-9-CM codes may have an exact match, approximate match, or multiple matches in ICD-10-CM. Approximately one-fourth of ICD-9-CM codes have an exact match in ICD-10-CM, meaning that the codes in both manuals describe exactly the same condition. Examples of these are primary pulmonary hypertension, acute gastritis with hemorrhage, and malignant neoplasm of the head of the pancreas.

Roughly half of ICD-9-CM codes have an approximate match in ICD-10-CM, meaning that the ICD-10-CM code is similar to, but not an exact duplicate of, the ICD-9-CM code. Examples are malignant neoplasm of islets of Langerhas in ICD-9-CM and malignant neoplasm of endocrine pancreas in ICD-10-CM; idiopathic myocarditis in ICD-9-CM and isolated myocarditis in ICD-10-CM.

Most remaining ICD-9-CM codes have one-to-many forward mappings, meaning there are several ICD-10-CM codes for conditions that are described by only one code in ICD-9-CM. One-to-many forward mappings include examples discussed earlier in this chapter for coma, postmenopausal osteoporosis, Down syndrome, as well as most codes describing bilateral sites, injuries, and many external cause codes. Without reference to a patient's medical record, it is not possible to determine which ICD-10-CM code is the single best translation.

Some ICD-9-CM codes have a many-to-one forward mapping, meaning there is only one ICD-10-CM code that correlates with several ICD-9-CM codes. Hypertension is an example of a many-to-one forward match in which three ICD-9-CM codes—Malignant, Benign, and Unspecified hypertension—correspond with a single ICD-10-CM code, Essential hypertension. A few ICD-9-CM codes have no match at all in ICD-10-CM.

Working in reverse, the relationships are different. Only a few ICD-10-CM codes have an exact match in ICD-9-CM. Others are approximate or many-to-one backward mappings, meaning that several ICD-10-CM codes compare to one ICD-9-CM code. Some ICD-10-CM to ICD-9-CM GEMs are one-to-many backward mappings, meaning that for a given ICD-10-CM code, there are several possible corresponding codes in ICD-9-CM, such as those cited above for hypertension.

In the case of ICD-10-CM combination code, a many-to-one backward mapping occurs because several ICD-9-CM codes are required to convey the complete meaning of one ICD-10-CM, as is the case with diabetes with manifestations. It should be understood that using GEMs to find exact code matches is approximate and should be used only for research and trending purposes, not actual code assignment to patient encounters for billing purposes.

● **ONLINE INFORMATION:** For further information on GEMs, see the "ICD-10-CMS/PCS to ICD-9-CM Reimbursement Mappings: 2009 Version, Documentation and User's Guide" available at www.cms.gov/ICD10/Downloads/reimbmapguide2009.pdf.

▶ **CRITICAL THINKING QUESTION:** Imagine that you are working in a medical office. The physician says that to save time and money, rather than having you take intensive training to learn ICD-10-CM coding, you should use GEM files to find the codes. Do you think this is a good idea? Why or why not?

CHAPTER REVIEW

Summary

- ICD-9-CM, which has been used for diagnosis coding in the United States since 1979, is being replaced by a new diagnosis code set, ICD-10-CM, which is mandatory for dates of service, or dates of discharge for inpatients, that occur on or after October 1, 2013.
- ICD-10-CM codes are more specific than ICD-9-CM codes and provide more consistent data regarding patients' medical conditions.
- Everyone who is part of the health care system or uses its data is impacted, including providers, payers, regulators, vendors, claims clearinghouses, medical billing services, researchers, educational institutions, and support staff in each of these settings.
- All computer systems that collect, transmit, receive, or store diagnostic data need updating by January 1, 2012 with Version 5010, a new standard for electronic transactions, due to the expanded length, format, and structure of codes.
- The overall process to plan for, implement, and monitor the ICD-10-CM transition requires approximately five years.

- Because ICD-10-CM provides for a greater level of granularity and specificity, providers need to be sure that their documentation provides the needed information and that they record it in a way that is easy for coders to abstract.
- Coder training involves learning the new code set, coding guidelines, and new or updated software.
- Terminology and coding concepts used in ICD-9-CM are replaced with more current clinical terminology and updated coding concepts.
- Many of the "Official Guidelines for Coding and Reporting" are similar between ICD-9-CM and ICD-10-CM, but coders must be alert for those that are different.
- AHIMA and AAPC, the two leading professional organizations for coders, have specific requirements for coders to upgrade their skills to ICD-10-CM.
- GEMs are public domain electronic files designed to give all sectors of the health care industry that use coded data a tool to convert and test systems, link data in long-term clinical studies, develop application-specific mappings, and analyze data collected during the transition period and beyond.
- An exact one-to-one matching of the ICD-9-CM and ICD-10-CM codes is not possible due to the changes in structure and concepts in ICD-10.

Review Questions

Directions: Answer the following questions without looking back at the material covered in this chapter. Write your answers in the space provided.

1. State five benefits of ICD-10-CM.

    a. _____

    b. _____

    c. _____

    d. _____

    e. _____

2. State five ways in which ICD-10-CM is similar to ICD-9-CM.

    a. _____

    b. _____

    c. _____

    d. _____

    e. _____

3. State five ways in which ICD-10-CM differs from ICD-9-CM.

    a. _____

    b. _____

    c. _____

    d. _____

    e. _____

4. When is ICD-10-CM code set mandatory?

    a. January 1, 2012

    b. January 1, 2013

    c. October 1, 2013

    d. Whenever the computer systems are ready.

5. Name three types of HIPAA-mandated electronic transactions that are impacted by the Version 5010 standard.

   a. _____

   b. _____

   c. _____

6. Which of the following is not a change in provider documentation expected under ICD-10-CM?

   a. Glasgow Coma Scale

   b. Down's Syndrome

   c. Pathologic fractures

   d. Version 5010

7. State five ways a coder can obtain training in ICD-10-CM.

   a. _____

   b. _____

   c. _____

   d. _____

   e. _____

8. Cite three examples of medical terms that have new definitions under ICD-10-CM.

   a. _____

   b. _____

   c. _____

9. Which of the following areas will impact coders? Check all that apply.

   a. Learning new software

   b. Updating encounter forms

   c. Enhanced data entry skills

   d. Expanded medical terminology

   e. Reprogramming electronic transactions

10. Which is the most accurate description of GEMs?

    a. An exact one-to-one matching of the ICD-9-CM and ICD-10-CM codes

    b. An authoritative guide to assign ICD-10-CM codes to patient records for billing

    c. A mapping of relationships between ICD-9-CM and ICD-10-CM codes

    d. Electronic software that provides a definitive translation of ICD-9-CM code to ICD-10-CM codes

Activity #5: Identifying Key Deadlines and Activities

Directions: Review all references to key dates in the ICD-10-CM implementation process throughout the chapter, then match each of the following dates with the activity due on that date.

1. 2009 (ongoing) _____

2. January 1, 2010 _____

a. All electronic claims must use Version 5010.

b. Payers and providers begin internal testing of Version 5010 standards for electronic claims.

3. January 1, 2011 _____   c. ICD-10-CM codes are used on all health care claims.

4. January 1, 2012 _____   d. Regular updates to ICD-10-CM begin.

5. Early 2013 _____   e. Ongoing follow-up identifies and resolves claim errors and denials related to ICD-10-CM.

6. October 1, 2013 _____   f. Long-range organization and communication begins in health care organizations.

7. 2014 (ongoing) _____   g. CMS begins accepting Version 5010 claims.

8. October 1, 2014 _____   h. Intensive education of coders begins.

Activity #6: Defining Key Words

Directions: Match each key word with its definition.

1. Granular _____   a. Mapping ICD-9-CM code(s) to the closest equivalent ICD-10-CM code

2. Professional organization _____   b. Occurring on the right or left side

3. Backward mapping _____   c. Programming specifications

4. Laterality _____   d. Detail

5. Electronic transaction _____   e. New electronic standards for transmitting ICD-10-CM and related data

6. Forward mapping _____   f. Independent company or not-for-profit organization that provides support and information to specific types of businesses

7. Health care administrators _____   g. A single code has several possible equivalents in the other code set.

8. One-to-many _____   h. Mapping ICD-10-CM code(s) to the closest equivalent ICD-9-CM code

9. Version 5010 _____   i. Data transmitted via computers

10. Transaction standard _____   j. Individuals in each health care organization responsible for managing the organization

Activity #7: Determining the Definition of the Abbreviations

Directions: Write out the full meaning of each abbreviation.

1. OGCR _____

2. NCPDP _____

3. NCHS _____

4. ICD-10-CM _____

5. GCS _____

6. AHIMA _____

7. AAPC _____

8. ASC _____

9. CMS _____

10. ICD-10-PCS _____

Activity #8: ICD-10-CM Abstracting Challenges

Directions: Briefly describe how abstracting will change for each of the following conditions.

1. Obstetrics _____

2. Injury to right eye _____

3. Falls _____

4. Place of occurrence—private dwelling _____

5. Immunization _____

6. Diabetes type 2 with diabetic cataract _____

7. Anemia in neoplastic disease _____

8. Time frame for AMI _____

9. Coma _____

10. First visit for a traumatic fracture _____

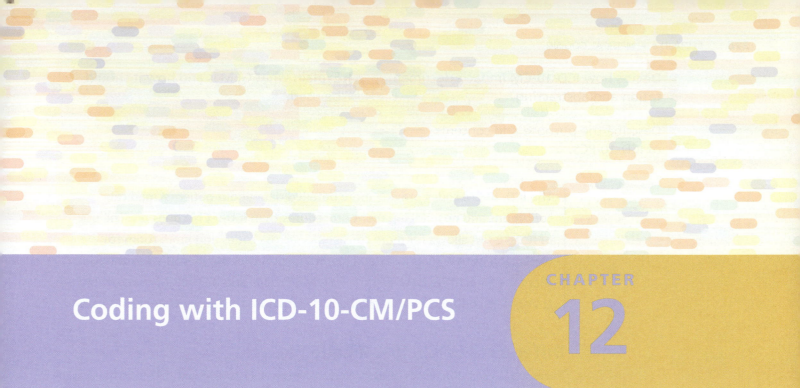

Coding with ICD-10-CM/PCS

After completion of this chapter you should be able to:

Describe the differences in code features between ICD-9-CM and ICD-10-CM.

Explain the contents and organization of ICD-10-CM.

Identify the conventions that are the same between ICD-9-CM and ICD-10-CM.

Discuss the new conventions and guidelines used in ICD-10-CM.

Demonstrate how to select the condition(s) to be coded.

Demonstrate how to locate and use main terms in the index.

Demonstrate how to verify codes in the tabular list.

Explain the guidelines for sequencing diagnosis codes.

Demonstrate how to accurately assign ICD-10-CM codes to patient encounters.

Key Words and Concepts you will learn in this chapter:

Block
Category
Code
Combination codes
Conventions
Default
Default code
Excludes1
Excludes2
Extension
First-listed diagnosis
Multiple coding
Nonessential modifiers
Placeholder
Principal diagnosis
Sequela
Short dash
Subcategory

Discuss how ICD-10-CM impacts documentation and abstracting.

Explain what GEM is and how it should be used.

Describe the purpose and contents of ICD-10-PCS.

> The ICD-10-CM codes provide more detailed data about patients' medical conditions and hospital inpatient procedures than ICD-9-CM codes do. The use of ICD-10-CM allows for more consistency across codes and more room for expansion as new diagnoses and medical procedures are identified. Although there are similarities between the ICD-9-CM codes and ICD-10-CM codes, there are changes to coding conventions and code structure that coders might understand.

Differences in ICD-10-CM Code Features

There are several differences in the features between ICD-10-CM and ICD-9-CM codes: the number of codes, code organization and structure, code composition, and level of detail. The number of codes increased from 14,000 diagnosis codes in the ICD-9-CM volumes to more than 68,000 in the ICD-10-CM manual. Table 12-1 ● summarizes major differences between codes in the two coding systems.

● **ONLINE INFORMATION:** Additional information about ICD-10-CM can be found on the Centers for Medicare & Medicaid Services (CMS) Web site:
www.cms.hhs.gov/ICD10

▶ **CRITICAL THINKING QUESTION:** As a student, why is it important to study both ICD-9-CM and ICD-10-CM coding when ICD-10-CM is likely to be the system used in the field?

TABLE 12-1 Comparison of Codes in ICD-9-CM and ICD-10-CM

Feature	ICD-9-CM	ICD-10-CM
Number of codes	14,000	68,000+
Code length	3 to 5 digits	3 to 7 characters
Code structure	3-digit category	3-digit category
	4th and 5th digits for etiology, anatomic site, manifestation	4th, 5th, 6th characters for etiology, anatomic site, severity 7th-digit extension
First character	Always numeric, except E codes and V codes	Used for additional information
Subsequent characters	All numeric	2nd character is always numeric
Decimal point	Mandatory after 3rd character, except E codes where decimal point is after 4th character	Mandatory after 3rd character on all codes
Extensions	None	Some codes (such as obstetrics and injuries) use a 7th character as an extension. Codes less than 6 characters that require a 7th character extension must contain placeholder "x" to fill the missing digits. The 7th character must always be a valid 7th character for that code (not "x".)
Placeholders	None	Character "x" is used as a 5th character placeholder in certain 6-character codes to allow for future expansion. The placeholder is also used to fill in other empty characters (e.g., character 5 and/or 6) when a code that is less than 6 characters in length requires a 7th character (extension). Do not use "x" to fill out a code that does not require a valid character as its last character.

Contents and Organization of the ICD-10-CM

The ICD-10-CM manual (2010 Draft) is a single volume and is not separated into volumes as is the ICD-9-CM. It is organized as follows:

- Introductory matter
  - Preface
  - Introduction
  - How to Use the ICD-10-CM (Draft 2010)
  - ICD-10-CM Draft Conventions
- ICD-10-CM Draft Official Guidelines for Coding and Reporting 2010
- ICD-10-CM Index to Diseases and Injuries
- ICD-10-CM Neoplasm Table
- ICD-10-CM Table of Drugs and Chemicals
- ICD-10-CM Index to External Causes
- ICD-10-CM Tabular List of Diseases and Injuries

Table 12-2 ● shows the chapters in the tabular list and summarizes the nature of the changes made to each chapter in ICD-10-CM. Each chapter uses codes beginning with a unique letter of the alphabet, except for the letter D, which is used in Chapters 2 and 3, and the letter H, which is used in Chapters 7 and 8. The 2010 Draft ICD-10-CM does not contain any appendices.

TABLE 12-2 Organization of ICD-10-CM Tabular List

Chapter Number and Name	Code Range	Nature of Revisions
1. Certain infectious and parasitic diseases	A00–B99	Received codes from other chapters; new sections
2. Neoplasms	C00–D48	Received codes from other chapters
3. Diseases of the blood and blood-forming organs and certain disorders involving the immune mechanism	D50–D89	Received codes from other chapters
4. Endocrine, nutritional and metabolic diseases	E00–E90	Major changes to diabetes codes
5. Mental and behavioral disorders	F01–F99	Reorganized
6. Diseases of the nervous system	G00–G99	Divided into three chapters
7. Diseases of the eye and adnexa	H00–H59	New chapter
8. Diseases of the ear and mastoid process	H60–H95	New chapter
9. Diseases of the circulatory system	I00–I99	Received codes from other chapters
10. Diseases of the respiratory system	J00–J99	Received codes from other chapters
11. Diseases of the digestive system	K00–K93	Received codes from other chapters
12. Diseases of the skin and subcutaneous tissue	L00–L99	Major restructuring
13. Diseases of the musculoskeletal system and connective tissue	M00–M99	Received codes from other chapters; major expansion of codes
14. Diseases of the genitourinary system	N00–N99	Received codes from other chapters
15. Pregnancy, childbirth and the puerperium	O00–O99	Received codes from other chapters; trimester codes added
16. Certain conditions originating in the perinatal period	P00–P96	Title changes
17. Congenital malformations, deformations, and chromosomal abnormalities	Q00-Q99	Title changes
18. Symptoms, signs, and abnormal clinical and laboratory findings, not elsewhere classified	R00–R99	Received codes from other chapters
19. Injury, poisoning, and certain other consequences of external causes	S00–T98	Major reorganization and code expansion
20. External causes of morbidity	V01–Y99	Major revisions
21. Factors influencing health status and contact with health services	Z00–Z99	Received codes from other chapters

TABLE 12-3 Organizational Hierarchy of ICD-10-CM Tabular List

Level	Example
Chapter	Chapter 15. Pregnancy, Childbirth and the Puerperium (O00-O9a)
Block	Pregnancy with abortive outcome (O00-O08)
Category	O03 Spontaneous abortion
Subcategory	O03.3 Other and unspecified complications following incomplete spontaneous abortion
Code	O03.31 Shock following incomplete spontaneous abortion

Each chapter contains codes for a body system or related diseases. Any instructional notes at the beginning of the chapter apply to all codes within that chapter. Within each chapter, codes are subdivided into blocks, categories, subcategories, and codes.

- A **block** in ICD-10-CM is comparable to a section in ICD-9-CM. It is a contiguous range of codes within a chapter. Instructional notes at the beginning of the block apply to all codes within that block.
- A **category** is three characters in length. A three-character category that has no further subdivision is equivalent to a code. Instructional notes at the beginning of the category apply to all codes within that category.
- A **subcategory** is either four or five characters in length. Each level of subdivision after a category and before a code is a subcategory. Instructional notes at the beginning of the subcategory apply to all codes within that subcategory.
- The final level of subdivision is a **code**. Codes may be three, four, five, six, or seven characters in length. All codes in the tabular list of the official version of the ICD-10-CM are in bold. Codes that have applicable 7th characters are still referred to as codes, not subcategories. Instructional notes under a code apply only to that specific code.

Table 12-3 ● illustrates the organizational hierarchy within the tabular list.

PRACTICE **PITFALLS**

Be on the watch for letters that can be easily confused with numbers. The capital letter I can be confused with the number 1. The letter S can be confused with the number 5. The capital letter O can be confused with the number 0. In the ICD-10-CM manual, the number zero is written as Ø to help distinguish it from the capital letter O.

ACTIVITY #1

Identifying the Organization of ICD-10-CM

Directions: Look up the following entries in the ICD-10-CM manual. Determine if each entry is a block, category, subcategory, or code, and write the appropriate answer next to each entry.

1. D56 Thalassemia _____
2. F20.0 Paranoid schizophrenia _____
3. Diseases of esophagus, stomach, and duodenum (K20-K31) _____
4. O60.12 Preterm labor second trimester with preterm delivery second trimester _____
5. O48.1 Prolonged pregnancy _____
6. S37.0 Injury of kidney _____
7. S67 Crushing injury of wrists, hand, and fingers _____
8. T20.1xxS Burn of esophagus, sequela _____
9. Visual disturbances and blindness (H53–H54) _____
10. M48.44 Fatigue fracture of vertebra, thoracic region _____

E codes and V codes in ICD-9-CM have undergone some changes in ICD-10-CM. Although these classifications exist in ICD-10-CM, they are no longer called E codes and V codes. ICD-9-CM E-codes are now reported in ICD-10-CM using codes beginning with the letter V, W, X and Y in Chapter 20: External Causes of Morbidity. External causes of morbidity have a separate index, the ICD-10-CM Index to External Causes, which follows the Table of Drugs and Chemicals. This is similar to the E-code index in ICD-9-CM.

ICD-9-CM V codes are reported in ICD-10-CM using codes beginning with the letter Z in Chapter 21: Factors Influencing Health Status, and Contact with Health Services. The main terms for these codes are indexed in the main alphabetic index of diseases of ICD-10-CM, similar to ICD-9-CM.

ICD-10-CM Conventions and Guidelines

ICD-10-CM is accompanied by "Official Guidelines for Coding and Reporting" (OGCR), just as ICD-9-CM is. The organization of OGCR is similar:

Section I. Conventions, General Coding Guidelines and Chapter-Specific Guidelines

A. Conventions for the ICD-10-CM
B. General Coding Guidelines
C. Chapter-Specific Coding Guidelines

Section II. Selection of Principal Diagnosis

Section III. Reporting Additional Diagnoses

Section IV. Diagnostic Coding and Reporting Guidelines for Outpatient Services.

Many of the guidelines in Sections I.B., II, III, and IV are similar in both the ICD-9-CM and ICD-10-CM manuals. Changes in these sections are related to differences in code structure, such as additional characters, 7th-character extensions, and laterality. Guidelines in Section I.A. reflect new and updated **conventions** (use of symbols, typeface, and layout features.) Guidelines in Section C reflect changes in chapter organization and updated clinical terminology, definitions, and practice.

Similar Conventions and Guidelines in ICD-9-CM and ICD-10-CM

Many ICD-9-CM and ICD-10-CM conventions are similar. In the ICD-10-CM manual, the conventions are listed in introductory matter, preceding the OGCR. Prior to performing actual coding, it is important to recognize and understand the conventions, as these are crucial to interpreting ICD-10-CM instructions and assigning the accurate code(s). Table 12-4 ● summarizes the conventions that are similar in both the ICD-9-CM and ICD-10-CM codes.

New Conventions and Guidelines in ICD-10-CM

ICD-10-CM introduces the use of some new conventions and OGCR. See Table 12-5 ● for a summary of the new conventions.

EXCLUSION NOTES Instead of the single Excludes note used in ICD-9-CM, the ICD-10-CM tabular list utilizes two exclusion notes: Excludes1 and Excludes2. Exclusion notes may appear at the block, category, subcategory, or code level. Notes at the category or subcategory level apply to all codes that follow, so it is important to check not only the code itself but also the preceding headings. For example, K55, *Vascular disorder of intestine,* has a note for Excludes1, *necrotizing enterocolitis of newborn (P77.-).* This note applies to all the subsequent codes, K55.0 through K55.9. If the coder were to read only the notes for one code, such as K55.1, the coder would miss the added instruction at the K55 category level.

Excludes1 indicates that the condition represented by the code and the condition excluded are mutually exclusive and should not be coded together, such as the acquired and congenital forms of the same condition. When an Excludes1 note appears under a code, none of the codes that appear after it should be used with the original code itself. Continuing with the same example,

TABLE 12-4 Conventions That Are the Same for ICD-9-CM and ICD-10-CM

Convention	Meaning/Use
[ ] Square brackets	Tabular: Synonyms, alternative wording, explanatory phrases
	Index: Indicates sequencing on manifestation codes or other paired codes. The code in square brackets [ ] should be sequenced second.
( ) Parentheses	Tabular and index: nonessential modifiers
: Colon	Tabular: Appears after an incomplete term that requires one or more modifiers following the colon to be classified to that code or category
NEC	Tabular and index: Not Elsewhere Classifiable. The medical record contains additional details about the condition, but no more specific code is available to use.
NOS	Tabular: Not Otherwise Specified. Information to assign a more specific code is not available in the medical record.
Boldface	Tabular: Code titles
Heavy type	Index: Main terms
Italics *Slanted type*	Tabular: Exclusion notes, manifestation codes
Includes notes	Tabular: Begin with "Includes" and further define, clarify, or give examples
Inclusion terms	Tabular: A list of synonyms or conditions included within a classification
See	Index: It is necessary to reference another main term or condition to locate the correct code.
See Also	Index: Coder may refer to an alternative or additional main term if the desired entry is not found under the original main term.
And	Tabular: Means "and/or"
With	In a code title, means "both" or "together"
Code First/Use Additional Code	Tabular: Provides sequencing instructions for conditions that have both an underlying etiology and multiple body system manifestations and certain other codes that have sequencing requirements.
Code Also	Tabular: More than one code may be required to fully describe the condition.

TABLE 12-5 New Conventions in ICD-10-CM

ICD-10-CM Convention	Meaning/Use
Excludes1	Mutually exclusive codes. None of the codes that appear after it should be used with the original code itself.
Excludes2	The condition excluded is not part of the condition represented by the code, but may be reported together if documented.
✓4th ✓5th ✓6th ✓7th ✓x7th	Used in front of a code to indicate that an additional digit is needed for the code to be complete.
x	A placeholder in codes with less than six characters that require a 7th character extension. The x itself has no meaning and is not replaced with an actual number or letter. In some codes, the x is used to reserve room for future expansion.
- Short dash	Additional characters should be assigned in place of the -. The additional characters may be number or letters, depending on the code.
With/Without	Within a set of alternative codes, describe options for final character.

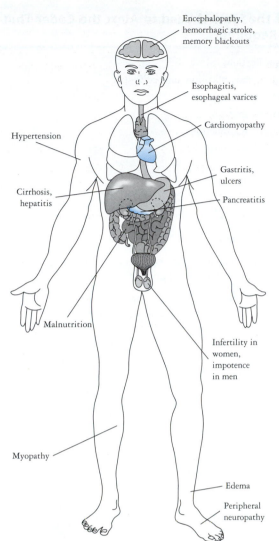

FIGURE 12-1

Physiologic effects of alcoholism

© Pearson Education

Encephalopathy, hemorrhagic stroke, memory blackouts

Esophagitis, esophageal varices

Cardiomyopathy

Hypertension

Gastritis, ulcers

Cirrhosis, hepatitis

Pancreatitis

Malnutrition

Infertility in women, impotence in men

Myopathy

Edema

Peripheral neuropathy

the Excludes1 note under K55 means that *necrotizing enterocolitis of newborn (P77.-)* should not be reported with any of the codes within the K55 category.

Excludes2 indicates that the condition excluded is not part of the condition represented by the code but that the patient may have both conditions at the same time. These conditions are not mutually exclusive. When an Excludes2 note appears under a code, it is acceptable to use the main code and the excluded code if the patient is documented to have both conditions. For example, K86.0, *Alcohol induced chronic pancreatitis,* has an Excludes2 note for *alcohol induced acute pancreatitis* (K85.2.) The second condition is not included in code K86.0, but it may be reported together with it if the documentation states that the patient has both conditions. Other conditions associated with alcoholism are noted in Figure 12-1 ●.

Some codes may have both Excludes1 and Excludes2 notes. For example, the block *Diseases of liver* (K70–K77) has an Excludes1 note for *jaundice NOS* (R17), meaning that R17 should not be reported with any of the codes from K70 through K77. The same block also has several Excludes2 notes. The conditions listed under Excludes 2 are not included in any of the codes K70 through K77, but they may be reported together with them if the patient is documented to have both conditions. K77 may appear on a different physical page than the block heading, so the coder who failed to review the beginning of the category would not be aware of these instructions.

If a code doesn't have any exclusion notes, then it can be used with any other code that is supported by the medical record and the official guidelines.

TABLE 12-6 Illustration of the Symbol Used to Alert the Coder That Additional Characters Are Required

✓5th	K94.2	Gastrostomy complications
	K94.20	Gastrostomy complication, unspecified
	K94.21	Gastrostomy hemorrhage
	K94.20	Gastrostomy infection
	K94.20	Gastrostomy malfunction

ACTIVITY #2

Interpreting Exclusion Notes

Directions: For each pair of codes, indicate if they can or cannot be used together based on the exclusion notes. Circle the correct answer.

1.	G43.004 & G43.709	OK	Don't use together
2.	D56.1 & D57.411	OK	Don't use together
3.	H71.00 & H95.131	OK	Don't use together
4.	M21.532 & M21.721	OK	Don't use together
5.	O070 & O4.84	OK	Don't use together
6.	R22.2 & R19.01	OK	Don't use together
7.	R29.890 & M79.62	OK	Don't use together
8.	M80.012 & M89.712	OK	Don't use together
9.	S83.015A & M23.204	OK	Don't use together
10.	T38.0x5D & T490x5D	OK	Don't use together

USE ADDITIONAL CHARACTERS. ICD-10-CM has two ways of alerting the user to use additional characters on a code: a symbol containing ✓4th, ✓5th, ✓6th, ✓7th, or ✓x7th in front of a code, or a short dash (-) at the end of a code number. Most editions of ICD-9-CM use an octagon symbol or a colored box with 4th or 5th preceding a code in the tabular list to indicate that a subcategory needs additional characters and the coder should look to the next level down for more specificity. In ICD-10-CM this practice is continued, but with more choices because ICD-10-CM codes may have as many as seven characters and ICD-9-CM codes have, at the most, five characters. In ICD-10-CM the additional characters for characters 4 through 6 are listed below the subcategory. Table 12-6 ● illustrates the symbol used to alert the coder that additional characters are required.

EXTENSIONS AND PLACEHOLDERS. An **extension** is the seventh character of a code that must appear in that position, regardless of the length of the code. The addition of an extension is indicated by the symbol ✓7th preceding a subcategory. Definitions for the extension character appear in a colored box preceding the code entry, often at a preceding block, category, or subcategory level. When a code less than six characters requires an extension, the symbol ✓x7th is used. ✓x7th means that the code requires a seventh character and the **placeholder** X must fill the empty position(s) on a code less than six characters in length. The X itself has no meaning and is not replaced with an actual number or letter. For example, the OGCR for Chapter 12: Diseases of Skin and Subcutaneous Tissue (L00-L99), item a.2 states, "Assignment of the code for Unstageable pressure ulcer (L89.--0) should be based on the clinical documentation."

The designation means that this guideline applies to all codes beginning with L89 and ending in Ø, such as L89.000, L89.010, L89.130, etc. Earlier we looked at Excludes1 *necrotizing*

FIGURE 12-2

A pressure ulcer

© CaptureIt/Alamy

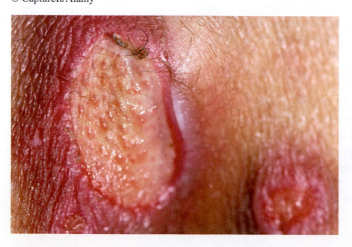

enterocolitis of newborn (P77.-). The code designation P77.- uses the "-" to indicate all codes beginning with P77.

The extension must appear in the 7th position, regardless of the length of the code itself. The range of codes the extension characters apply to is dictated by where the characters and definitions appear within the organizational hierarchy. Codes that require a 7th-digit extension are considered to be invalid if it is omitted.

PRACTICE **PITFALLS**

It is important to notice exactly where a set of extension definitions appears within the organizational hierarchy. When the extension characters and definitions are listed at the beginning of a chapter, they are used with all subsequent codes in the chapter; when they appear at the beginning of a block, they are used with all codes in the block; when they appear at the beginning of a category or subcategory, they are used with all codes in the category or subcategory, respectively.

Use of extensions is common in Chapter 19: Injury, Poisoning, and Certain Other Consequences of External Causes (S00–T98) and selected categories in Chapter 13: Diseases of the Musculoskeletal System and Connective Tissue (M00–M99) to denote whether the current encounter is the *initial* encounter (A), *subsequent* encounter (D), or *sequela* (S). **Sequela** is a late effect or delayed healing. Extensions are also common in Chapter 15: Pregnancy, Childbirth, and the Puerperium (O00–O9A) to identify each fetus in a multiple-gestation pregnancy.

Table 12-7 ● illustrates a sample entry in the tabular list that requires an extension and a placeholder.

PRACTICE **PITFALLS**

In ICD-9-CM discussions and instructions, it is common to use the X to indicate that a code needs a 4th or 5th character to be complete. For example, 250.xx means that category 250 requires a 4th and 5th character and the coder should assign numbers in place of the X. ICD-10-CM uses the **short dash** (-) in a different manner. When an ICD-10-CM code has a "-" after it, additional characters should be assigned. The additional characters may be numbers or letters, depending on the code.

TABLE 12-7 A Sample Entry in the Tabular List That Requires an Extension and a Placeholder

✓4th S01 Open wound of head

The appropriate 7th character is to be added to each code from category S01.

A   initial encounter
D   subsequent encounter
S   sequela

✓5th S01.0 Open wound of scalp

✓x7th S01.00 Unspecified open wound of scalp

- To assign a code for *unspecified open wound of scalp, initial encounter*, select the code S01.00.
- Because the code is only five characters in length, the symbol ✓x7th reminds you to add the placeholder x to make it six characters long.
- Finally, add the extension A to designate the initial encounter.
- The final code is S01.00xA

ACTIVITY #3

Assigning the Correct Number of Characters

Directions: Look up the following codes in the tabular list and determine if each is correct, needs additional characters, needs a placeholder, and/or needs an extension. Some codes may need more than one of these items. If the code is correct, write "Correct" in the space provided. If the code is incorrect, write the correct code for the stated condition in the space provided.

1. E65 Localized adiposity_____

2. E66 Morbid obesity due to excess calories _____

3. G43.1 Migraine with aura, not intractable, with status migrainosus _____

4. I48.0 Atrial fibrillation _____

5. O31.00 Papyraceous fetus, first trimester, fetus 1 _____

6. O29.8x2 Other complications of anesthesia during pregnancy, second trimester _____

7. S71.151 Bite, right thigh, sequela _____

8. S84.22 Injury of cutaneous sensory nerve at lower leg level, left leg, initial encounter _____

9. S72.02 Displaced fracture of epiphysis, left femur, subsequent encounter for closed fracture with nonunion _____

10. T59.6x Toxic effect of hydrogen sulfide, accidental, subsequent encounter _____

WITH AND WITHOUT. For some codes, the options "with" and "without" represent alternatives for the final character. The **default** is always "without," meaning that if the documentation does not specifically state "with" or "without," the code for "without" should be assigned. The final character is assigned differently for five- vs. six- character codes.

For five-character codes, the final character is as follows:

0   without

1   with

For example, under K72.1- *Chronic hepatic failure,* a fifth character designates the presence or absence of coma:

K72.1**0** Chronic hepatic failure, **without** coma

K72.1**1** Chronic hepatic failure, **with** coma

For six-character codes, the final digit is as follows:

1   with

9   without

For example, under G43.10- *Migraine with aura, not intractable,* a sixth character designates the presence or absence of status migrainosus:

G43.101   Migraine with aura, not intractable, **with** status migrainosus

G43.10**9**   Migraine with aura, not intractable, **without** status migrainosus

In both examples, "without" is the default, but the character that designates "without" is different. Be aware that the numbers Ø, 1, and 9 do not always carry the meaning of "with" or "without." Coders should not assume they know what a code number represents without detailed reading of the code description.

LATERALITY. ICD-10-CM contains a new OGCR, Section I.B.13, Laterality, which describes how to designate the side of the body affected when bilateral sites exist. For bilateral sites, such as eyes, ears, arms, legs, the final character of the code indicates right or left side. Some of

FIGURE 12-3

Conjunctivitis

© Dorling Kindersley

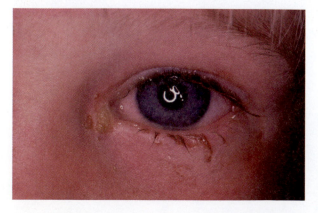

TABLE 12-8 Example of Laterality in ICD-10-CM

ICD-10-CM code	Description	
H16.04	Marginal corneal ulcer	subcategory
H16.041	Marginal corneal ulcer, **right** eye	code
H16.042	Marginal corneal ulcer, **left** eye	code
H16.043	Marginal corneal ulcer, **bilateral**	code
H16.049	Marginal corneal ulcer, **unspecified** eye	code

these codes also provide an option for bilateral, both sides affected. If there is no designation for bilateral, separate codes would be assigned for the right side and the left side. If the site is unspecified, the code for unspecified would be assigned. The implementation of laterality is one example of why ICD-10-CM has many times the number of codes as ICD-9-CM does. In ICD-9-CM a condition such as *Marginal corneal ulcer* has one code number, 370.01, whereas ICD-10-CM has four codes plus a subcategory heading (five entries total) for the same condition. Table 12-8 ● illustrates laterality for *Marginal corneal ulcer.*

▶ **CRITICAL THINKING QUESTION:** What are some ways a coder can remember the differences between the guidelines and conventions found in the ICD-10-CM manual compared to the ICD-9-CM code book?

Selecting Diagnoses to Be Coded

The first step in coding with ICD-10-CM is the same as ICD-9-CM: identify the diagnosis (diagnoses) to be coded, based on the documentation. The OGCR provide guidelines for this task in Section I.B. as well as Section IV for *outpatient* services and Sections II and III for *inpatient* services. Chapter-specific guidelines in Section I.C. provide more detailed guidance for selected conditions.

Selecting Outpatient Diagnoses

For outpatient coding, the coder needs to identify the main reason for the services provided, which is called the **first-listed diagnosis**. This is the "diagnosis, condition, problem, or other reason for the encounter visit shown in the medical record to be chiefly responsible for the services provided" (OGCR IV.A.). Coding conventions and the general (OGCR I. B.) and chapter-specific (OCGR I.C.) guidelines take precedence over Section IV outpatient guidelines. Signs or symptoms that are an integral part of the disease process should not be coded when the diagnosis has been established. Additional conditions, signs, or symptoms not part of the confirmed disease process should be coded in addition to the first-listed diagnosis when they are managed during the encounter. Conditions that are resolved, not treated, or have no bearing on the current encounter should not be coded.

When the diagnosis is uncertain, as indicated in the medical record by terms such as *probable, possible, suspected, questionable, rule out,* or *working diagnosis,* do not code the uncertain diagnosis. Instead, code the presenting signs and symptoms. This guideline for outpatient services is different from the guideline for uncertain diagnoses for inpatient services.

Codes exist for encounters due to reasons other than a disease or injury. These may be routine health screenings, preventive care, diagnostic services only, therapeutic services only, preoperative evaluations, prenatal visits, and similar situations (Figure 12-4 ●). Codes for most of these situations are classified under Factors Influencing Health Status and Contact with Health Services (Z00–99.) Detailed guidelines appear in OGCR IV, and codes can be located in the Index to Diseases and Injuries.

Selecting Inpatient Diagnoses

For inpatient services, the main reason that services were provided is called the **principal diagnosis** (Figure 12-5 ●). This is the "condition established after study to be chiefly responsible for occasioning

FIGURE 12-4

Woman having an ultrasound during a prenatal exam

© Monkey Business Images/ Shutterstock.com

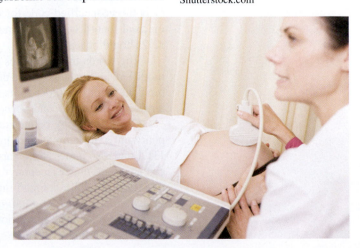

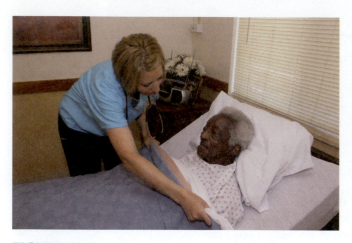

FIGURE 12-5

Caring for a patient in an inpatient care setting

© Pat Watson/Pearson Education

the admission of the patient to the hospital for care" (OGCR Section II). Coding conventions and the general (OGCR I.B) and chapter-specific (OGCR I.C) guidelines take precedence over Sections II and III inpatient guidelines. Signs or symptoms that are an integral part of the disease process should not be coded when the diagnosis has been established. Additional conditions, signs, or symptoms that are not part of the confirmed disease process should be coded in addition to the principal diagnosis when they are relevant to the current admission. This is defined as "all conditions that coexist at the time of admission, that develop subsequently, or that affect the treatment received and/or the length of stay. Diagnoses that relate to an earlier episode which have no bearing on the current hospital stay are to be excluded" (OGCR III).

The guideline for coding uncertain diagnoses is different for inpatient than for outpatient services. For inpatients, when the diagnosis is uncertain, as indicated in the medical record by words such as *probable, possible, suspected, questionable, rule out,* or *working diagnosis,* code the uncertain diagnosis as if it exists. This diagnosis is the reason for the hospital admission, and any diagnostic and therapeutic services provided. (OGCR II.H.)

Locating the Main Term

After identifying the first-listed diagnosis or principal diagnosis, the first step in assigning the code is to locate the main term in the ICD-10-CM Index to Diseases and Injuries. The condition is listed as the main term, usually in the form of a noun. Anatomical sites or organs are generally not indexed as main terms. Main terms appear in boldface type in the index.

For example, when coding for a sprained ankle, the main term is *sprain,* not *ankle.* The entry for Ankle states "*see* condition." This means to look up the term that describes the condition affecting the ankle. Do not look up the word *condition.*

Subterms, those words indented under the main term in roman type (not boldface), describe the main term in greater detail, such as anatomical location or other disease variation.

For example, under the main term *Sprain,* subterms describe the anatomical site of the sprain, such as *ankle.* Under the subterm *ankle,* additional subterms further describe the anatomical site within the ankle, such as *deltoid ligament* S93.42-.

Some subterms provide cross-referencing instructions. When the instruction following the word *see* is capitalized, the coder should look under the entry listed for the correct code. For example, under Sprain, ankle, the subterm *internal collateral ligament* provides cross-referencing instructions to "*see* Sprain, ankle, specified ligament NEC." This means that a sprain of the internal collateral ligament should be reported with the code S93.49- *Sprain, ankle, specified ligament NEC.* There is no separate code specifically for sprain of the internal collateral ligament.

A code listed next to a main term in the ICD-10-CM index is referred to as a default code. The **default code** represents that condition that is most commonly associated with the main term, or is the unspecified code for the condition. For example, if appendicitis is documented in the medical record without any additional information, such as acute or chronic, the default code K37 should be assigned.

The words in parentheses ( ) after the main term are **nonessential modifiers**. Nonessential modifiers are included in the default description of the code and do not need to be present in the medical record in order to use the code. For example, under the main term *Appendicitis,* the terms *pneumococcal* and *retrocecal* are by default included in the default appendicitis code K37.

Conditions may be indexed under more than one main term. For example, chronic rhinopharyngitis (inflammation of the nose and throat) can be located under Rhinopharyngitis, chronic J31.1 and also under Nasopharyngitis, chronic J31.1. If the coder cannot locate a main term, she can also look under an eponym (a condition named after a person) a synonym, or other alternative term. In addition, broad-ranging main terms can be referenced, such as *Abnormal, Anomaly, Complication, Disease, Findings, Infection, Injury,* or *Syndrome.* In some cases, the coder may need to look in several locations under different main terms, to identify multiple code options before proceeding.

When an instruction beginning with *see* is the only information listed beside a main term, it is necessary to reference another main term or condition to locate the correct code. When a specific main term is to be referenced, it is always capitalized, as in "Atopy - *see* History, allergy." The coder will not find a code under Atopy but should look up the main term *History* and the subterm *allergy*. The note "*see* condition" means to look up the name of the condition as the main term. For example, "Ankle - *see* condition." Do not look up the word "condition" but, rather, the name of the condition that is affecting the ankle, such as Sprain.

Specialized Index Locations

Although most conditions and reasons for the encounter are located in the Index to Diseases and Injuries, ICD-10-CM has three additional references for specialized purposes:

- *Neoplasms* are indexed on the Neoplasm Table, located immediately after the Index to Diseases and Injuries. The location differs from the ICD-9-CM neoplasm table, which is located under "N" in the Alphabetic Index.
- *Poisonings, adverse effects, and underdosing* are indexed on the ICD-10-CM Table of Drugs and Chemicals, which is located immediately following the Neoplasm Table. This is similar to the ICD-9-CM.
- *External causes of illness and injury* are located in a separate index, the ICD-10-CM Index to External Causes, which follows the Table of Drugs and Chemicals. This is similar to the E-code Index in ICD-9-CM. External causes reported under E codes in ICD-9-CM are generally reported using codes beginning with the letter V in ICD-10-CM.

Verifying Codes in the Tabular List

After identifying the potential code(s) in the index, the next step in assigning a code is to verify it in the tabular list. This is an essential step because the index does not always provide the full code or full information about how to use the code.

A short dash (-) at the end of an index entry indicates that additional characters are required. Even if a dash is not included at the index entry, it is necessary to refer to the tabular list to verify that no 7th character is required and to review the instructional notes. Characters for laterality and the 7th position extension can only be assigned in the tabular list. The tabular list also includes instructional notes that must be followed, such as those for sequencing, multiple coding, and inclusion and exclusion notes, as discussed earlier in this chapter.

ACTIVITY #4

Finding the Main Term and Determining the Correct ICD-10-CM Code

Directions: In Chapter 10 you coded these conditions using the ICD-9-CM code book. Now follow the same process of identifying main terms in the index and verifying them in the tabular list to assign the correct ICD-10-CM code. Based on the condition, look up the appropriate ICD-10-CM code and write it in the space provided. Also underline the main term.

1. Complicated open wound of left ear, initial encounter _____
2. Deprivation of water, subsequent encounter _____
3. Stuttering _____
4. Chicken pox _____
5. Blackwater fever _____
6. Patella fracture, right knee, subsequent encounter _____
7. Quartan malaria _____
8. Hemophilia C _____
9. Congestive heart failure _____
10. Type 1 diabetes _____

To verify a code, look up the code number in the tabular list and follow these steps:

- Read the code title to confirm that the code accurately describes the intended condition.
- Read the instructional notes under the code.
- Check for any symbols indicating that additional characters are required.
- Read the title of the three-character category and read any instructional notes under the category title.
- Read the title of the block and the chapter headings, and read any instructional notes under those titles.
- Compare and contrast any other codes being considered for first-listed or principal diagnosis.
- Assign all required digits and write down the code, taking time to double-check for transcription or typographical errors.
- Repeat this process for each code required.

Combination Codes and Multiple Coding

Combination codes are codes that describe multiple conditions with one code. As discussed in Chapter 11, ICD-10-CM has more combination codes than ICD-9-CM. Conditions that ICD-9-CM classifies using multiple codes may be classified in ICD-10-CM with a combination code. Coders need to give special attention to the direction in the index and instructional notes in the tabular list to determine when a combination code is available and when **multiple coding** (using two or more codes to fully describe a condition) is required. For example, diabetes type 2 with diabetic cataract is classified using two codes in ICD-9-CM but a single combination code in ICD-10-CM. Table 12-9 ● shows examples of ICD-9-CM multiple coding replaced by ICD-10-CM combination codes.

Not all possible conditions have combination codes in ICD-10-CM. Multiple coding is the use of more than one code to fully describe a condition. ICD-10-CM uses conventions in both the index and the tabular list to alert the coder to the need for multiple coding. When multiple codes are required to fully describe an encounter, the final step in assigning codes is to sequence them properly. Sequencing instructions may be found in any or all of several locations.

In the index, sequencing of etiology/manifestation codes is indicated by use of square brackets [ ]. The code in brackets, the manifestation, should be sequenced second. For example, dementia in Parkinson's disease is indexed under the main term *Dementia,* and the subterms in *Parkinson's disease* G20 [F02.80] (Figure 12-6 ●). The square brackets around [F02.80] indicate that G20 *Parkinson's disease* should be sequenced first, followed by F02.80 *Dementia in other diseases classified elsewhere, without behavioral disturbance.*

In the tabular list, sequencing may be indicated by instructions to "Code first" or "Use additional code." These conventions provide sequencing instructions for conditions that have both an underlying etiology and multiple body system manifestations and certain other codes that have sequencing requirements. "Code first" appears under the manifestation code, indicating that the etiology should be sequenced first. "Use additional code" appears under the etiology code, indicating that the manifestation should be sequenced second.

TABLE 12-9 Examples of ICD-9-CM Multiple Coding Replaced by ICD-10-CM Combination Codes

ICD-9-CM Code	ICD-9-CM Title	ICD-10-CM Code	ICD-10-CM Title
250.50	Diabetes mellitus, type 2, not stated as uncontrolled, with ophthalmic manifestations	E11.36	Type 2 diabetes mellitus with diabetic cataract
366.41	Diabetic cataract		
292.12	Drug induced psychotic disorder with hallucinations	F14.251	Cocaine dependence with cocaine induced psychotic disorder with hallucinations
304.20	Cocaine dependence, unspecified		

The convention "Code also" appears in the tabular list and indicates that more than one code may be required to fully describe the condition. The "Code also" instruction does not dictate the sequence. Sequence is determined by the circumstances of the encounter or admission. For example, under the block heading "Glomerular diseases (N00–N08)" the coder is instructed to "Code also any associated kidney failure (N17–N19)." This note means that for any condition coded as N00–N08, the coder should also code associated kidney failure, if it exists. However, the sequencing is not dictated by this note. The coder will sequence according to the reason for the encounter.

In the OGCR, sequencing may be described in the general coding guidelines (I.B); inpatient (Sections II and III) or outpatient guidelines (Section IV), respectively; or in the chapter-specific guidelines (I.C.1–21).

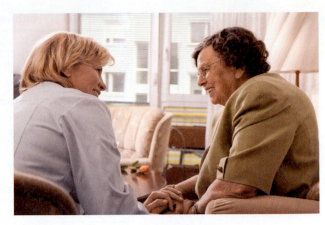

FIGURE 12-6

A patient with dementia being comforted

© Alexander Raths/Shutterstock.com

PRACTICE **PITFALLS**

Be alert for new or modified instructions in the official guidelines. Anemia in malignant neoplasm has different sequencing in ICD-10-CM compared to ICD-9-CM. In ICD-9-CM, the circumstances of the encounter dictate whether the neoplasm or the anemia is sequenced first (ICD-9-CM OGCR I.C.2.c.1). In ICD-10-CM, neoplasm is always coded first and associated anemia is sequenced second, even when the primary reason for the encounter is treatment directed towards the anemia (ICD-10-CM OGCR I.C.2.c.1).

ACTIVITY #5

Assigning Combination Codes and Multiple Codes

Directions: Based on the condition, look up the appropriate ICD-10-CM codes and write them in the space provided. Sequence multiple codes in correct order.

1. Toxic shock syndrome due to streptococcus A _____ _____

2. Anemia in tuberculosis of the lung _____ _____

3. Wilson's disease with Kayser-Fleischer ring in the right eye _____ _____

4. Chronic combined systolic and diastolic heart failure, due to hypertension _____ _____

5. Acute deep phlebothrombosis in the popliteal vein in the right leg in third trimester of pregnancy _____ _____

General Equivalency Mapping

GEM files were developed to give health care data users a tool to convert and test systems and to compare data collected before and after the ICD-10-CM transition period. GEMs are not intended to be used by coders to assign codes for specific patient encounters. The general purpose and use of GEMs was discussed in Chapter 11. This chapter provides coded examples of the various types of GEM mappings.

An exact match is one in which the ICD-9-CM code is described exactly like the ICD-10-CM code. Table 12-10 ● shows examples of a GEM exact match.

An approximate match is one in which the ICD-10-CM code is similar to, but not an exact duplicate of, the ICD-9-CM code. Table 12-11 ● shows examples of a GEM approximate match.

A one-to-many forward mapping is one in which there are several ICD-10-CM codes for conditions that are described by only one code in ICD-9-CM. Without reference to a patient's medical record, it is not possible to determine which ICD-10-CM code is the single best translation. Table 12-12 ● shows examples of GEM one-to-many forward mapping.

TABLE 12-10 Examples of GEM Exact Match

ICD-9-CM	ICD-10-CM
416.0 Primary pulmonary hypertension	I27.0 Primary pulmonary hypertension
427.31 Atrial fibrillation	I48.0 Atrial fibrillation
157.0 Malignant neoplasm of the head of the pancreas	C25.0 Malignant neoplasm of the head of the pancreas
274.9 Gout, unspecified	M10.9 Gout, unspecified

TABLE 12-11 Examples of GEM Approximate Match

ICD-9-CM	ICD-10-CM
154.4 Malignant neoplasm of islets of Langerhans	C25.4 Malignant neoplasm of endocrine pancreas
422.91 Idiopathic myocarditis	I40.1 Isolated myocarditis
535.01 Acute gastritis with hemorrhage	K29.00 Acute gastritis without bleeding

TABLE 12-12 Examples of GEM One-to-Many Forward Mapping

ICD-9-CM	ICD-10-CM
379.21 Vitreous degeneration	H43.811 Vitreous degeneration, right eye
	H43.812 Vitreous degeneration, left eye
	H43.813 Vitreous degeneration, bilateral
	H43.819 Vitreous degeneration, unspecified eye
182.0 Malignant neoplasm of corpus uteri, except isthmus	C54.1 Malignant neoplasm of endometrium
	C54.2 Malignant neoplasm of myometrium
	C54.3 Malignant neoplasm of fundus uteri
	C54.9 Malignant neoplasm of corpus uteri, unspecified
424.0 Mitral valve disorders	I34.0 Nonrheumatic mitral (valve) insufficiency
	I34.1 Nonrheumatic mitral (valve) prolapse
	I34.2 Nonrheumatic mitral (valve) stenosis
	I34.8 Other nonrheumatic mitral valve disorders
	I34.9 Nonrheumatic mitral valve disorder, unspecified

TABLE 12-13 Examples of GEM Many-to-One Forward Mapping

ICD-9-CM	ICD-10-CM
401.0 Malignant hypertension	I10 Essential hypertension
401.1 Benign hypertension	
401.9 Unspecified hypertension	
250.01 Diabetes, type 1, not stated as uncontrolled	E10.9 Type 1 diabetes mellitus without complications
250.03 Diabetes, type 1, uncontrolled	
250.40 Diabetes with renal manifestations, type II or unspecified type, not stated as uncontrolled	E11.21 Type 2 diabetes mellitus with diabetic nephropathy
581.81 Kimmelstiel-Wilson syndrome	
295.70 Schizoaffective disorder, unspecified	F25.9 Schizoaffective disorder, unspecified
295.71 Schizoaffective disorder, subchronic	
295.72 Schizoaffective disorder, chronic	
295.73 Schizoaffective disorder, subchronic with acute exacerbation	
295.74 Schizoaffective disorder, chronic with acute exacerbation	

TABLE 12-14 **Example of ICD-9-CM and ICD-10-CM Coding for Down Syndrome**

ICD-9-CM	ICD-10-CM Tabular List
758.0 Down syndrome	Q90.0 Trisomy 21, nonmosaicism (meiotic nondisjunction)
	Q90.1 Trisomy 21, mosaicism (mitotic nondisjunction)
	Q90.2 Trisomy 21, translocation
	Q90.9 Down's syndrome, unspecified

A many-to-one forward mapping is one in which multiple ICD-9-CM codes are described by a single ICD-10-CM code. Table 12-13 ● shows examples of GEM many-to-one forward mapping.

Due to the inability of ICD-9-CM codes to capture all the required detail in ICD-10-CM, in many cases more ICD-10-CM codes exist than are mapped in the GEM files. Down syndrome is an example of when additional documentation or genetic testing may be needed. GEMs forward mapping from ICD-9-CM to ICD-10-CM shows a mapping to a single code, Q90.9 *Down syndrome, unspecified*. In the tabular list, additional codes with greater specificity are listed as shown in Table 12-14 ●.

Coma is an example of a condition that requires additional documentation and abstracting for complete ICD-10-CM code assignment. ICD-9-CM classifies coma with one code, 780.01 *Coma*, which is mapped to R40.20 *Unspecified coma*. This would appear to be a one-to-one approximate map. However, the ICD-10-CM tabular list includes additional options not reflected in GEMs. An adult with documented coma assessment of GCS on arrival to the emergency department could be documented as E2-V3-M3 = 8 and would be coded as shown in Table 12-15 ●. The fifth and sixth characters of the ICD-10-CM code classify the GCS Response and Points. The seventh digit classifies the time of the assessment, in this example, on arrival to the emergency department.

PRACTICE **PITFALLS**

GEM files do not contain exact matches in ICD-10-CM for most ICD-9-CM codes. Whenever specific patient encounters need ICD-10-CM codes, they should be coded directly from the medical record using the ICD-10-CM index and tabular list. If a patient is assigned a code for a condition using ICD-9-CM prior to the transition date and the patient is seen again after ICD-10-CM implementation, the record should be fully recoded using ICD-10-CM. GEMs are not to be used to assign codes to patient records.

When no exact match exists between ICD-9-CM and ICD-10-CM codes, project managers for data conversion or research projects define how GEMs are applied. Translating data from one code set to the other represents a series of compromises, depending on how the data are used. Data used for reimbursement can be mapped differently than data used for research or statistical purposes. Two unequal codes are mapped for reimbursement purposes as long as they both fall

TABLE 12-15 **Example of ICD-10-CM Coma Coding**

Response	GCS	Points	ICD-10-CM
Eye opening	Opens to pain, not applied to face	2	R40.1212 Coma scale, eyes open, to pain
Verbal	Inappropriate responses, words discernible	3	R40.2232 Coma scale, best verbal response, inappropriate words
Motor	Abnormal (spastic) flexion	3	R40.2332 Coma scale, best motor response, withdraws to pain

TABLE 12-16 Example of ICD-10-PCS Code Structure

0PHC3BZ Insertion of a monopolar external fixation device on the head of the right humerus						
Position → Description →	**1** Section	**2** Body system	**3** Root operation	**4** Body part	**5** Surgical approach	**6** Implanted devices	**7** Qualifying circumstance
Example → Meaning →	**0** Medical & surgical	**P** Upper bones	**H** Insertion	**C** Humeral head, right	**3** Percutaneous	**B** External fixation device, monoplanar	**Z** No qualifier

into the same general reimbursement group. Maps for research purposes are designed to capture the greatest level of detail related to the study's purpose.

For example, ICD-10-CM classifies obstetric codes by trimester rather than the episode of care used in ICD-9-CM. A map used for research can be defined based on the location of services. When working with hospital inpatient data, ICD-10-CM encounters coded for patients in the third trimester can be mapped to the ICD-9-CM code with the episode of care for delivered. When working with physician office data, ICD-10-CM encounters coded for patients in the third trimester might be mapped to the ICD-9-CM code with the episode of care for antepartum.

As with all data conversion projects, any use involving the trending or tracking of ICD-9-CM to ICD-10-CM needs to be done with full awareness of the approximations and potential distortions. GEMs provide a tool for working with data that would otherwise be cumbersome and nearly impossible to correlate.

ICD-10-PCS

ICD-10-PCS is the United States' replacement for the ICD-9-CM Procedure Coding System, which has been used in the United States since 1979 for reporting hospital inpatient procedures (health services provided to patients to diagnose, treat, or prevent a condition). ICD-10-PCS has over 72,000 codes compared to 4,000 in ICD-9-CM. ICD-9-CM procedure codes comprised Volume 3 of the ICD-9-CM coding manual, and ICD-10-PCS is published as a separate book.

Coding under ICD-10-PCS is much more specific and substantially different from ICD-9-CM procedure coding. Codes are seven alphanumeric characters in length and follow a prescribed structure where each character of the code describes particular criteria. An example of the code structure is shown in Table 12-16 ●. Coders first look up the procedure in the alphabetic index, where the first three to four characters of the code are identified. Then they refer to a corresponding grid in the tabular list where the remaining digits are assigned based on the details of the procedure. Detailed instruction on ICD-10-PCS is beyond the scope of this text.

CHAPTER REVIEW

Summary

- ICD-10-CM codes have several differences from ICD-9-CM codes, including the number of codes, code organization and structure, code composition, and level of detail.
- Many of the official guidelines in Sections I.B., II, III, and IV are similar for both ICD-10-CM and ICD-9-CM codes. Changes in these sections are related to differences in code structure, such as additional characters, 7th-character extensions, and laterality.
- New conventions in ICD-10-CM include exclusion notes, additional digit symbols, extensions, placeholder characters, short dash, and with/without options for the final character.
- The process for assigning a code in ICD-10-CM is similar to doing so for ICD-9-CM: select the diagnoses to be coded, locate the main term and verify it in the tabular list, reading all instructional notes and conventions.
- ICD-10-CM uses more combination codes where multiple codes were used in ICD-9-CM, but multiple coding is still required in ICD-10-CM.

- GEM files were developed to give health care data users a tool to convert and test systems, and compare data collected before and after the ICD-10-CM transition period, but are not intended to be used by coders to assign codes for specific patient encounters.
- Coding under ICD-10-PCS is much more specific and is substantially different from ICD-9-CM procedure coding. Codes are seven alphanumeric characters in length and follow a prescribed structure where each character of the code describes particular criteria.

Review Questions

Directions: Answer the following questions without looking back at the material covered in this chapter. Write your answers in the space provided. If you are unable to answer any of these questions, refer back to that section in the chapter, and then fill in the answers.

1. Which of the following statements about ICD-10-CM are TRUE?

    a. All codes are 7 characters long.

    b. There are over 68,000 codes.

    c. All codes begin with a letter.

    d. The placeholder character is x.

    e. The placeholder is used with all codes less than seven characters.

2. Sequence the order in which the following sections of the manual appear:

    a. Neoplasm Table _____

    b. Index to Diseases and Injuries _____

    c. Tabular list of diseases and injuries _____

    d. Table of Drugs and Chemicals _____

    e. Official Guidelines for Coding and Reporting _____

    f. Index to External Causes _____

3. What is a block in ICD-10-CM?

    a. A contiguous range of codes within a chapter whose instructional notes apply to all codes within that block.

    b. A three-character category that has no further subdivision.

    c. A group of seven-character codes that begin with the same three characters.

    d. The final level of subdivision in the tabular list.

4. Name five conventions that are the same in ICD-9-CM and ICD-10-CM

    a. _____

    b. _____

    c. _____

    d. _____

    e. _____

5. What does the new ICD-10-CM convention Excludes1 mean?

    a. The condition excluded is not part of the condition represented by the code, but may be reported together if documented.

    b. The codes that appear after it are mutually exclusive codes and should not be used with the original code itself.

    c. An additional digit is needed for the code to be complete.

    d. There are several options for the final character, within a set of alternative codes.

6. For outpatient coding, when should signs and symptoms should be coded?

    a. When the patient describes them to the provider

    b. When the patient has never had them before

    c. When the diagnosis is uncertain as indicated in the medical record

    d. When a confirmed diagnosis is stated in the medical record

7. What should a coder do when searching for a main term in the index?

    a. Look for the anatomical site or organ.

    b. Start with the tabular list.

    c. Look for the condition or disease.

    d. Disregard cross-referencing instructions.

8. When verifying a code in the tabular list, the coder should do all of the following except:

    a. Read the instructional notes under the code.

    b. Check for any symbols indicating that additional characters are required.

    c. Read the title of the three-character category, and read any instructional notes under the category title.

    d. Assign the code that was printed in the index.

9. When sequencing multiple codes in ICD-10-CM, the coder should:

    a. Follow the same sequencing rules as in ICD-9-CM.

    b. Check the ICD-10-CM guidelines for sequencing rules.

    c. Sequence according to the reason for the encounter.

    d. Code first the manifestation.

10. Name an ICD-9-CM code that meets the criteria for each type of GEM mapping.

    a. One-to many _____

    b. Exact match _____

    c. Many-to-one _____

    d. Approximate match _____

Activity #6: Defining Key Words

Directions: Match the following terms with the proper definition by writing the letter of the correct definition in the space next to the term.

1. _____ Block

    a. Describes multiple conditions with one code

2. _____ First-listed diagnosis

    b. The condition established after study to be chiefly responsible for occasioning the admission of the patient to the hospital for care

3. _____ Conventions

    c. A late effect or delayed healing

4. _____ Combination code

    d. A subdivision of three characters in length that is further subdivided

5. _____ Principal diagnosis

    e. Each subdivision after a category and before a code, containing four or five characters

6. _____ Excludes1

    f. The use of symbols, typeface, and layout features

7. _____ Extension

    g. A contiguous range of codes within a chapter, comparable to a section in ICD-9-CM

8. _____ Sequela

    h. The letter *x,* which must fill the empty positions on a code less than six characters in length that requires an extension

9. _____ Code

    i. The 7th character of a code, which must appear in that position, regardless of the length of the code

10. _____ Placeholder

    j. The main reason for the outpatient services provided

11. _____ Multiple coding

    k. A convention indicating that additional characters should be assigned

12. _____ Dash

    l. The condition excluded is not part of the condition represented by the code, but the patient may have both conditions at the same time and the conditions are not mutually exclusive

13. _____ Category

    m. Using two or more codes to fully describe a condition

14. _____ Excludes2

    n. The condition represented by the code and the condition excluded are mutually exclusive and should not be coded together.

15. _____ Subcategory

    o. The final level of subdivision containing three, four, five, six or seven characters

Activity #7: Assigning ICD-10-CM Codes for Diseases, Disorders, and Symptoms

Directions: In Chapter 10 you coded these conditions using ICD-9-CM. Now follow the same process of identifying main terms in the index and verifying them in the tabular list to assign the correct ICD-10-CM code. Based on the condition, look up the appropriate ICD-10-CM code and write it in the space provided. Also underline the main term.

1. Gangrene of the tunica vaginalis _____

2. Hypercholesterolemia _____

3. Sudden infant death syndrome (SIDS) _____

4. Glomerulohyalinosis diabetic syndrome _____

5. Bladder neck stricture _____

6. Popliteal thrombophlebitis _____

7. Ulcerative colitis _____

8. Superior mesenteric artery syndrome _____

9. Renal artery thrombosis _____

10. Recurrent urethritis _____

11. Diabetes mellitus _____

12. Endogenous obesity _____

13. Essential hypertension _____

14. Inguinal hernia _____

15. Borderline glaucoma, both eyes _____

16. Ulcerative gastroenteritis _____

17. Hallux valgus, left foot _____

18. Epidural hematoma of the brain _____

19. Internal hemorrhoids _____

20. Endocrine imbalance _____

21. Nausea and vomiting _____

22. Fever due to heat _____

23. Low back pain _____

24. Difficulty walking _____

25. Postnasal discharge _____

Activity #8: Assigning ICD-10-CM Codes for Injuries

Directions: Based on the condition, look up the appropriate ICD-10-CM code and write it in the space provided. Also underline the main term.

1. Lateral dislocation of right patella, first visit _____

2. Dislocated jaw, subsequent encounter _____

3. Sprained left great toe, interphalangeal joint, initial encounter _____

4. Low back strain, sequela _____

5. Open wound of pharynx, third visit _____

6. Traumatic dislocation of right ulnohumeral joint, subsequent encounter _____

7. First visit for a displaced comminuted fracture to the left tibia _____

8. Third-degree burn of forearm, initial encounter _____

9. Initial visit for third-degree burn on the head _____

10. Second visit to check on a second-degree burn to the back _____

11. Traumatic tear to the left rotator cuff capsule, initial encounter _____

12. Late effect of tear right lateral meniscus _____

13. Subsequent encounter for delayed healing of a Type I occipital condyle fracture of the skull _____

14. Colles' fracture of right radius, initial encounter _____

15. Crushed left heel, subsequent encounter _____

Activity #9: Assigning ICD-10-CM Codes for Neoplasms

Directions: In Chapter 10 you coded these conditions using ICD-9-CM. Now follow the same process of identifying main terms in the Index and verifying them in the tabular list to assign the correct ICD-10-CM code. Based on the condition, look up the appropriate ICD-10-CM code and write it in the space provided.

1. Benign breast tumor _____

2. Ca in situ, uterus _____

3. Lung tumor _____

4. Secondary ca, pancreas _____

5. Primary ca, pylorus _____

6. Prostate cancer _____

7. Ependymoblastoma, spinal cord _____

8. Femur osteofibroma _____

9. Melanoma _____

10. Benign brain tumor _____

11. Intramuscular lipoma _____

12. Leukemia _____

13. Papillary hydradenoma _____

14. Leydig cell tumor (male) _____

15. Sebaceous cyst _____

16. Mucoid adenoma of the auricle _____

17. Aldosteronoma _____

18. Plasmacytoma, esophagus _____

19. Papillary intraductal carcinoma, salivary duct _____

20. Wrist disgerminoma _____

Activity #10: Assigning ICD-10-CM Codes for Complications of Pregnancy, Delivery, and Puerperium

Directions: Based on the condition, look up the appropriate ICD-10-CM codes and write them in the space provided. Underline the main term. Sequence the codes correctly.

1. Severe hyperemesis with electrolyte imbalance in 12th week of gestation _____

2. Primary uterine inertia in intrauterine pregnancy, delivered single liveborn at 39 weeks
   _____ _____

3. Cesarean delivery of single stillborn at 38 weeks gestation due to placental infarction
   _____ _____ _____

4. Intrauterine pregnancy at 13 weeks, with pernicious anemia _____ _____

5. Patient in 36th week of pregnancy has premature rupture of membranes with delivery beginning 28 hours later, producing a healthy girl _____

6. Spontaneous delivery of premature twins in 32nd week of pregnancy, both liveborn
   _____ _____

7. Postpartum pulmonary thromboembolism _____

8. Cesarean delivery during 37th week of gestation due to breech presentation, single live-born female _____ _____ _____

9. First-degree tear of vaginal wall during delivery resulting in a liveborn boy _____

10. Gestational diabetes _____

Activity #11: Assigning ICD-10-CM Codes for Diseases, Disorders, and Conditions of Newborns

Directions: Based on the condition, look up the appropriate ICD-10-CM codes and write them in the space provided. Underline the main term. Sequence the codes correctly.

1. Newborn with hemolytic disease due to ABO isoimmunization _____ _____

2. Baby girl born in hospital at 33 weeks gestation, weighs only 1,850 grams and has withdrawal syndrome due to mother's material heroin addiction _____ _____ _____

3. Normal male infant delivered by cesarean when it was noted early in labor that he was experiencing fetal distress due to cord compression _____ _____ _____

4. Neonatal hypoglycemia _____

5. Intrauterine growth retardation of newborn _____ _____

Activity #12: Assigning ICD-10-CM Codes for Factors Influencing Health Status and Contact with Health Services

Directions: In Chapter 10 you coded these conditions using ICD-9-CM. Now follow the same process of identifying main terms in the index and verifying them in the tabular list to assign the correct ICD-10-CM code. Based on the condition, look up the appropriate ICD-10-CM code and write it in the space provided. Also underline the main term.

1. Personal history of breast cancer _____

2. Family history of colon cancer _____

3. Long term use of insulin _____

4. Osteoporosis screening _____

5. Eye examination _____

6. Insertion of intrauterine contraceptive device _____

7. Admission for radiotherapy _____

8. Tracheostomy status _____

9. Absence of leg below the knee _____

10. Fitting of cardiac pacemaker _____

11. Encounter for vaccination _____

12. Bone marrow donor _____

13. Newborn, born in hospital, by cesarean section _____

14. Preoperative laboratory test _____

15. Annual physical examination _____

16. Routine newborn checkup, 8 to 28 days old _____

17. Screening for colon cancer _____

18. Genetic susceptibility to breast cancer _____

19. Routine postpartum follow-up for observation _____

20. Exposure to hepatitis _____

Activity #13: Assigning ICD-10-CM Codes for External Causes

Directions: Use the External Cause Index to look up the appropriate ICD-10-CM code and write it in the space provided. Also underline the main term.

1. Driver of van injured in traffic collision with automobile on a public highway, initial encounter _____

2. Car passenger injured in traffic collision with a pickup truck on a public highway, subsequent encounter _____

3. Pedestrian on foot injured by moving automobile on a public highway, initial encounter _____

4. Bicycle rider injured in traffic collision with pickup truck, sequela _____

5. Motorcycle driver injured upon running into a light pole, subsequent encounter _____

6. Bus driver injured when the bus collided with railway train, sequela _____

7. Drowning and submersion due to fishing boat overturning, sequela _____

8. Fall due to ice and snow on steps, initial encounter _____

9. Fall on sidewalk curb, initial encounter _____

10. Injury from fall into swimming pool and striking wall, sequela _____

11. Drowning from fall in full bathtub, initial encounter _____

12. Assault by handgun discharge, subsequent encounter _____

13. Suicide attempt by jumping from a ten-story building, sequela _____

14. Dog bite, initial encounter _____

15. Woman seen for injuries inflicted by husband as perpetrator, subsequent encounter _____

16. Soldier injured by fragments of improvised explosive device (IED) during war, initial encounter _____

17. Poisoning, bee sting, sequela _____

18. Adverse effect of penicillin, initial encounter _____

19. Poisoning, heroin, subsequent encounter _____

20. Performance of correct procedure on wrong side or body part due to medical error, initial encounter _____

Activity #14: Assigning ICD-10-CM Combination Codes and Multiple Codes

Directions: Based on the condition, look up the appropriate ICD-10-CM codes and write them in the space provided. Sequence multiple codes in correct order.

1. Normal delivery, single liveborn infant _____ _____

2. Type 1 diabetes with diabetic moderate chronic kidney disease _____ _____

3. Acute cystitis due to *E. coli* _____ _____

4. Dermatitis on hand and arm due to contact with insecticide _____ _____

5. Mucositis of vagina and vulva due to radiotherapy _____ _____

6. Acute bronchitis due to *Hemophilus influenzae* _____

7. Type 2 diabetes with diabetic polyneuropathy _____

8. Arteriosclerotic heart disease of autologous artery coronary artery bypass graft with unstable angina pectoris _____

9. Stage II pressure ulcer of right buttock _____

10. Crohn's disease of large intestine with fistula _____

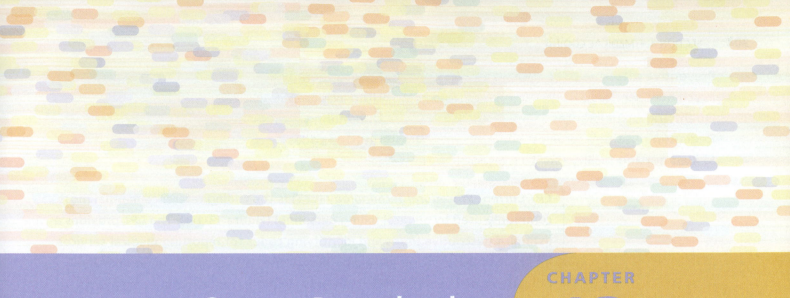

Current Procedural Terminology (CPT) Coding

After completion of this chapter you should be able to:

Name the six sections of the CPT and RVS manuals.

Use the CPT to properly code procedures and services.

Key Words and Concepts you will learn in this chapter:

Bilateral procedures

Biofeedback

Block procedures

Consultation

CT (computed tomography) scan

Custodial care

Diagnostic x-rays

Dialysis

Emergency

Established patient

Evaluation and management (E/M) codes

Follow-up days

Global period

Hospital inpatient services

Home services

Laboratory examinations

Modifiers

Multiple procedures

New patient

Nuclear medicine

Occupational therapy

Physical medicine and rehabilitation

Physical therapy

CPT/Current Procedural Terminology (CPT) is the coding reference manual most commonly used by medical billing personnel (Figure 13-1 ●). The CPT provides a listing of descriptive terms and identifying codes for reporting medical services and procedures performed by providers. It uses a five-digit code to identify procedures and services, which not only simplifies reporting but also allows for compilation of data. The purpose of the CPT is to provide a uniform system that accurately describes medical, surgical, and diagnostic services.

The CPT was originally created by the American Medical Association in 1966. Since that time, it has undergone extensive revisions. Revisions are made every year with additional updates as needed. Because of the extensive changes that sometimes appear, it is important to use the correct version of the CPT. Using an outdated CPT may result in using codes that have been changed or deleted, and it may cause a delay or denial of a claim payment.

The CPT manual has six major sections (Table 13-1 ●). In addition to the sections, the manual contains fourteen appendices that contain further information on coding, including the use of modifiers. Although the CPT manual tends to be divided by medical specialty, any qualified provider may use a code from any section of the manual.

Using the CPT

To properly code using the CPT, choose the numerical code associated with the English-language description of the procedure performed. Sometimes the procedure is phrased in different terminology (e.g., testectomy is found under orchiectomy even though both are legitimate medical terms). Therefore, it is important to check all related codes and alternate terminology for a procedure. It also may be necessary to consult a medical dictionary for alternate terminology for a specified procedure.

Each section of the CPT contains specific instructions relating to that section before the code listing. It is important to read each of these instructions in order to properly code the procedures contained in that section.

Semicolons in the CPT

Some descriptions in the CPT are subprocedures of other descriptions. These subheading descriptions will be indented under the main procedure. To properly understand an indented procedure, read the description of the main procedure (the one not indented) up to the semicolon. Next, add the remaining description found in the indented wording. For example, codes 21208 and 21209 read as follows:

21208   Osteoplasty, facial bones; augmentation (autograft, allograft, or prosthetic implant)

21209   reduction

Therefore, the correct description for 21209 is Osteoplasty, facial bones; reduction (autograft, allograft, or prosthetic implant). It is important to carefully read the full

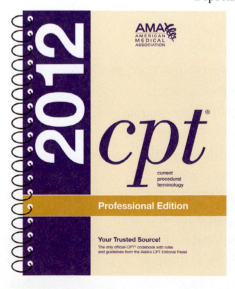

TABLE 13-1 The Six Major Divisions of the CPT Manual

Evaluation and Management	99201–99499
Anesthesia	00100–01999
Surgery	10021–69990
Radiology/Nuclear Medicine	70010–79999
Pathology and Laboratory Tests	80047–89398
Medicine	90281–99199

description of all related procedures before choosing the one that best describes the procedure performed. A slight change in the main description can significantly alter the meaning of the indented procedure.

Signs and Symbols Used in the CPT

Most coding manuals have signs and symbols to alert you to specific situations with codes. However, different versions of the coding manuals may have different signs and symbols, or none indicated at all.

Listed below are some of the common signs and symbols used in the CPT:

- • This code is new to this edition of the CPT. It has just been added to the list of CPT codes.
- ▲ This code has been changed from last year's edition of the CPT.
- + This is an add-on code. This code cannot be used alone but must be used in addition to another code. This procedure is performed in addition to or in conjunction with another procedure.
- # This code identifies out-of-numerical-sequence codes.
- Ø This code is exempt from the use of modifier -51 (modifier -51 indicates multiple surgical procedures).

Many CPT manuals also contain signs or symbols for nonspecific codes or unspecified codes often indicated by color blocks. These codes should only be used as a last resort when no other code is appropriate.

The details of the signs and symbols used in your version of the CPT should appear at the beginning of the book. You should read this section carefully before coding.

Using the CPT Index

The CPT index lists all main procedures, often with a choice of several codes. Again, some procedures are indented, indicating that the unindented procedure listed directly above them is part of the description.

Listings in the CPT manual are arranged by the procedure done, then by the site of the procedure. For example, the heading "Amputation" then lists numerous parts of the body that can be amputated and their related codes. Some parts of the body also have their own heading elsewhere in the index.

When coding, it is always important to first look up the procedure in the index and then verify the code by referring to the tabular list.

Modifiers

Modifiers are two-digit codes that can be added to CPT codes to denote unusual circumstances. These modifiers more fully describe the procedure that was performed. In addition, modifiers alter the valuation of procedure by increasing or decreasing the allowed amount.

For example: Modifier -80 denotes the use of an assistant surgeon. Because the assistant surgeon is merely assisting and is not responsible for the primary care of the patient, he is paid substantially less than the primary surgeon (Figure 13-2 ●).

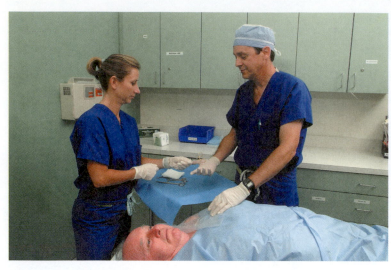

Some commonly used modifiers include the following:

-*22* Increased procedural services

-*24* Unrelated evaluation and management service by the same provider during a postoperative period

-*26* Professional component

-*32* Mandated services

-*47* Anesthesia by surgeon

-*50* Bilateral procedure

-*51* Multiple procedures

-*52* Reduced services

-*57* Decision for surgery

-*62* Two surgeons

-*80* Assistant surgeon

FIGURE 13-2

An assistant surgeon helping the primary surgeon during a surgical procedure

© Michal Heron/Pearson Education

Unlisted Codes

Listed at the end of each CPT section and subsection are **unlisted codes**. These are the codes that end in "99." Procedures that are unusual or new and, therefore, do not have a designated code to describe them are coded by the appropriate unlisted code (based on body section or type of service). These codes are to be used only when no other appropriate code is available.

The following coding sections deal specifically with using the CPT manual. Only those sections that need additional explanation are included. Because the CPT is the main reference manual used by medical billing personnel, it is vitally important that its usage be thoroughly understood. You also should go through the general guidelines listed in the CPT manual to assist in coding each section.

Evaluation and Management Codes

Evaluation and management (E/M) codes designate services provided in the provider's office, outpatient or ambulatory facility (Table 13-2 ●). These services are casually referred to as office visits, but specific criteria must be met in order to assign E/M codes.

To code E/M services it is important to first be able to define the terms *new patient* and *established patient*. A **new patient** is one who has not received any professional services from the provider, or another provider of the same specialty who belongs to the same group practice, within the past three years. An **established patient** is one who has received professional services from the provider, or another provider of the same specialty who belongs to the same group practice, within the past three years.

Usually the provider determines the overall level of E/M service, but medical billers and coders need to verify that the level assigned by the provider meets the official criteria. If they do not, the office could lose reimbursement. The key components in selecting a level of E/M services are

- history,
- examination, and
- medical decision making.

The history includes all or some of these elements: the chief complaint; history of present illness; review of systems; and past history, family history, or social history (Figure 13-3 ●). The extent of the history is based on the provider's clinical judgment and on the nature of the presenting problems. The levels of E/M services recognize four types of examination. These are defined as follows:

- *Problem focused.* A limited examination of the affected body area or organ system.
- *Expanded problem focused.* A limited examination of the affected body area or organ system and other symptomatic or related organ system(s).

TABLE 13-2 **Evaluation and Management Codes Subsections**

Office or Other Outpatient Services	99201–99215
Hospital Observation Services	99217–99226
Hospital Inpatient Services	99221–99239
Consultations	99241–99255
Emergency Department Services	99281–99288
Critical Care Services	99291–99292
Nursing Facility Services	99304–99318
Domiciliary, Rest Home, or Custodial Care Services	99324–99337
Domiciliary, Rest Home, or Home Care Plan Oversight	99339–99340
Home Services	99341–99350
Prolonged Services	99354–99360
Case Management Services	99363–99368
Care Plan Oversight Services	99374–99380
Preventive Medicine Services	99381–99429
Non–Face-to-Face Physician Services	99441–99444
Special Evaluation and Management Services	99450–99456
Newborn Care Services	99460–99465
Inpatient Neonatal Intensive Care Services and Pediatric and Neonatal Critical Care Services	99466–99480
Other Evaluation and Management Services	99499

- *Detailed.* An extended examination of the affected body area(s) and other symptomatic or related organ system(s).
- *Comprehensive.* A general multisystem examination or a complete examination of a single organ system.

Medical decision making refers to the complexity of establishing a diagnosis and/or selecting a management option. The following are the four types of medical decision making:

- Straightforward
- Low complexity
- Moderate complexity
- High complexity

In addition to the key components in selecting a level of E/M services, other components must be considered. These are counseling, coordination of care, the nature of the presenting problem, and time. These components, other than time, are considered contributory factors in the majority of encounters.

For further instructions regarding selecting the proper E/M code, see the E/M Services Guidelines in the CPT manual. The following subsections describe coding of some evaluation and management services.

Office or Other Outpatient Services 99201–99215

Office visits are the evaluation and management of a patient's condition in a provider's office, clinic, or hospital outpatient department. This category is used for problem-oriented visits during which the provider manages an active illness or disease. There are separate categories of E/M codes used for preventive services and work or disability evaluations.

If care is provided outside of normal office hours, codes 99050 through 99060 are used in addition to the regular office visit code. This

FIGURE 13-3

Obtaining information on the patient's history

© Michal Heron/Pearson Education

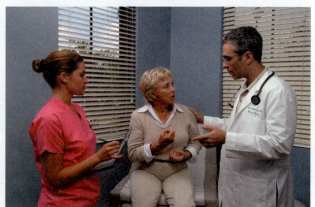

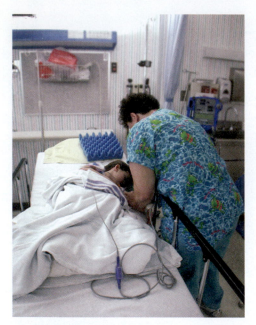

FIGURE 13-4

Caring for a patient in a hospital setting

© Jyn Meyer/Shutterstock.com

allows the provider to possibly obtain extra compensation for the inconvenience of providing care outside the usual business hours.

Hospital Inpatient Services: 99221–99239

Hospital inpatient services are the evaluation and management of a patient provided in an inpatient hospital setting. This means the patient has been formally admitted to an inpatient hospital. Some services provided at the hospital building are outpatient services, including emergency department and observation care. In addition, not all services provided to inpatients are coded from this category. For example, critical care for adults, neonates, and children, as well as inpatient consultations, are coded from other E/M categories.

Coding for these services is not based on whether the patient is a new or established patient but, rather, whether it is the first service for that admission or a subsequent service. In addition, the time and the complexity of the case are considered (Figure 13-4 ●).

Consultations: 99241–99255

A **consultation** is an opinion provided by a specialist at the request of another provider. The specialist may request diagnostic services and may make therapeutic recommendations to the referring provider. However, the specialist does not usually take over the day-to-day treatment or management of the patient. In fact, for the service to qualify as a consultation, the provider cannot be responsible for the regular management of the patient. Consultation codes are divided based on whether the service is outpatient or inpatient.

If the consulting provider subsequently assumes responsibility for the routine care of the patient's condition, the subsequent services should be coded as visits and not consultations. If the consultant is seeing the patient in addition to the regular attending provider, 99231–99233 or 99251–99255 should be used, as appropriate.

Emergency Department Services: 99281–99288

When a patient goes to the outpatient or emergency department of a hospital, there usually is a provider in attendance who provides professional care at the facility. The provider's charges may appear on the hospital bill or may be billed separately (Figure 13-5 ●).

Many hospitals have two types of outpatient departments: (1) the emergency room (ER) and (2) ambulatory medical clinics. All emergency department services are considered to be outpatient, even if the patient is subsequently admitted as an inpatient. When the same physician provides the emergency department care and does the admission, all services are bundled into the code for Initial Inpatient Services.

FIGURE 13-5

An emergency department physician at work

© David Mager/Pearson Education

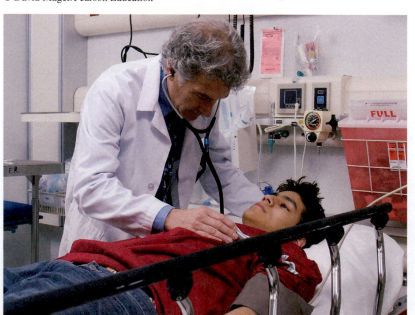

If the patient wants to have his or her regular provider in attendance and the provider is called in from outside the hospital to provide services, code 99056 should be used.

If the patient visits the outpatient clinic of a facility, regular office visit coding should be used because a clinic is conceptually the same as an office.

Nursing Facility Services: 99304–99318

A **skilled nursing facility (SNF)** is primarily engaged in providing skilled nursing care and related services for residents who require medical or nursing care; or rehabilitation services for the rehabilitation of injured, disabled, or sick persons (Figure 13-6 ●).

An individual is often admitted to an SNF from an acute care facility. This may occur because the acuteness of the patient's condition has been stabilized and only time and continued noncritical treatments are required.

Domiciliary, Rest Home, or Custodial Care Services: 99324–99337

Custodial care is primarily for the purpose of meeting the personal daily needs of the patient and could be provided by personnel without medical care skills or training. For example, custodial care includes assistance with walking, bathing, dressing, eating, and other activities. Skilled nursing personnel are not required for this nonmedical type of care, which is commonly referred to as "assisting with the activities of daily living" of the patient.

Home Services: 99341–99350

As the name implies, **home services** are visits performed by a provider in the patient's home. The coding of these services is based on the same factors as office visits.

Preventive Medicine: 99381–99429

Preventive medicine is, as the name implies, routine well care provided when there is not an active illness or disease. If there is any credible diagnosis indicated, do not code as preventive. These codes are assigned based on the age of the patient and whether the patient is new or established. Some services provided as part of preventive care, such as immunizations, are billed in addition to the E/M code. If an identifiable medical problem is found during the preventive care visit and requires significant additional work, the appropriate E/M code from the Office or Other Outpatient Services category may be assigned. The modifier -25 should be added to the Office or Other Outpatient Services E/M code. If the visit is primarily for the management of an active illness or disease, do not code it as preventive.

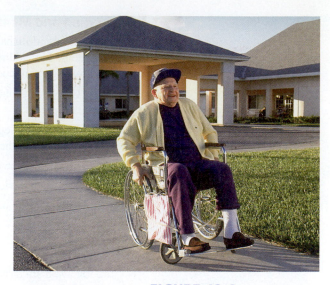

FIGURE 13-6

Skilled nursing facilities provide care for individuals who require longer stays than hospitals allow.

© Michal Heron/Pearson Education

ACTIVITY #1

E/M CPT Coding

Directions: Based on the service description, look up the appropriate E/M CPT code and write it in the space provided.

Description	Code
1. Office visit, evaluation of established patient medical decision low complexity, expanded problem-focused history	1. _____
2. Rest home visit, evaluation of new patient, medical decision making straightforward, problem-focused history, and problem-focused exam	2. _____
3. Initial hospital visit, new or established patient, detailed or comprehensive history, and detailed or comprehensive exam, straightforward or low-complexity medical decision	3. _____
4. Subsequent hospital care, medical decision of moderate complexity, expanded problem-focused history	4. _____
5. Initial nursing facility care, established patient, medical decision of low complexity, detailed history, comprehensive exam	5. _____
6. Rest home visit, established patient, straightforward medical decision, problem-focused interval history, and problem-focused exam	6. _____
7. Emergency department care, minimal care, straightforward medical decision, problem-focused history, and problem-focused exam	7. _____
8. Initial inpatient consultation, new patient, medical decision of moderate low complexity, comprehensive history, and comprehensive exam	8. _____
9. Initial office consultation, medical decision of high complexity, comprehensive history, and comprehensive examination.	9. _____
10. Follow-up minimal consultation, office, straightforward medical decision making, problem-focused history, and problem-focused exam	10. _____

Evaluation and Management Modifiers

All evaluation and management services are billed by use of the five-digit CPT code; the code may be detailed by adding a modifier to it. Some of the modifiers that may be used with evaluation and management codes are these:

-24 Unrelated evaluation and management service by the same provider during a postoperative period

-25 Significant, separately identifiable evaluation and management service by the same provider on the same day of the procedure or other service

-32 Mandated service.

-52 Reduced services.

-57 Decision for surgery.

PRACTICE **PITFALLS**

The following are billing tips on using the CPT:

1. When counseling and coordination of care consume more than 50 percent of a visit, you can bill for the higher level E/M codes (and receive the higher reimbursement). The provider must be certain to document the time spent and the reason why.

2. Make sure the diagnosis code you submit is consistent with the level of the visit for which you are billing.

3. If the code you are submitting is a high-level code or is unusual, include documentation to support the services when the claim is submitted.

Anesthesia

Services involving the administration of anesthesia are reported by using five-digit procedure codes from the anesthesia section in the CPT manual. The CPT code range for anesthesia is 00100–01999 (Table 13-3 ●). Types of care reported using anesthesia codes include general, regional, and supplementation of local anesthesia. In addition to anesthesia, services such as the

TABLE 13-3 Anesthesia Codes Subsections

Head	00100–00222
Neck	00300–00352
Thorax	00400–00474
Intrathoracic	00500–00580
Spine and Spinal Cord	00600–00670
Upper Abdomen	00700–00797
Lower Abdomen	00800–00882
Perineum	00902–00952
Pelvis (Except Hip)	01112–01190
Upper Leg (Except Knee)	01200–01274
Knee and Popliteal Area	01320–01444
Lower Leg (Below Knee, Includes Ankle and Foot)	01462–01522
Shoulder and Axilla	01610–01682
Upper Arm and Elbow	01710–01782
Forearm, Wrist, and Hand	01810–01860
Radiological Procedures	01916–01936
Burn Excisions or Debridement	01951–01953
Obstetric	01958–01969
Other Procedures	01990–01999

usual preoperative and postoperative visits, anesthesia care during a procedure, the administration of fluids and/or blood, and the usual monitoring services during anesthesia are coded using the codes found in the anesthesia section of the CPT manual. These codes are generally reported by anesthesiologists. When the surgeon provides anesthesia, modifier -47 is appended to the surgical procedure code. Anesthesia codes are assigned based on the type of surgical procedure being performed and one anesthesia code may be used for several related surgical procedures. In other words, there is not a separate anesthesia code for every single CPT surgical procedure. To locate anesthesia codes in the CPT index, look up the main term *Anesthesia,* then the type of procedure. If you look up the name of the procedure as the main term, you will be directed to the code for the surgical procedure itself, not the anesthesia.

CPT codes marked with the Moderate Sedation symbol (⊙) include this type of anesthesia in the procedure code. Reimbursement for anesthesia services is typically based on a formula known as B+T+M, which stands for Base units, Time units, and Modifying units.

Anesthesia Base Units

Anesthesia base units are designed to allow for the preparation for anesthesia, the administration of the anesthetic, and the administration of fluids and blood incident to the anesthesia or surgery. The value of the base unit for each procedure is established by the American Society of Anesthesiologists (ASA). The Relative Value Unit (RVU) for the surgical procedure code includes surgery, local infiltration, digital block, or topical anesthesia.

Anesthesia Time Units

The length of time that a patient is under anesthesia determines the amount of money that will be allowed for the procedure. Anesthesia time begins when the anesthesiologist starts to prepare the patient for the induction of anesthesia in the operating room area (or its equivalent). The time ends when the anesthesiologist is no longer in constant attendance, usually when the patient is ready for postoperative supervision. This time should always be indicated on the claim form when billing for anesthesia services.

Actual anesthesia time should be reported in minutes. Usually you will convert the minutes to quarter-hour (15-minute) increments and enter this value in block 24G on the CMS-1500. Some insurers may require that you report the time using minutes or hours, so it is important to know what is required by each insurance company.

ACTIVITY #2

Anesthesia CPT Coding: Never-Ending Circle Challenge

Directions: Starting with the marked line, look up the codes and enter one digit on each line. Use the last number of the previous code as the first number of the following code (e.g., codes 00133, 38405, and 50023 would be written 0 0 1 3 3 8 4 0 5 0 0 2 3).

Never-Ending Circle

1. Insertion of tissue expander(s) for other than breast, including subsequent expansion

2. Anesthesia for all procedures on esophagus, thyroid, larynx, trachea, and lymphatic system of neck; not otherwise specified, age one year or older

3. Anesthesia for intracranial procedures; not otherwise specified procedures in sitting position

4. Molecular diagnostics; molecular isolation or extraction interpretation and report

5. Percutaneous skeletal fixation of humeral epicondylar fracture, medial or lateral, with manipulation

6. Repair of dural/cerebrospinal fluid leak, not requiring laminectomy

7. Radiologic examination, ribs, bilateral; three views including posteroanterior chest, minimum of four views

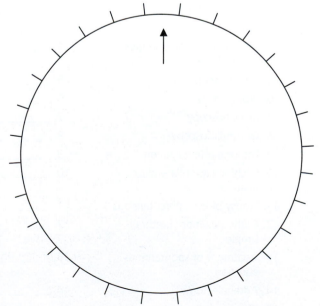

Anesthesia Modifiers

All anesthesia services are billed by use of the anesthesia five-digit CPT code plus the addition of a physical status modifier. The physical status modifier describes the condition of the patient at the time anesthesia is administered. This is determined by the anesthesiologist based on definitions established by the ASA. The use of other optional modifiers may be appropriate.

Physical status modifiers are represented by the initial P followed by a single digit from 1 through 6, as follows:

P1   A normal healthy patient

P2   A patient with mild systemic disease

P3   A patient with severe systemic disease

P4   A patient with severe systemic disease that is a constant threat to life

P5   A moribund patient who is not expected to survive without the operation

P6   A declared brain-dead patient whose organs are being removed for donor purposes

Under certain circumstances, it may be necessary to use other modifiers for anesthesia services as follows:

-22   Increased procedural services

-23   Unusual anesthesia

-32   Mandated services

-51   Multiple procedures

Qualifying Circumstances

Many anesthesia services are provided under particularly difficult circumstances because of factors such as extraordinary condition of the patient, notable operative conditions, or unusual risk factors. This section includes a list of important **qualifying circumstances** that significantly

ACTIVITY #3

Anesthesia CPT Coding

Directions: Based on the service description, look up the appropriate anesthesia CPT code and write it in the space provided.

Description	Code	Description	Code
1. Routine obstetric care w/antepartum care, vaginal	1. _____	16. Laminectomy, sitting position	16. _____
2. Excision of tonsil tags	2. _____	17. Sigmoidoscopy	17. _____
3. Anoscopy	3. _____	18. Renal biopsy, percutaneous	18. _____
4. Arthroscopy, ankle surgical removal of FB	4. _____	19. Liver transplant (recipient)	19. _____
5. Laryngoscopy	5. _____	20. Myringotomy	20. _____
6. Proctoscopy	6. _____	21. Thoracoplasty	21. _____
7. Bronchoscopy	7. _____	22. Repair blood vessel, direct; neck	22. _____
8. Ophthalmoscopy	8. _____	23. Pneumocentesis	23. _____
9. Femoral artery ligation	9. _____	24. Circumcision, using clamp; newborn	24. _____
10. Orchiopexy, unilateral or bilateral	10. _____	25. Salpingo-oophorectomy; complete	25. _____
11. Biopsy of liver, percutaneous	11. _____	26. Bronchoplasty, graft repair	26. _____
12. Catheterization, urethra; simple	12. _____	27. Tracheoplasty, cervical	27. _____
13. Treatment of spontaneous abortion	13. _____	28. Treatment of closed metacarpal fracture; single	28. _____
14. Adrenalectomy	14. _____	29. Cryotherapy	29. _____
15. Urethroplasty; first stage	15. _____	30. Treatment of closed distal tibial fracture	30. _____

impact on the character of the anesthetic service provided. These procedures would not be reported alone but would be reported as additional procedure numbers qualifying an anesthesia procedure or service. More than one code may be selected.

99100 Anesthesia for patient of extreme age, under 1 year or over 70 years

99116 Anesthesia complicated by utilization of total body hypothermia

99135 Anesthesia complicated by utilization of controlled hypotension

99140 Anesthesia complicated by emergency conditions

In some instances information contained in the modifiers is part of the anesthesia code description. For example, some anesthesia codes include the age of the patient. In these cases, the CPT manual includes a note under the code that says, "Do not report this code in conjunction with 99100." This means that the medical biller should list only the anesthesia code and not the qualifying circumstance code. Emergency conditions need to be specified. An **emergency** is defined as existing when delay in treatment of the patient would lead to a significant increase in the threat to life or body part.

Surgery

The surgery section of the CPT book is arranged according to body systems (e.g., integumentary, respiratory, etc.) (Table 13-4 ●). Within each body system, surgeries are arranged according to their anatomic position from the head downward toward the feet.

Surgery Modifiers

Surgical procedures are billed by use of the five-digit CPT code, and the code may be detailed by adding a modifier to it. Some of the modifiers that may be used with surgical CPT codes are as follows:

-22 Increased Procedural Services

-26 Professional Component

-32 Mandated Services

-47 Anesthesia by Surgeon

TABLE 13-4 **Surgery Codes Subsections**

General	10021–10022
Integumentary System	10040–19499
Musculosketal System	20005–29999
Respiratory System	30000–32999
Cardiovascular System	33010–37799
Hemic and Lymphatic Systems	38100–38999
Mediastinum and Diaphragm	39000–39599
Digestive System	40490–49999
Urinary System	50010–53899
Male Genital System	54000–55899
Reproductive System Procedures	55920
Intersex Surgery	55970–55980
Female Genital System	56405–58999
Maternity Care and Delivery	59000–59899
Endocrine System	60000–60699
Nervous System	61000–64999
Eye and Ocular Adnexa	65091–68899
Auditory System	69000–69979
Operating Microscope	69990

-50 Bilateral Procedure

-51 Multiple Procedures

-52 Reduced Services

-54 Surgical Care Only

-62 Two Surgeons

-66 Surgical Team

-76 Repeat Procedure by Same Provider

-77 Repeat Procedure by Another Provider

-80 Assistant Surgeon

-81 Minimum Assistant Surgeon

-90 Reference (Outside) Laboratory

-99 Multiple Modifiers

Multiple or Bilateral Procedures

Multiple procedures comprise more than one surgical procedure performed during the same operative session. The first procedure to be listed when reporting multiple surgical procedures is the procedure with the highest fee. All additional surgical procedures should be listed in descending fee order followed by modifier -51. The provider's full fee should be listed for each procedure billed.

Block procedures are multiple surgical procedures performed during the same operative session, in the same operative area, usually in the integumentary system. The objective of these codes is to handle multiple repetitions of the same service. A block procedure consists of a primary code and subsequent modifying codes.

For example:

11100 Biopsy of skin, subcutaneous tissue or mucous membrane; single lesion

11101 Each separate additional lesion

11200 Removal of skin tags, up to 15 lesions

11201 Each additional 10 lesions

Procedure	Billed Amt	Allowed
Tonsillectomy (42821)	$600	$600
Eustachian Tube Inflation	$300	$200

Bilateral procedures are surgeries that involve a pair of similar body parts (e.g., breasts, eyes). There are two main types of operative sessions for multiple or bilateral procedures.

Same Time, Different Operative Field, Incision, or Orifice

When more than one surgery is performed during the same operative session but in a different operative field or through a different incision or orifice (opening), code each procedure separately with the primary procedure listed on the insurance claim form first. Bilateral procedures follow the same rules as multiple procedures performed through different incisions.

Same Time, Same Operative Field, Incision, or Orifice

Sometimes, when multiple procedures are performed during the same operative session through the same operative field, incision, or orifice the additional procedures are considered to be incidental.

An incidental procedure is one that does not add significant time or complexity to the operative session. In this case, the allowable amount would be that of the primary procedure only. No additional amount would be allowed for the extra procedures. However, if the additional procedures are not incidental, then the rules for handling multiple procedures explained earlier would be applied.

Following the rules previously indicated, the payer would allow 100 percent of the primary procedure plus 50 percent of the secondary procedure. Therefore, in this example, the allowable amount would be 100 percent of $600 + 50 percent of $200 for a total allowance of $700.

ACTIVITY #4

Surgery CPT Coding Crossword Puzzle

Directions: Based on the service description, look up the appropriate CPT code and write it in the crossword puzzle space provided.

Across

1. Ventriculocisternostomy, third ventricle; stereotactic, neuroendoscopic method
2. Thoracentesis with insertion of tube with or without water seal
3. Laminotomy with decompression of nerve root(s), including partial facetectomy, foraminotomy and/or excision of herniated intervertebral disk; one interspace, cervical, one interspace, lumbar
4. Treatment of superficial wound dehiscence; simple closure
5. Conization of cervix, with or without fulguration, with or without dilation and curettage, with or without repair; cold knife or laser, loop electrode excision

Down

1. Stereotactic biopsy, aspiration, or excision of lesion, spinal cord
2. Open treatment and reduction of vertebral fracture, posterior approach, one segment, thoracic
3. Incision of soft tissue abscess; superficial, deep or complicated
4. Anesthesia for all procedures on esophagus, thyroid, larynx, trachea, and lymphatic system of neck; not otherwise specified, age one year or older, needle biopsy of thyroid
5. Simple repair of superficial wounds of scalp, neck, axillae, external genitalia, trunk, and/or extremities 2.6 cm to 7.5 cm

PRACTICE PITFALLS

It is important to understand which procedure is the primary procedure and which is the secondary procedure.

For example, let's look at the same procedures as those just reviewed, billed as follows:

Procedure	Billed Amt	Allowed
Tonsillectomy (42821)	$300	$600
Eustachian Tube Inflation	$600	$100
Total	$900	$700

The primary procedure is the tonsillectomy, and the inflation is the secondary procedure. Therefore, using the multiple surgery rules but following the provider's billing, the allowed amount would be as follows:

100 percent of $600 up to the actual charge	$300
50 percent of $200 or the actual charge, whichever is less	+100
Total Allowance would be	$400

As you can see, incorrect billing would substantially reduce the claim payment amount.

Assistant Surgeon

As mentioned briefly in the modifiers section, some surgical procedures require an assistant surgeon. When billing for assistant surgeon services, modifier -80 or -81 should be added to the appropriate CPT code. You will know when an assistant is used by reading the operative report.

Unbundling

Unbundling is the idea of using two or more CPT codes rather than one inclusive code. For example, a surgeon performs a total abdominal hysterectomy with bilateral salpingo-oophorectomy. The procedure should be charged as an inclusive code, but the provider submits a charge for a total abdominal hysterectomy and a separate charge for the salpingo-oophorectomy. CMS considers unbundling to be fraudulent behavior.

Global Period

The **global period** is defined as the days immediately following a surgical procedure for which a provider must monitor a patient's condition in regard to that particular procedure. Surgical procedures include the surgery, local anesthesia, and the normal, uncomplicated follow-up care associated with the procedure.

Complications or other circumstances requiring additional or unusual services concurrent with the procedure or procedures, or during the listed period of normal follow-up care, may warrant additional charges on a fee-for-service basis. All visits occurring within the listed **follow-up days** should be combined with the surgical charge. There are two categories for follow-up care:

Follow-up care for diagnostic procedures (e.g., endoscopy, injection procedures for radiology). Includes only care that is related to recovery from the diagnostic procedure itself. Care of the underlying condition for which the diagnostic procedure was performed or other accompanying conditions is not included and may be charged separately in accordance with the services rendered.

Follow-up care for therapeutic procedures. Generally includes all normal postoperative care. Complications, exacerbations, recurrence, or the presence of other diseases or injuries requiring additional services concurrent with the surgical procedure(s) or during the indicated period of normal follow-up care may warrant additional charges coded and allowable separately.

PRACTICE **PITFALLS**

1. Two codes are reported, but one of the codes includes both services and should have been the only code reported. Claim is billed as follows.
   a. 11750 Excision of nail and nail matrix, partial or complete for permanent removal
   b. 11752 Excision of nail and nail matrix, partial or complete for permanent removal; with amputation of tuft of distal phalanx

Since the excision of nail and nail matrix is part of 11752, only 11752 should be reported. Payment for 11752 includes payment for both the excision and the amputation.

2. Two or more CPT codes for distinct services are reported, but there is a single code that combines the two. Claim is billed as follows:
   a. 43453 Dilation of esophagus, over guide wire or string
   b. 43200 Esophagoscopy, rigid or flexible fiber optic; diagnostic procedure

A dilation of the esophagus via an esophagoscope could be reported correctly with a single code or incorrectly with two codes. The following is the correct billing for these services:

43226 Esophagoscopy, rigid or flexible fiberoptic; with insertion of guide wire followed by dilation over guide wire

FIGURE 13-7

Visualizing a fetus in utero through the use of an ultrasound

© Moreno Soppelsa/Shutterstock

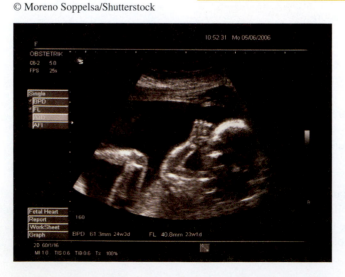

When additional surgical procedure(s) are carried out within the listed period of follow-up care for a previous surgery, the follow-up periods will run concurrently through their normal termination.

Maternity Expenses

The services normally provided in maternity cases include all routine, antepartum care (prior to delivery), delivery, and all routine, postpartum care (after delivery). The maternity procedure codes are based on this premise unless the specific code indicates otherwise (Figure 13-7 ●).

Antepartum care (prenatal) includes:

• Initial and subsequent history
• Provider's exams, usually one per month for the first eight months, then weekly during the ninth month

- Weight, blood pressure, urinalysis (monthly or weekly)
- Fetal heart tones
- Maternity counseling on food requirements, vitamins, and related items

Delivery includes:

- Vaginal delivery (with or without episiotomy, forceps, or breech delivery)
- Cesarean delivery

Postpartum care (after delivery) includes:

- Postdelivery hospital visits
- Postdelivery office visits (usually one or two routine checkups) during the first six weeks following delivery

Cosmetic Surgery

Although some procedures are cosmetic in nature and are performed solely to improve the appearance, they may also be performed for functional reasons. For instance, a blepharoplasty is the removal of excessive skin and fat from the eyelids. Certainly, removal of excessive skin and fat improves the person's appearance. However, most plans cover blepharoplasty when the skin overhang is so extensive that it interferes with the patient's vision. Therefore, the fact that a cosmetic procedure is performed does not necessarily mean that it is considered solely cosmetic.

When the restorative or cosmetic nature of the procedure is not obvious, billers should include documentation to verify the need for services. This documentation often includes the following:

- Hospital admission history and physical
- Operative report
- Pathology report
- Pre- and postoperative photographs
- A narrative report from a referring provider, if available

ACTIVITY #5

Surgery CPT Coding: Never-Ending Circle Challenge

Directions: Starting with the marked line, look up the codes and enter one digit on each line. Use the last number of the previous code as the first number of the following code (for example, codes 00133, 38405, and 50023 would be written 0 0 1 3 3 8 4 5 0 0 2 3).

Never-Ending Circle

1. Chemosurgery for second stage, fixed or fresh tissue, up to five specimens

2. Cystourethroscopy, with steroid injection into stricture

3. Rhinoplasty for nasal deformity secondary to congenital cleft lip or palate, including columellar lengthening; tip, septum, osteotomies

4. Radical resection for tumor, radial head or neck

5. Closed treatment of carpal scaphoid fracture; without manipulation

6. Open treatment of rib fracture without fixation, each

7. Renal endoscopy through established nephrostomy or pyelostomy, with or without irrigation, instillation, or ureteropyelography, exclusive of radiologic service; with removal of foreign body or calculus

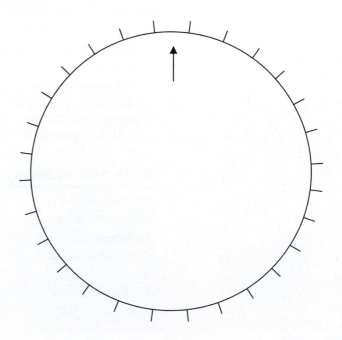

ACTIVITY #6

Surgery CPT Coding

Directions: Based on the surgery service description, look up the appropriate surgical CPT code and write it in the space provided. Be as specific as possible with descriptions. Use modifiers when necessary.

Description	Code
1. Excision of mediastinal cyst	1. _____
2. Pyelotomy; with exploration	2. _____
3. Repair, laceration of palate; up to 1.25 cm	3. _____
4. Resection of external cardiac tumor	4. _____
5. Wedging of clubfoot cast	5. _____
6. Puncture aspiration of cyst of breast	6. _____
7. Removal of foreign body; intraocular, anterior chamber	7. _____
8. Mastoidectomy; complete, radical	8. _____
9. Open treatment of ankle dislocation	9. _____
10. Nipple/areola reconstruction	10. _____
11. Hysterotomy, abdominal	11. _____
12. Cholecystectomy	12. _____
13. Amniocentesis, any method	13. _____
14. Spinal puncture, lumbar, diagnostic	14. _____
15. Acne surgery, removal of comedones	15. _____
16. Routine obstetric care w/antepartum care, vaginal	16. _____
17. Excision of tonsil tags	17. _____
18. Direct repair of aneurysm, carotid—use of assistant	18. _____
19. Arthroscopy, ankle surgical removal of FB	19. _____
20. Excision of lesion of pancreas—use of assistant	20. _____

Radiology/X-ray

The radiology section of the CPT is arranged according to the anatomic position and the body part, starting at the head and moving downward toward the feet (Table 13-5 ●). Knowledge of anatomy will make it much easier to locate to which area of the radiology section to refer. The radiology section is divided into four main areas:

Diagnostic x-rays are all uses of radiant energy in medical diagnosis and therapeutic procedures.

CT (computed tomography) scans are 365-degree pictures of specific body areas. This scan provides a three-dimensional picture of the area and is used to help identify tumors and cancers located in an organ. CT scans are much more definitive than x-rays (Figure 13-8 ●).

TABLE 13-5 Radiology and X-ray Codes Subsection

Diagnostic Radiology	70010–76499
Diagnostic Ultrasound	76506–76999
Radiologic Guidance	77001–77032
Breast, Mammography	77051–77059
Bone/Joints	77071–77084
Radiation Oncology	77261–77799
Nuclear Medicine	78000–79999

Ultrasonography is a radiological technique in which deep structures of the body are visualized by recording the reflections of ultrasonic waves directed into the tissue.

Radiation oncology services involve the use of radiation to treat a condition. This treatment is used in conjunction with chemotherapy to treat malignant cancers. Normally, radiation therapy is composed of multiple treatments and does not include a "picture" of the body part. It is done for treatment purposes only, not for diagnostic reasons.

Nuclear medicine combines use of radioactive elements and x-rays to image an organ or body part. Certain radioactive elements collect in different organs. Therefore, to see whether an organ is working effectively or to determine whether it is enlarged, a radioactive element is injected into the patient, and pictures are taken of the organ at specified intervals to determine how, where, and how much of the element collects in that specific organ.

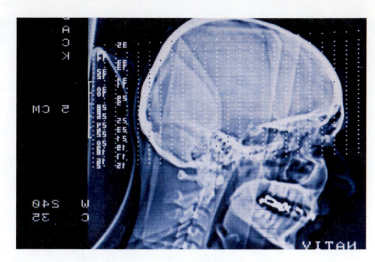

FIGURE 13-8

Three-dimensional CT scan of the skull

© Oliver Sved/Shutterstock.com

ACTIVITY #7

Radiology CPT Coding

Directions: Based on the service description, look up the appropriate radiology CPT code and write it in the space provided.

Description	Code
1. Platelet survival study	1. _____
2. Intermediate radiology therapeutic treatment planning	2. _____
3. CT, lumbar spine w/o contrast	3. _____
4. A/P abdominal x-ray, single view	4. _____
5. Intravenous pyelography with KUB	5. _____
6. Ultrasound, retroperitoneal, real time w/image documentation; limited	6. _____
7. Infusion of radio-element solution	7. _____
8. Salivary gland function study	8. _____
9. X-ray knee, A/P and lateral	9. _____
10. Cephalogram, orthodontic (professional component)	10. _____
11. X-ray hand; three views	11. _____
12. Duodenography, hypotonic	12. _____
13. Pelvimetry, with or without placental localization	13. _____
14. X-ray forearm, A/P and lateral (professional component)	14. _____

Pathology/Laboratory

Laboratory examinations are the analyses of body substances to determine their chemical or tissue makeup. Body fluids or tissues are collected and then either run through analyzing machines or viewed under a microscope to identify any abnormal substances or tissues. CPT codes for this section are arranged by the type of testing or service (Table 13-6 ●). Pathology/Laboratory codes are reported by the entity that performs the actual test. Do not use one of these codes to indicate that a test was ordered or a specimen was collected. When a blood specimen is collected and sent out, report the code 36415, Venipuncture.

TABLE 13-6 Pathology/Laboratory Codes Subsection

Organ or Disease-Oriented Panels	80047–80076
Drug Testing	80100–80104
Therapeutic Drug Assays	80150–80299
Evocative/Suppression Testing	80400–80440
Consultations (Clinical Pathology)	80500–80502
Urinalysis	81000–81099
Chemistry	82000–84999
Hematology and Coagulation	85002–85999
Immunology	86000–86849
Transfusion Medicine	86850–86999
Microbiology	87001–87999
Anatomic Pathology	88000–88099
Cytopathology	88104–88199
Cytogenetic Studies	88230–88299
Surgical Pathology	88300–88399
In Vivo (e.g.,Transcutaneous) Laboratory Procedures	88720–88749
Other Procedures	89049–89240
Reproductive Medicine Procedures	89250–89398

CPT codes 80047–80076 refer to various types of panel tests. Panel tests are composed of multiple tests that are combined and run from one specimen. The number of tests determines which code to use. When a charge slip is received from the provider listing numerous lab tests, the biller should check to ensure that the tests are not all part of a single-panel test.

ACTIVITY #8

Bundled CPT Codes

Directions: Please indicate the bundled CPT code and the charge for the services listed below.

Bill from Provider	CPT Code	Charge
Calcium	82310	$ 25
Carbon dioxide	82374	$ 25
Chloride	82435	$ 25
Creatinine	82565	$ 15
Glucose	82947	$ 10
Potassium	84132	$ 15
Sodium	84295	$ 15
Urea Nitrogen	84520	$ 30

CPT Code _____   **Charge** _____

Component Charges

Whenever a lab or x-ray test is performed, two distinct services are actually completed. The first service is the taking of the specimen or x-ray. This charge should include the expense for the personnel performing the test and the cost of the necessary equipment. This is called the Technical Component (TC).

The second service is for the interpretation or reading of the results of the test. This is called the Professional Component (PC) and is denoted by adding modifier -26 to the CPT code.

PRACTICE **PITFALLS**

Many different laboratory tests are commonly ordered by most providers. Following is a list of some of these services with general coding and billing guidelines:

Urinalysis. If unspecified, use code 81000.

Glucose. If unspecified, use 82947.

Pregnancy testing. If unspecified, use 84702.

TB test. If unspecified, use 86480.

Pap smears. 88142 for routine Pap smears; usually, a covered expense if the patient is being treated for vaginitis, pelvic pain, or dysmenorrhea.

Handling/conveyance charges. Normally coded 99000–99002; these charges are usually billed when the specimen is obtained in the provider's office but sent to an outside laboratory for analysis (99000), or when the specimen is obtained somewhere other than the provider's office and sent to the laboratory for analysis (99001).

ACTIVITY #9

Laboratory CPT Coding

Directions: Based on the service description, look up the appropriate laboratory CPT code and write it in the space provided.

Description	Code
1. Wet mount for ova and parasites	1. _____
2. Huhner test and semen analysis	2. _____
3. Comprehensive metabolic panel	3. _____
4. Serum cholesterol, total	4. _____
5. Blood ethchlorvynol	5. _____
6. Feces screening for lipids, qualitative	6. _____
7. Ascorbic acid (vitamin C), blood	7. _____
8. Desipramine, assay	8. _____
9. Digoxin, RIA (reduced services)	9. _____
10. Histamine test	10. _____
11. Galactose test (reference laboratory)	11. _____

Medicine

This area of the CPT includes nonsurgical and medical care services (Table 13-7 ●). Nonsurgical services include optometry care, chiropractic care, acupuncture treatment, physical therapy, and hospital care. The following subsections describe coding of some of these services.

Immunization Administration for Vaccines/Toxoids: 90460–90749

Immunizations are considered to be preventive treatment. Therefore, an active illness or disease is usually not present.

Psychiatry 90801–90899

Psychiatric services include treatment for psychotic and neurotic disorders, organic brain dysfunction, alcoholism, and chemical dependency.

The language description generally indicates psychotherapy, individual therapy, or group therapy. The ICD-9 coding is usually in the range of 290.00 to 319.00. The providers of service are usually an M.D. (often a psychiatrist) or a clinical psychologist. Most benefit plans require a referral by an M.D. if one of the following providers is indicated: MFCC (Marriage, Family, and Child Counselor), LCSW (Licensed Clinical Social Worker), or MSW (Master of Social Work).

TABLE 13-7 Medicine Codes Subsections

Immune Globulins, Serum or Recombinant Procedures	90281–90399
Immunization Administration for Vaccines/Toxoids	90460–90474
Vaccines/Toxoids	90476–90749
Psychiatry	90801–90899
Biofeedback	90901–90911
Dialysis	90935–90999
Gastroenterology	91010–91299
Ophthalmology	92002–92499
Special Otorhinolaryngologic Services	92502–92700
Cardiovascular	92950–93799
Non-Invasive Vascular Diagnostic Studies	93875–93990
Pulmonary	94002–94799
Allergy and Clinical Immunology	95004–95199
Endocrinology	95250–95251
Neurology and Neuromuscular Procedures	95800–96020
Medical Genetics and Genetic Counseling Services	96040
Central Nervous System Assessments/Tests	96101–96125
Health and Behavior Assessment/Intervention	96150–96155
Hydration, Therapeutic, Prophylactic, Diagnostic Injections and Infusions, and Chemotherapy and Other Highly Complex Drug or Highly Complex Biologic Agent Administration	96360–96549
Photodynamic Therapy	96567–96571
Special Dermatological Procedures	96900–96999
Physical Medicine and Rehabilitation	97001–97799
Medical Nutrition Therapy	97802–97804
Acupuncture	97810–97814
Osteopathic Manipulative Treatment	98925–98929
Chiropractic Manipulative Treatment	98940–98943
Education and Training for Patient Self-Management	98960–98962
Non-Face-to-Face Nonphysician Services	98966–98969
Special Services, Procedures, and Reports	99000–99091
Qualifying Circumstances for Anesthesia	99100–99140
Moderate (Conscious) Sedation	99143–99150
Other Services and Procedures	99170–99199
Home Health Procedures/Services	99500–99602
Medication Therapy Management Services	99605–99607

Psychiatric care may be reported without time dimensions using CPT code 90845, or with time dimensions using CPT codes 90804–90815, based on practices customary in the local area. Modifiers -52 or -22 may be used to report reduced or unusual service time.

Biofeedback: 90901–90911

Biofeedback training teaches a person to consciously control automatic, internal body functions. For instance, through conscious control, some body rhythms that control the constriction of blood vessels and beating of the heart can be increased or decreased. This type of treatment can be used for a variety of illnesses or symptoms. A common use is for the control of intractable pain.

Dialysis: 90935–90999

Dialysis is a maintenance procedure used for end-stage renal disease when the kidneys cease functioning. The fees for dialysis are usually billed on a monthly basis. When coding, the actual dates of service should be indicated, or a monthly from/through date should be used. Normally, the insurance carrier provides coverage only for the first thirty months of treatment. After that time, Medicare becomes the primary payer. If the dialysis is performed in an acute facility, the patient may be billed separately for the facility fees and the provider fees. Remember, the CPT codes are only to be used on provider services.

Ophthalmology: 92002–92499

Optometry or ophthalmology care is provided by either an optometrist (O.D.) or an ophthalmologist (M.D.). Most health plans do not cover routine vision care services related to the refraction and subsequent prescription of glasses or contact lenses.

Special Otorhinolaryngologic Services: 92502–92700 (Ear, Nose, and Throat)

Otorhinolaryngologic services are for the care and treatment of the nerves of the special senses. Some of the services entail regular hearing tests.

Cardiovascular: 92950–93799

The cardiovascular section is very large, and it is heavily used by the medical biller. Following are some of the more commonly billed services:

93000   EKG

93010   EKG Interpretation and Report Only

93015   Cardiovascular Stress Test

93224   48-Hour EKG Monitoring

Physical Medicine and Rehabilitation: 97001–97799

Physical medicine and rehabilitation (also known as physiatry or rehabilitation medicine) is the manipulation and therapy associated with the nonsurgical care and treatment of the patient.

This therapy often follows surgery or an injury to a joint or muscle. When either of these events occurs, the muscles attaching to the affected joint become weak or atrophied. Consequently, to restore full movement, concentrated therapy to the affected area may be required. Physical therapy treatments may include functional activities, mobility training, manipulation, physical modalities, assessment, instruction, and specialized testing or therapeutic exercises.

Physical therapy is the science of physical or corrective rehabilitation or treatment of abnormal conditions of the musculoskeletal system through the use of heat; light; water; electricity; sound; massage; and active, passive, or restrictive exercise. Physical therapy is usually performed by a registered physical therapist (RPT), although it is not uncommon for chiropractors (DC), podiatrists (DPM) and osteopathic physicians (DO) to bill for these services as well (Figure 13-9 ●).

The objective of **occupational therapy** is to either restore normal movement, or, in the case of paralysis, to teach the patient alternative ways of dealing with his or her handicap to meet the demands of everyday living. Occupational therapy is normally billed by an occupational therapist (OT), a hospital, or a rehabilitative facility.

Speech therapy is focused on improving speech and verbal communication skills. It is usually performed by a speech and language therapist.

FIGURE 13-9

A physical therapist helping a patient perform her required exercises

AVAVA/Shutterstock.com

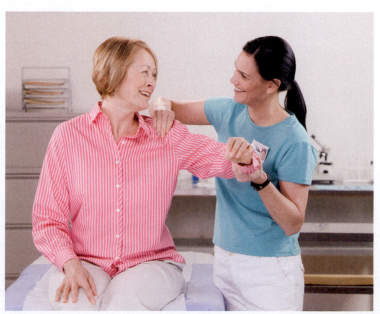

ACTIVITY #10

Medicine CPT Coding

Directions: Based on the service description, look up the appropriate medicine CPT code and write it in the space provided.

Description	Code
1. Diathermy with paraffin bath	1. _____
2. Tar and ultraviolet treatment, dermatology	2. _____
3. Manipulation for physical therapy by provider, one area	3. _____
4. Electrocardiogram, complete	4. _____
5. Provocative testing, for allergies	5. _____
6. Elective cardioversion	6. _____
7. Gonioscopy	7. _____
8. Psychoanalysis	8. _____
9. Biofeedback training for high blood pressure	9. _____
10. Intramuscular, Hep-B vaccine, adult	10. _____
11. Informational book of diabetes care	11. _____
12. Specimen handling fee	12. _____
13. Home visit for postnatal assessment and follow-up care	13. _____
14. Subsequent hospital visit, detailed interval history, detailed examination	14. _____
15. Group psychotherapy by a provider	15. _____
16. Emergency department care at hospital, problem-focused history, problem-focused exam, straightforward medical decision making; tetanus toxoid injection	16. _____
17. Supplies, office	17. _____
18. 25 minutes, standby, for EEG monitoring	18. _____
19. Rapid desensitization, 45 min, insulin	19. _____
20. Cardiopulmonary resuscitation	20. _____
21. New patient consultation for complications of diabetes/inpatient, comprehensive history, comprehensive exam, high-complexity medical decision making	21. _____
22. IV hydration, 45 minutes	22. _____
23. Problem-focused history; problem-focused exam; initial emergency room exam for severe congestion, straightforward decision making	23. _____
24. Comprehensive exam and history for new patient with severe arthritis, office, moderate complexity	24. _____
25. Contact lens prescription	25. _____

Specialist Services

The remaining part of this section of the CPT is composed of services that are usually billed only by specialists within a given field. It is important to take the time to look through this section and to become aware of what services are listed. A brief explanation of some of these sections is provided below.

Gastroenterology: 91010–91299

Gastroenterology procedures are those services related to the digestive system, including the esophagus, stomach, and intestines.

Pulmonary: 94002–94799

Pulmonary services include treatment and testing of the respiratory system in relation to lung function.

Allergy and Clinical Immunology: 95004–95199

This section includes allergy testing and desensitization (allergy shots).

Neurology and Neuromuscular Procedures: 95800–96020

Neurology includes nerve and muscle testing. These services may be considered lab or medical.

Hydrations, Infusions, Chemotherapy Administration: 96360–96549

Chemotherapy includes administration of chemotherapy agents, usually for treatment of cancer. These codes do not include the cost of the chemical.

Special Dermatological Procedures: 96900–96999

Dermatological procedures are procedures to treat the skin.

Special Services, Procedures, and Reports: 99000–99091

This section includes miscellaneous services not covered elsewhere. It also includes critical care services that are usually considered to be hospital or emergency care.

Some sections of the CPT Medicine section may be considered diagnostic testing (DXL), medical, or surgical (this varies from payer to payer).

CHAPTER REVIEW

Summary

- The CPT is used for coding procedures and services rendered by a provider. It provides a uniform means of reporting.
- The CPT reference book has six major sections. The correct code is located according to the section that pertains to the service or procedure performed.
- Modifiers are two-digit codes that can be added to CPT codes to denote unusual circumstances. These modifiers more fully describe the procedure that was performed. In addition, modifiers alter the valuation of the procedure by increasing or decreasing the allowed amount.
- CPT coding is one of the most vital functions that a medical biller performs. Without proper CPT coding, claims may be denied, delayed, or returned for correction.

Review Questions

Directions: Answer the following questions without looking back into the material just covered. Write your answers in the space provided.

1. What are evaluation and management codes? _____

_____

2. What is physical medicine? _____

_____

3. In what order is the CPT surgical section arranged? _____

_____

4. When is modifier -80 used? _____

_____

5. (True or False?) Modifier -50 is used when billing for preoperative care only. _____

If you are unable to answer any of these questions, refer back to that section in the chapter, and then fill in the answers.

Activity #11: CPT Coding—Part 1

Directions: Based on the service description, look up the appropriate CPT code and write it in the space provided.

Description	Code
1. Pulmonary stress testing	1. _____
2. 45-minute individual psychotherapy	2. _____
3. Color vision exam	3. _____
4. Evaluation and management, critical care, 1 hour	4. _____
5. Prosthetic training, 35 minutes	5. _____
6. Peritoneal dialysis for May, age 35	6. _____
7. Psychological testing, 5 hours	7. _____
8. Infusion of calcium, 1.5 hours	8. _____
9. Gonioscopy	9. _____
10. Tetanus injection, intramuscular, for cut due to rusty can	10. _____
11. Intermediate ophthalmologic exam and evaluation for continued care	11. _____
12. Pediatric pneumogram	12. _____
13. Typhoid vaccination, oral	13. _____
14. Initial comprehensive consultation, office, moderate complexity, comprehensive history, comprehensive exam	14. _____
15. ER problem-focused exam, problem-focused history, straightforward	15. _____
16. Initial hospital visit, normal newborn	16. _____
17. Allergy injection	17. _____
18. Allergen serum, one vial, single antigen	18. _____
19. Hearing aid exam, monaural	19. _____
20. Initial consultation, problem-focused history, problem-focused exam, straightforward, office	20. _____
21. Pulmonary stress testing	21. _____
22. Psychiatric diagnostic interview examination	22. _____
23. Hospital discharge day management, 20 minutes	23. _____
24. Office visit, established patient, detailed history, expanded exam, moderate complexity; initial hospital admission, comprehensive history, comprehensive exam, low complexity	24. _____
25. Minimal office visit, established patient	25. _____

Activity #12: CPT Coding Crossword Puzzle

Directions: Based on the service description, look up the appropriate CPT code and write it in the crossword puzzle space provided.

Across

1. Full thickness graft, free, including direct closure of donor site, trunk; 20 sq cm or less

2. Ureterotomy with exploration or drainage

3. Established office visit, expanded, low complexity

4. Dilation of urethral stricture by passage of sound or urethral dilator; male; initial

5. Anesthesia for procedures on external, middle, and inner ear including biopsy; not otherwise specified

Down

1. Excision, trochanteric pressure ulcer, with primary suture

2. Closure of ureterovisceral fistula

3. Radical resection of tumor, distal phalanx of finger

4. Anesthesia for procedures on plastic repair of cleft lip

5. Anesthesia for all procedures on the integumentary system, muscles and nerves of head, neck, and posterior trunk, not otherwise specified

Activity #13: CPT Coding—Part 2

Directions: Based on the service description, look up the appropriate CPT code and write it in the space provided.

Description	Code
1. Urinalysis	1. _____
2. Complete chest x-ray	2. _____
3. ECG, complete	3. _____
4. CBC with differential	4. _____
5. MRI of left hip joint	5. _____
6. Lipid panel	6. _____
7. Erythropoietin bioassay	7. _____
8. CT scan of the abdomen with contrast	8. _____
9. Cardiovascular stress test with exercise, interpretation and report only	9. _____
10. Cholecystography with oral contrast	10. _____
11. Streptokinase, antibody	11. _____
12. HIV-1 antigen	12. _____
13. Ultrasound for gestational age, limited	13. _____
14. Transesophageal echocardiography for congenital cardiac anomalies; Doppler echocardiography, pulsed wave	14. _____
15. Facial nerve function study	15. _____
16. Ova and parasites, concentration and identification	16. _____
17. Blood potassium	17. _____
18. Estradiol, RIA (placental)	18. _____
19. General toxicology screen	19. _____
20. Cyanocobalamin bioassay (vitamin B-12)	20. _____
21. Lithium levels, interpretation and report only	21. _____
22. Serum albumin	22. _____
23. Needle biopsy ultrasonic guidance, complete	23. _____
24. Unilateral renal venography, complete	24. _____
25. MRI w/contrast, brain	25. _____

Activity #14: CPT Coding—Part 3

Directions: Based on the service description, look up the appropriate CPT code and write it in the space provided.

Description	Code
1. Radiologic exam, hand: two views	1. _____
2. Bone age studies	2. _____
3. Radiological examination, surgical specimen	3. _____
4. Mammography; unilateral	4. _____
5. Ultrasound, spinal canal and contents	5. _____
6. Skin test, tuberculosis, intradermal	6. _____
7. Theophylline, assay	7. _____
8. Urinalysis, qualitative	8. _____
9. Obstetric panel	9. _____
10. Iron binding capacity, serum; chemical	10. _____
11. Radiologic examination, abdomen single view	11. _____
12. Radiologic exam, hip; unilateral	12. _____
13. Glucose tolerance test, three specimens	13. _____
14. FSH	14. _____
15. Hepatitis panel	15. _____
16. Entire spine, myelography, super. & inter.	16. _____
17. Cervicocerebral angiography, w/catheter including vessel origin, supervision and interpretation	17. _____
18. Basic dosimetry, radiation therapy	18. _____
19. Laryngography w/contrast	19. _____
20. Protozoa	20. _____
21. Gases, blood PO2	21. _____
22. Heparin assay	22. _____
23. Hepatitis Be antigen (HBeAg)	23. _____
24. Necropsy (autopsy); forensic examination	24. _____
25. Russell viper venom time, diluted	25. _____
26. Ureterectomy, with bladder cuff (separate procedure)	26. _____
27. Radical abdominal hysterectomy—assistant	27. _____
28. Tenotomy, percutaneous, toe, single tendon	28. _____
29. Synovectomy, foot, flexor	29. _____
30. Pericardiocentesis; initial	30. _____

Activity #15: CPT Coding—Part 4

Directions: Based on the service description, look up the appropriate CPT code and write it in the space provided.

Description	Code
1. Excision or curettage of bone cyst or benign tumor, talus or calcaneus	1. _____
2. Removal of permanent pacemaker generator	2. _____
3. Renal biopsy, percutaneous by trocar	3. _____

4. Partial hymenectomy or revision of hymenal ring   4. _____

5. Myringotomy with aspiration   5. _____

6. Thoracoplasty   6. _____

7. Repair blood vessel, direct; neck   7. _____

8. Colostomy or skin level cecostomy   8. _____

9. Circumcision, using clamp; newborn   9. _____

10. Salpingo-oophorectomy; complete   10. _____

11. Bronchoplasty, graft repair—assistant   11. _____

12. Tracheoplasty, cervical   12. _____

13. Closed treatment of metacarpal fracture; single w/o manipulation   13. _____

14. Cryotherapy for acne   14. _____

15. Open treatment, internal fixation of distal tibial fracture of fibula only   15. _____

16. Vaginal hysterectomy, for uterus greater than 250 grams   16. _____

17. Ankle fusion   17. _____

18. Anesthesia for tympanotomy   18. _____

19. Percutaneous, transluminal angioplasty; coronary balloon, single vessel   19. _____

20. Lithotripsy, extracorporeal shock wave with water bath   20. _____

21. Radial orchiectomy, inguinal approach   21. _____

22. Repair, laceration of palate, complex   22. _____

23. Vulvectomy   23. _____

24. Venous thrombectomy, direct, femoropopliteal vein, by leg incision or catheter   24. _____

25. Complete amputation of penis   25. _____

Activity #16: CPT and ICD-9-CM Coding

Directions: Based on the service description, look up the appropriate ICD-9-CM and CPT codes and write them in the spaces provided.

Description	ICD-9-CM code	CPT code
1. Glaucoma provocative test	1. _____	_____
2. Diabetic minimal checkup, established	2. _____	_____
3. Hearing loss; comprehensive audiometry evaluation and speech recognition	3. _____	_____
4. Allergen immunotherapy, single injection for grass allergy	4. _____	_____
5. Physical therapy for skeletal pain, 45 minutes	5. _____	_____
6. Initial hospital care of a normal newborn	6. _____	_____
7. Problem-focused interval history, problem-focused exam, follow-up visit to Shady Oaks Rest Home, advanced senility	7. _____	_____
8. Emergency high-complexity comprehensive history, comprehensive exam, admit to Hoag Memorial Hospital; pulmonary edema	8. _____	_____

9. Manipulation with hot packs and traction and ultrasound, physical therapy for low back pain   9. _____   _____

10. Therapeutic phlebotomy for URI   10. _____   _____

Activity #17: CPT Coding: Never-Ending Circle Challenge

Directions: Starting with the marked line, look up the codes and enter one digit on each line. Use the last number of the previous code as the first number of the following code (for example, codes 00133, 38405, and 50023 would be written 0 0 1 3 3 8 4 0 5 0 0 2 3).

Never-Ending Circle

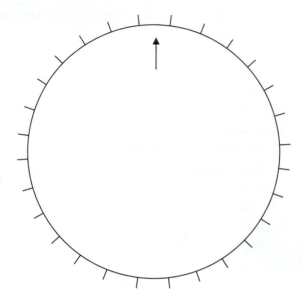

1. Detailed office visit, moderate complexity

2. Exploration, repair, and presacral drainage for rectal injury; with colostomy

3. Telangiectasia injection, trunk

4. Folic acid; serum RBC

5. Thyroid uptake; single determination

6. Anesthesia for vaginal procedures; vaginal hysterectomy

7. Excision of frenum, labial or buccal

SECTION 5

MEDICAL BILLING

The CMS-1500 Form and Medical Billing Procedures

Key Words and Concepts you will learn in this chapter:

Acknowledgment reports

Claim attachment

Claims register

Defense Enrollment Eligibility Reporting System (DEERS)

Electronic claims

Electronic claims submission

Group plan

Incomplete data master list

Insurance claims register

Optical Character Recognition (OCR)

Overinsurance

Primary plan

Professional courtesy

Prompt payment laws

Secondary plan

Self-funded plan

State insurance commissioner

Superbills

TRICARE

TRICARE-certified (authorized) provider

TRICARE-contracted provider

After completion of this chapter you should be able to:

Properly complete the CMS-1500 Claim Form.

Explain the types of services that should be billed on a CMS-1500 Form.

Describe the use of the charge slip and the information it contains.

List procedures or situations when delayed billing is appropriate.

Describe items that may affect the billing amount of a service or procedure.

State the most common billing forms used and their applicability.

List the guidelines that can facilitate the quickest possible payment of a claim.

Describe how follow-up days, maternity bundling, unbundling, diagnosis related groups, and ambulatory patient groups can affect the procedures and amounts billed.

Properly calculate the patient's portion of a bill using a given scenario.

- Describe the purpose of the patient claim form, and list the information it contains.

- Properly define the terms used in coordination of benefits.

- Use the Order of Benefit Determination (OBD) rules to determine the proper primary, secondary, and tertiary payers on a given claim.

- Discuss how benefits are coordinated with an HMO.

- Explain what a clean claim is and why it is important to submit clean claims.

- Explain the reason for the incomplete data master list and the information entered on it.

- Explain what submission time limits are and how they can affect claim payment.

- List the optical scanning guidelines.

- Explain electronic claims submission and the benefits of using it.

- List the common billing reports that are used, and explain their purpose.

- Explain how to handle denied claims.

- Explain how to handle the resubmission of a claim.

- Explain how to appeal the decision on a claim.

- Explain how to make an adjustment on a claim.

- Discuss the role of the state insurance commissioner.

Professional services billing forms usually come in three types: the superbill (also known as a charge slip), the CMS-1500, and the patient claim form.

The medical biller is be required to use several types of billing forms, depending on the type of services rendered and to whom the bill is being submitted for payment.

Superbill

Superbills (Figure 14-1 ●) are internal billing forms used by many providers of service and suppliers. This form serves as a charging slip to expedite the process of billing medical insurance. The standard form has a list of common diagnostic and procedural codes from which the practitioner can choose to indicate the services provided at the encounter.

A charge slip is an invoice and, as such, is subject to the same accountability requirements as other standard billing forms. Superbills and charge slips may be different, depending on the provider of service and the form he or she chooses to use. However, the type of information required by payers is generally the same.

CMS-1500 Form

The CMS-1500 is a standardized form approved by both the American Medical Association and the Centers for Medicare and Medicaid Services (CMS) for use as a "universal" form for billing professional services (Figures 14-2 ● and 14-3 ●).

This is the only form acceptable for billing Medicare and Medicaid programs for provider's services or medical supplies (the UB-04 is allowed for use when billing hospital services).

Paul Provider, M.D.
5858 Peppermint Place
Anytown, USA 12345
(765) 555-6768

Superbill/Charge Slip

Date of Service: _____ Account Number: _____

Name (Last, First): _____

X	Code	Description	Fee	X	Code	Description	Fee	X	Code	Description	Fee
Initial				**Established**				**Special Procedures**			
	99202	Expanded Exam	60.00		99211	Minimal Exam	35.00				
	99203	Detailed Low Complexity	100.00		99212	Brief Straightforward Exam	40.00				
	99204	Comp Moderate Complexity Exam	140.00		99213	Expanded Low Complexity Exam	45.00				
	99205	Comp High Complexity Exam	160.00		99214	Detailed Moderate Complexity Exam	60.00				
					99215	Comp High Complexity Exam	90.00				
Consultations				**Laboratory**				**Prescriptions**			
	99244	Comprehensive	150.00		36415	Venipuncture	20.00				
					81000	Urinalysis	30.00				
					82948	Glucose Fingerstick	18.00				
					93000	EKG	55.00				

X	Code	Diagnosis	X	Code	Diagnosis	X	Code	Diagnosis
	466	Bronchitis, Acute		401	Hypertension		460	Upper Resp Tract Infection
	428	Congestive Heart Failure		414	Ischemic Heart Disease		599.0	Urinary Tract Infection
	431	CVA		724.2	Low Back Syndrome		616	Vaginitis
	250.0	Diabetes Mellitus		278.0	Obesity		490	Bronchitis
	625.3	Dysmenorrhea		715	Osteoarthritis		244	Acquired Hypothyroidism
	345	Epilepsy		462	Pharyngitis. Acute		**ICD-9-CM**	**Other Diagnosis**
	0009.0	Gastroenteritis		714	Rheumatoid Arthritis			

Remarks/Special Instructions	New Appointment	Statement of Account	
		Old Balance	
		Today's Fee	
Referring Physician	Recall	Payment	
		New Balance	

CPI® codes, descriptions, and two-digit numeric modifiers are copyrighted 2005 American Medical Association. All Rights Reserved

FIGURE 14-1

Sample superbill

SAMPLE

1500

HEALTH INSURANCE CLAIM FORM

APPROVED BY NATIONAL UNIFORM CLAIM COMMITTEE 08/05

PICA | PICA

CARRIER

1. MEDICARE (Medicare #) | MEDICAID (Medicaid #) | TRICARE CHAMPUS (Sponsor's SSN) | CHAMPVA (Member ID#) | GROUP HEALTH PLAN (SSN or ID) | FECA BLK LUNG (SSN) | OTHER (ID)

1a. INSURED'S I.D. NUMBER (For Program in Item 1)

2. PATIENT'S NAME (Last Name, First Name, Middle Initial)

3. PATIENT'S BIRTH DATE MM DD YY SEX M F

4. INSURED'S NAME (Last Name, First Name, Middle Initial)

5. PATIENT'S ADDRESS (No., Street)

6. PATIENT RELATIONSHIP TO INSURED Self Spouse Child Other

7. INSURED'S ADDRESS (No., Street)

CITY STATE

8. PATIENT STATUS Single Married Other

CITY STATE

ZIP CODE TELEPHONE (Include Area Code) ( )

Employed Full-Time Student Part-Time Student

ZIP CODE TELEPHONE (Include Area Code) ( )

9. OTHER INSURED'S NAME (Last Name, First Name, Middle Initial)

10. IS PATIENT'S CONDITION RELATED TO:

11. INSURED'S POLICY GROUP OR FECA NUMBER

a. OTHER INSURED'S POLICY OR GROUP NUMBER

a. EMPLOYMENT? (Current or Previous) YES NO

a. INSURED'S DATE OF BIRTH MM DD YY SEX M F

b. OTHER INSURED'S DATE OF BIRTH MM DD YY SEX M F

b. AUTO ACCIDENT? YES NO PLACE (State)

b. EMPLOYER'S NAME OR SCHOOL NAME

c. EMPLOYER'S NAME OR SCHOOL NAME

c. OTHER ACCIDENT? YES NO

c. INSURANCE PLAN NAME OR PROGRAM NAME

d. INSURANCE PLAN NAME OR PROGRAM NAME

10d. RESERVED FOR LOCAL USE

d. IS THERE ANOTHER HEALTH BENEFIT PLAN? YES NO *If yes,* return to and complete item 9 a-d.

READ BACK OF FORM BEFORE COMPLETING & SIGNING THIS FORM.

12. PATIENT'S OR AUTHORIZED PERSON'S SIGNATURE I authorize the release of any medical or other information necessary to process this claim. I also request payment of government benefits either to myself or to the party who accepts assignment below.

SIGNED ______ DATE ______

13. INSURED'S OR AUTHORIZED PERSON'S SIGNATURE I authorize payment of medical benefits to the undersigned physician or supplier for services described below.

SIGNED ______

PATIENT AND INSURED INFORMATION

14. DATE OF CURRENT: MM DD YY ILLNESS (First symptom) OR INJURY (Accident) OR PREGNANCY(LMP)

15. IF PATIENT HAS HAD SAME OR SIMILAR ILLNESS. GIVE FIRST DATE MM DD YY

16. DATES PATIENT UNABLE TO WORK IN CURRENT OCCUPATION FROM MM DD YY TO MM DD YY

17. NAME OF REFERRING PROVIDER OR OTHER SOURCE

17a.

17b. NPI

18. HOSPITALIZATION DATES RELATED TO CURRENT SERVICES FROM MM DD YY TO MM DD YY

19. RESERVED FOR LOCAL USE

20. OUTSIDE LAB? YES NO $ CHARGES

21. DIAGNOSIS OR NATURE OF ILLNESS OR INJURY (Relate Items 1, 2, 3 or 4 to Item 24E by Line)

1. ___ . ___ 3. ___ . ___

2. ___ . ___ 4. ___ . ___

22. MEDICAID RESUBMISSION CODE ORIGINAL REF. NO.

23. PRIOR AUTHORIZATION NUMBER

24. A. DATE(S) OF SERVICE From MM DD YY To MM DD YY	B. PLACE OF SERVICE	C. EMG	D. PROCEDURES, SERVICES, OR SUPPLIES (Explain Unusual Circumstances) CPT/HCPCS MODIFIER	E. DIAGNOSIS POINTER	F. $ CHARGES	G. DAYS OR UNITS	H. EPSDT Family Plan	I. ID. QUAL.	J. RENDERING PROVIDER ID. #
1								NPI	
2								NPI	
3								NPI	
4								NPI	
5								NPI	
6								NPI	

PHYSICIAN OR SUPPLIER INFORMATION

25. FEDERAL TAX I.D. NUMBER SSN EIN

26. PATIENT'S ACCOUNT NO.

27. ACCEPT ASSIGNMENT? (For govt. claims, see back) YES NO

28. TOTAL CHARGE $

29. AMOUNT PAID $

30. BALANCE DUE $

31. SIGNATURE OF PHYSICIAN OR SUPPLIER INCLUDING DEGREES OR CREDENTIALS (I certify that the statements on the reverse apply to this bill and are made a part thereof.)

SIGNED DATE

32. SERVICE FACILITY LOCATION INFORMATION

a. NPI b.

33. BILLING PROVIDER INFO & PH # ( )

a. NPI b.

NUCC Instruction Manual available at: www.nucc.org

OMB APPROVAL PENDING

FIGURE 14-2

CMS-1500 Claim Form

BECAUSE THIS FORM IS USED BY VARIOUS GOVERNMENT AND PRIVATE HEALTH PROGRAMS, SEE SEPARATE INSTRUCTIONS ISSUED BY APPLICABLE PROGRAMS.

NOTICE: Any person who knowingly files a statement of claim containing any misrepresentation or any false, incomplete or misleading information may be guilty of a criminal act punishable under law and may be subject to civil penalties.

REFERS TO GOVERNMENT PROGRAMS ONLY

MEDICARE AND CHAMPUS PAYMENTS: A patient's signature requests that payment be made and authorizes release of any information necessary to process the claim and certifies that the information provided in Blocks 1 through 12 is true, accurate and complete. In the case of a Medicare claim, the patient's signature authorizes any entity to release to Medicare medical and nonmedical information, including employment status, and whether the person has employer group health insurance, liability, no-fault, worker's compensation or other insurance which is responsible to pay for the services for which the Medicare claim is made. See 42 CFR 411.24(a). If item 9 is completed, the patient's signature authorizes release of the information to the health plan or agency shown. In Medicare assigned or CHAMPUS participation cases, the physician agrees to accept the charge determination of the Medicare carrier or CHAMPUS fiscal intermediary as the full charge, and the patient is responsible only for the deductible, coinsurance and noncovered services. Coinsurance and the deductible are based upon the charge determination of the Medicare carrier or CHAMPUS fiscal intermediary if this is less than the charge submitted. CHAMPUS is not a health insurance program but makes payment for health benefits provided through certain affiliations with the Uniformed Services. Information on the patient's sponsor should be provided in those items captioned in "Insured"; i.e., items 1a, 4, 6, 7, 9, and 11.

BLACK LUNG AND FECA CLAIMS

The provider agrees to accept the amount paid by the Government as payment in full. See Black Lung and FECA instructions regarding required procedure and diagnosis coding systems.

SIGNATURE OF PHYSICIAN OR SUPPLIER (MEDICARE, CHAMPUS, FECA AND BLACK LUNG)

I certify that the services shown on this form were medically indicated and necessary for the health of the patient and were personally furnished by me or were furnished incident to my professional service by my employee under my immediate personal supervision, except as otherwise expressly permitted by Medicare or CHAMPUS regulations.

For services to be considered as "incident" to a physician's professional service. 1) they must be rendered under the physician's immediate personal supervision by his/her employee, 2) they must be an integral, although incidental part of a covered physician's service, 3) they must be of kinds commonly furnished in physician's offices, and 4) the services of nonphysicians must be included on the physician's bills.

For CHAMPUS claims, I further certify that I (or any employee) who rendered services am not an active duty member of the Uniformed Services or a civilian employee of the United States Government or a contract employee of the United States Government, either civilian or military (refer to 5 USC 5536). For Black-Lung claims, I further certify that the services performed were for a Black Lung-related disorder.

No Part B Medicare benefits may be paid unless this form is received as required by existing law and regulations (42 CFR 424.32).

NOTICE: Any one who misrepresents or falsifies essential information to receive payment from Federal funds requested by this form may upon conviction be subject to fine and imprisonment under applicable Federal laws.

NOTICE TO PATIENT ABOUT THE COLLECTION AND USE OF MEDICARE, CHAMPUS, FECA, AND BLACK LUNG INFORMATION
(PRIVACY ACT STATEMENT)

We are authorized by CMS, CHAMPUS and OWCP to ask you for information needed in the administration of the Medicare, CHAMPUS, FECA, and Black Lung programs. Authority to collect information is in section 205(a), 1862, 1872 and 1874 of the Social Security Act as amended. 42 CFR 411.24(a) and 424.5(a) (6), and 44 USC 3101;41 CFR 101 et seq and 10 USC 1079 and 1086; 5 USC 8101 et seq; and 30 USC 901 et seq; 38 USC 613; E.O. 9397.

The information we obtain to complete claims under these programs is used to identify you and to determine your eligibility. It is also used to decide if the services and supplies you received are covered by these programs and to insure that proper payment is made.

The information may also be given to other providers of services, carriers, intermediaries, medical review boards, health plans, and other organizations or Federal agencies, for the effective administration of Federal provisions that require other third parties payers to pay primary to Federal program, and as otherwise necessary to administer these programs. For example, it may be necessary to disclose information about the benefits you have used to a hospital or doctor. Additional disclosures are made through routine uses for information contained in systems of records.

FOR MEDICARE CLAIMS: See the notice modifying system No. 09-70-0501, titled, 'Carrier Medicare Claims Record,' published in the Federal Register, Vol. 55 No. 177, page 37549, Wed. Sept. 12, 1990, or as updated and republished.

FOR OWCP CLAIMS: Department of Labor, Privacy Act of 1974, "Republication of Notice of Systems of Records," Federal Register Vol. 55 No. 40, Wed Feb. 28, 1990, See ESA-5, ESA-6, ESA-12, ESA-13, ESA-30, or as updated and republished.

FOR CHAMPUS CLAIMS: PRINCIPLE PURPOSE(S): To evaluate eligibility for medical care provided by civilian sources and to issue payment upon establishment of eligibility and determination that the services/supplies received are authorized by law.

ROUTINE USE(S): Information from claims and related documents may be given to the Dept. of Veterans Affairs, the Dept. of Health and Human Services and/or the Dept. of Transportation consistent with their statutory administrative responsibilities under CHAMPUS/CHAMPVA; to the Dept. of Justice for representation of the Secretary of Defense in civil actions; to the Internal Revenue Service, private collection agencies, and consumer reporting agencies in connection with recoupment claims; and to Congressional Offices in response to inquiries made at the request of the person to whom a record pertains. Appropriate disclosures may be made to other federal, state, local, foreign government agencies, private business entities, and individual providers of care, on matters relating to entitlement, claims adjudication, fraud, program abuse, utilization review, quality assurance, peer review, program integrity, third-party liability, coordination of benefits, and civil and criminal litigation related to the operation of CHAMPUS.

DISCLOSURES: Voluntary; however, failure to provide information will result in delay in payment or may result in denial of claim. With the one exception discussed below, there are no penalties under these programs for refusing to supply information. However, failure to furnish information regarding the medical services rendered or the amount charged would prevent payment of claims under these programs. Failure to furnish any other information, such as name or claim number, would delay payment of the claim. Failure to provide medical information under FECA could be deemed an obstruction.

It is mandatory that you tell us if you know that another party is responsible for paying for your treatment. Section 1128B of the Social Security Act and 31 USC 3801-3812 provide penalties for withholding this information.

You should be aware that P.L. 100-503, the "Computer Matching and Privacy Protection Act of 1988", permits the government to verify information by way of computer matches.

MEDICAID PAYMENTS (PROVIDER CERTIFICATION)

I hereby agree to keep such records as are necessary to disclose fully the extent of services provided to individuals under the State's Title XIX plan and to furnish information regarding any payments claimed for providing such services as the State Agency or Dept. of Health and Human Services may request.

I further agree to accept, as payment in full, the amount paid by the Medicaid program for those claims submitted for payment under that program, with the exception of authorized deductible, coinsurance, co-payment or similar cost-sharing charge.

SIGNATURE OF PHYSICIAN (OR SUPPLIER): I certify that the services listed above were medically indicated and necessary to the health of this patient and were personally furnished by me or my employee under my personal direction.

NOTICE: This is to certify that the foregoing information is true, accurate and complete. I understand that payment and satisfaction of this claim will be from Federal and State funds, and that any false claims, statements, or documents, or concealment of a material fact, may be prosecuted under applicable Federal or State laws.

According to the Paperwork Reduction Act of 1995, no persons are required to respond to a collection of information unless it displays a valid OMB control number. The valid OMB control number for this information collection is 0938-0008. The time required to complete this information collection is estimated to average 10 minutes per response, including the time to review instructions, search existing data resources, gather the data needed, and complete and review the information collection. If you have any comments concerning the accuracy of the time estimate(s) or suggestions for improving this form, please write to: CMS, Attn: PRA Reports Clearance Officer, 7500 Security Boulevard, Baltimore, Maryland 21244-1850. This address is for comments and/or suggestions only. DO NOT MAIL COMPLETED CLAIM FORMS TO THIS ADDRESS.

FIGURE 14-3

Back of CMS-1500 Claim Form

The following section ("CMS-1500 Block Explanations") will assist in explaining the uses of the various blocks on the form. It contains the block number along with the name of the block and a brief description of the information required for proper claim completion. The word "same" refers to a description that is the same as the title of the block.

The various sections of the CMS-1500 include information categorized as follows: patient, insured, secondary insurance, third-party liability, authorization signature, illness, procedures performed, and provider of services.

Following is a listing and explanation of the date codes used on the CMS-1500 form:

- *MM* Month (e.g., October = 10)
- *DD* Day (e.g., October 11 = 11)
- *CCYY* Four-Position Year (e.g., 2006 = 2006)
- *MM | DD | YY or MM | DD | CCYY* Indicates that a space must be reported between month, day, and year. This space is delineated by a dotted vertical line on the CMS-1500 Form. The year must always be written with four digits (e.g., 10 | 01 | 2006).

CMS-1500 Block Explanations

The CMS-1500 requires specific information entry in the various blocks. Refer to the CMS-1500 Matrix in Appendix B for a detailed explanation of the information required for the various blocks on the form.

The following list will assist in explaining the uses of the various blocks on the CMS-1500. It contains the block number along with the name of the block and a brief description of the information required. The word *same* refers to a description that is the same as the title of the block. Be aware that it is important to be sure and refer to any local rules that insurance companies may have regarding the completion of this form.

Information About the Patient

These blocks contain information about the patient.

1 Medicare, Medicaid, TRICARE (CHAMPUS), CHAMPVA, FECA Black Lung, or Other. Check the box of the organization to which you are submitting this claim for payment.

2 Patient's Name. Same.

3 Patient's Birth Date and Sex. All dates should be recorded as Month/Day/Year. Check the box for the appropriate sex.

5 Patient's Address and Phone Number. Same.

6 Patient's Relationship to Insured. Same.

8 Patient's Status. Check applicable boxes.

Information About the Insured

These blocks contain information on the insured, the insured's insurance, and the insured's employment.

1a Insured's ID Number. Social Security number, ID number, or policy number of insured.

4 Insured's Name. Subscriber's name.

7 Insured's Address and Phone Number. Same.

11 Insured's Policy Group or FECA Number. Subscriber's group number. This number refers to primary insured listed in 1a.

11a Insured's Date of Birth. Same.

11b Employer's Name or School Name. Employer or school name of insured party.

11c Insurance Plan Name or Program Name. Name of insurance company or group plan.

11d Is There Another Health Benefit Plan? Check appropriate box. If "YES" is checked, then items 9A–9D must be completed.

Information About the Secondary Insurance

These blocks contain information about a secondary insurance policy (if any), which may provide coverage on this patient.

9 Other Insured's Name. Other insured whose coverage may be responsible, in whole or in part, for the payment of this claim.

9a Other Insured's Policy or Group Number. Same.

9b Other Insured's Date of Birth and Sex. Same.

9c Employer's Name or School Name. Employer or School Name of other insured party.

9d Insurance Plan Name or Program Name. Name of insurance company or group plan for other insured.

Information About Third-Party Liability

These blocks contain information on whether a third party may be liable for payment on this claim.

10a Was Condition Related to: Employment? If "YES" is marked, then workers' compensation insurance is involved. If "NO" is marked, then workers' compensation is not involved. Circle whether employment is current or previous.

10b Was Condition Related to: Auto Accident? If "YES" is marked, then check for an injury date (item 14) and an injury diagnosis (item 21). The state the accident occurred in should also be indicated. If "NO" is marked, then the claim may not be for an auto accident injury.

10c Was Condition Related to: Other Accident? If "YES" is marked, then check for an injury date (item 14) and an injury diagnosis (item 21). If "NO" is marked, then the claim may not be for an accident injury.

10d Reserved for Local Use. Same.

Authorization Signatures

These blocks should be signed by the insured, or a permanent release of information and assignment of benefits should be kept on file. If a permanent release of information or assignment of benefits is on file, "Signature on File" should be placed in these boxes.

12 Patient's or Authorized Person's Signature. Patient's release of medical information.

13 Assignment of Benefits. This box should be signed by the patient in order to allow the insurer to pay the provider directly.

Information About the Illness

These blocks contain information about the current illness.

14 Date of Illness, Injury, Accident, or Pregnancy. All injury claims (e.g., injury diagnosis) must have an injury or accident date. If the patient's condition is a pregnancy, the date of the last menstrual period should be indicated.

15 If Patient Has Had Same or Similar Illness, Give First Date. Same.

16 Dates Patient Unable to Work in Current Occupation. Same.

17a and 17b Name of Referring Provider or Other Source. If this patient was referred to the current provider by another provider, hospital, or clinic, the referring party should be listed here. For claims billed by an assistant surgeon or anesthesiologist, the name and credentials of the attending surgeon should be listed here. For durable medical equipment (DME) claims, list the name of the prescribing provider. 17a is no longer reported. 17b is used to report the referring providers NPI number.

18 Hospitalization Dates Relating to Current Services. Same.

19 Reserved for Local Use. Leave blank.

20 Outside Lab. Was laboratory work performed outside your office? If so, check the "YES" box and indicate the total of the charges.

21 Diagnosis or Nature of Illness or Injury. The diagnosis indicates why the patient visited the provider. Both an ICD-9-CM code and a description should be indicated.

22 Medicaid Resubmission Code. Leave blank.

Information About the Procedures Performed

These blocks contain information about the procedures that were performed.

23 Prior Authorization Number. Authorization number for services that were approved before being rendered. Indicate the precertification or preauthorization number here. For DME claims indicate "Prescription on File," if applicable, and for claims requiring a second surgical opinion indicate "SSO Performed," if applicable.

24a Date of Service. The date service was rendered by the provider. A complete date must be given.

24b Place of Service. The location where the services were performed (see following section for further information).

24c Type of Service. Leave blank.

24d Procedures, Services, or Supplies. The five-digit procedure code as found in the CPT/RVS and HCPCS manuals. These are codes that have been assigned to each procedure that the provider can perform. By selecting the proper code, billers can describe the type of service performed with a few numbers. This eliminates the confusion that used to arise from various abbreviations and descriptions of a procedure. It also allows for easy computer tabulation of the different procedures performed.

24d Modifier Code. The two-digit modifier from the CPT/RVS further describing the procedure code.

24e Diagnosis Code. This is used in conjunction with item 21. The number placed in item 24E (e.g., 1, 2, 3, 4) refers to diagnosis 1, 2, 3, or 4, in item 21. In other words, the provider can perform different services for different illnesses or injuries on different dates and submit them all on one claim form.

24f Charges. The charge per line of service.

24g Days or Units. The number of times that a service was performed.

24h EPSDT Family Plan. Leave blank.

24i ID Qualifier. The ID qualifier number is placed in the shaded portion.

24j Providers' NPI. The provider's NPI is placed in the shaded portion.

28 Total Charge. The total charge of the claim.

29 Amount Paid. The amount paid by the patient or subscriber.

30 Balance Due. The difference between the total charge and the amount paid by the patient or subscriber (if any).

Information About the Provider of Services

These blocks contain information about the provider of services.

25 Federal Tax I.D. Number. If the provider of service is a provider or an individual, his or her Social Security or Taxpayer Identification Number should be used. If the provider of service is a facility, an Employer Identification Number should be indicated.

26 Patient's Account Number. Same.

27 Accept Assignment for Government Claims. Refers only to TRICARE or Medicare. Do not use to assign payment on this claim to the provider. Use item 13 only for your assignment of payment.

31 Signature of Provider or Supplier of Service Including Degrees or Credentials. Must be signed by the provider indicating that the said services have indeed been rendered. Degrees or credentials (e.g., M.D., D.O., etc.) should follow the name.

32 Name and Address of Facility Where Services Were Rendered. If this information is the same as item 33, it may be left blank. On some claims the NPI will be required to be placed in 32a and 32b.

33 Provider's/Supplier's Billing Name, Address, Zip Code, and Phone #. The name, address, and phone number of the provider or supplier of service. This is the address that payments will be addressed to if assignment of benefits was made in item 13. Some carriers require that the NPI be placed in 33a. As of 2008, 33b is not reported.

PRACTICE **PITFALLS**

Guidelines for Completing the CMS-1500

Properly completing the CMS-1500 form is vital to getting the proper reimbursement for the services that were rendered. The following guidelines will help to minimize errors and speed claims processing. (Refer to the CMS-1500 Matrix in Appendix B.)

1. Use all uppercase letters.
2. Do not go outside the box lines. Many forms are scanned by computer, and exceeding the box limits can cause errors.
3. Fill in all required blocks as appropriate for the claim submission.
4. Be sure that all diagnoses have related procedures and that all procedures have a related diagnosis.
5. Do not write on the form unless it is for the purpose of signing in block 12, 13, or 31.
6. Do not sign or write in red ink.
7. Do not use a highlighter on the form. Some scanners will pick up the highlighter and turn it into a black mark, thus obliterating the information in that item.
8. Substitute a space for dollar signs, decimal points, modifier dashes, and hyphens in Social Security numbers.
9. Include the hyphen in tax and employer identification numbers in block 25.
10. Do not place more than one service or code on each of the service code lines. If more than six procedures were performed, use an additional form.
11. Include only CPT and ICD-9-CM codes. Do not use narrative descriptions of services or diagnoses.
12. Do not use punctuation. Do not use special characters such as periods, parentheses, dollar signs, and ditto marks.
13. If it is necessary to add attachments, they should be on paper that is 8.5 × 11 inches.

Observing these guidelines will help ensure that claims are scanned in properly and will decrease the chance of errors and delays.

Patient Claim Form

In addition to the billing forms, a medical biller may occasionally receive a patient claim form (Figures 14-4 ● and 14-5 ●). This form is provided by self-funded plans. A **self-funded plan** is a company plan that insures the company and its own workers.

The information contained on this form is self-explanatory. The member should complete the information entitled "To Be Completed by Member," and the provider of services should complete the information entitled "To Be Completed by Provider."

Billing for Services

After the patient has been seen by the provider, the provider will complete a charge slip or fee ticket. The charge slip is a form used by the provider to indicate the services rendered, the diagnosis for the visit, and whether a return visit is required. This form usually contains a list of service descriptions along with the corresponding numeric billing codes and a list of diagnoses and diagnosis codes.

Patient Claim Form

Information must be printed or typewritten. Claim form must be completed and returned to us at the indicated address.

Medicare Patients: Submit this claim to Medicare FIRST! A copy of the Medicare Explanation of Benefits must be submitted with this claim form.

TO BE COMPLETED BY MEMBER

1. Information Pertaining to Member				
Name: Last, First, M.I.	Sex:	Date of Birth		Member ID #
Home Address: Street	City	State	Zip	Telephone Number
Marital Status	Name of Spouse	Spouse's Date of Birth		Member ID #
Is Spouse Employed?	If Yes, Name and Address of Employer			Employer Phone Number

2. Information Pertaining to Patient				
Patient Name: Last, First, M.I.	Sex	Date of Birth		Member ID #
Home Address: Street	City	State	Zip	Telephone Number
Is Patient Employed? Full-Time Part Time No	Relationship to Employee?	If Dependent Child Over 19, Name of School Where Full-time Student:		

3. Information Regarding Current Treatment			
Related to Illness?	Related to Pregnancy?	Related to Work?	Description of Illness or Injury
Date of Accident	Where Happened?	Describe Accident	

4. Information Regarding Insurance	
Are You, Your Spouse, or Dependent Children Covered by Any Other Insurance?	Name of Insured
If Yes, Name, and Address of Insurance	Insurance Phone Number

Patient's or Guardian's Signature

I certify that the above information is true and correct and I authorize the release of any medical information necessary to process this claim.

Signed: Date:

Assignment of Benefits:

I assign payment of benefits to the following provider:

Address: Street	City	State	Zip	Telephone Number

FIGURE 14-4

Patient claim form, side 1

The charge slip is given to the patient after the visit is complete. The patient, in turn, gives the charge slip to the receptionist for payment to be made and a return visit to be scheduled, if required. At that time, the receptionist collects any amount that the patient owes. For cash patients (those without insurance or responsibility by a third-party payer), the entire amount often is collected, or a payment plan is set up. For many patients covered by insurance, a small copayment will be required. The receptionist should issue a receipt for any monies collected and list the amount received and the form of payment (cash or check) on the charge slip.

TO BE COMPLETED BY PHYSICIAN

Patient's Name: Last, First, M.I.					

Home Address: Street	City	State	Zip	Telephone Number

Is Condition Due To Illness?	Injury?	Work Related?	Pregnancy?	If Yes, Date Of Last Menstrual Period

Diagnosis Or Nature Of Illness Or Injuries. Give Description And ICD-9 Code.

_____

_____

Date Of Service	Place Of Service	Description Of Medical Services Or Supplies Provided	CPT® Code	ICD-9-CM Code	Charge

Date Of First Symptoms	Date Of Accident	Date Patient First Seen		Total Charges	
Dates Patient Unable To Work From To:		If Still Disabled, Date Patient Should Return To Work		Amount Paid	
Patient Still Under Care For This Condition?	Date Of Same Or Similar Illness Or Condition		Does Patient Have Other Health Coverage?		

Under Section 6019 Of The Internal Revenue Code, Recipients Of Medical Payments Must Provide Identifying Numbers To Payors Who Must Report Such Payments To The Internal Revenue Service.   Taxpayer ID Number: _____ Social Security Number: _____

Physician's Name: _____   Signature: _____

_____

Street Address	City	State	Zip

INFORMATION REGARDING THIS CLAIM FORM

A Separate Claim Must Be Filed For Each Different Injury Or Illness.

A Claim Must Be Filed Within 90 Days of The Date Of Service Or Claim Benefits May Be Reduced.

If Patient Is Medicare Eligible, Claim Must First Be Submitted To Medicare For Payment. We Cannot Process Claim Without Information Regarding Medicare's Payment.

FIGURE 14-5

Patient claim form, side 2

The patient also should be given or sent a copy of the billing information. If the charge slip or superbill has carbon copies, one of these may be used as a bill for the patient. For patients covered by insurance plans, the medical biller prepares a claim to be sent to the insurance carrier.

Delayed Billing

If a procedure is expected to take an extended period of time (e.g., pregnancy, multiple surgeries), billing for the procedure should be delayed until the entire process is complete. The appropriate

ACTIVITY #1

Completing a Patient Claim Form

Directions: Based on the following scenarios, complete a patient claim form for the following patients. The provider of services is Paul Provider, M.D. Refer to the Patient Data Table and Provider Data Table in Appendix A for additional information.

1. The following services were billed for Abby Addison—Date of Service: 01/16/CCYY.

    Diagnosis: Hypertension

    99205—Comprehensive High-Complexity Exam ($160)

    81000—Urinalysis ($30)

    36415—Venipuncture ($20)

    Patient made a cash payment of $60 on this visit.

2. The following services were billed for Bobby Brumble—Date of Service: 01/16/CCYY.

    Diagnosis: Diabetes

    99211—Minimal Exam ($35)

    81000—Urinalysis ($30)

    82948—Glucose Fingerstick ($18)

    36415—Venipuncture ($20)

    Patient made a payment by check of $75 on this visit.

3. The following services were billed for Cathy Crenshaw—Date of Service: 01/16/CCYY.

    Diagnosis: Chronic Bronchitis

    99204—Comprehensive Moderate-Complexity Exam ($140)

    36415—Venipuncture ($20)

    Patient made a payment by check of $110 on this visit.

4. The following services were billed for Daisy Doolittle—Date of Service: 01/16/CCYY.

    Diagnosis: Congenital Hypothyroidism

    99203— Detailed Low-Complexity Exam ($100)

    36415—Venipuncture ($20)

    Patient made a cash payment of $15 on this visit.

5. The following services were billed for Edward Edmunds—Date of Service: 01/16/CCYY.

    Diagnosis: Coronary Artery Disease

    99214—Detailed Moderate-Complexity Exam ($60)

    93000—EKG ($55)

    81000—Urinalysis ($30)

    36415—Venipuncture ($20)

    Patient did not make a payment.

CPT code usually covers all services. For example, in the case of a pregnancy, all prenatal visits for nine months before the delivery, as well as the delivery of the baby and the postpartum care, are included under CPT code 59400. If the provider were to bill before the delivery, several scenarios could cause an error in billing. The patient could be rushed to the hospital in advanced labor and the baby could be delivered by another provider, or a complication could occur that requires the baby to be taken out by Cesarean section.

It is impossible to determine exactly what procedures a provider will perform until they are actually done, so billing should be postponed until all related services have been performed. Also, billing for procedures that have not been performed (even if you expect them to be performed in the future) is considered fraud.

Incomplete Data Master List

Incomplete patient data are a major source of delay in both billing for services and in payment for those services. Without complete patient data, it can be difficult to complete a billing form properly. In addition, many insurance carriers will refuse to pay a claim that is not completed properly. Problems of incomplete data often occur because of a discrepancy between the forms the patient completes and the information needed for proper patient chart maintenance.

An **incomplete data master list** is a complete listing of patients whose patient chart does not have properly filled out or completed patient forms. A master list for patients with incomplete data can help an office solve this problem quickly and efficiently.

A sample incomplete data master list is shown in Figure 14-6 ●. To complete the form, fill in data as detailed for the following fields:

Date. Indicate the date that you first noticed the information was missing.

Patient. Enter the patient's name.

Data Missing. List the data that are missing. Be sure to clearly list all items that are missing. Each piece of missing data should be placed on a separate line.

Why. List the reason why the data are missing. This can alert you to possible problems with your intake forms. For example, if a specific item is consistently overlooked by patients, perhaps it needs to be highlighted.

Disposition. When the information has been obtained, list the date obtained and the means by which the information was obtained.

Comp. Indicate the date the information was input into the computer.

Because of the limited amount of space on the form, standard abbreviations may need to be used. For example, the form shown in Figure 14-6 lists several codes. Any standard abbreviations created by the facility should be listed at the bottom of the form. This will eliminate confusion as to the proper abbreviation or its meaning.

FIGURE 14-6

Incomplete data master list

Incomplete Data Master List

Indicate below all the patients whose data is incomplete at the time the patient data is being put in the computer.

Date	Patient/Account	Data Missing	Why	Disposition	Data	Comp
1/1/ccyy	Kent Wright/12345	Birthdate	IL	PC – 1/10/ccyy	BD:03/15/63	1/10/ccyy
		Marital Status	PO	PC – 1/10/ccyy	Married	1/10/ccyy

Why Codes:
PO – Omitted or overlooked by patient
IL – Data was completed but is illegible
NI – Not included on forms

Disposition Codes:
PC – Phone Call
LS – Letter Sent
AP – Asked in person while patient was in office.

A letter should be sent to all patients on the incomplete data master list at least once a month, requesting needed information. This can be a simple form letter with space at the bottom for inserting the information requested. Include a self-addressed, stamped envelope with the letter.

Whenever you contact the patient to request missing or incomplete information, be sure to indicate that the information is needed to bill the insurance carrier.

An incomplete data master list also can alert you to information that is needed for your computer program. If several pieces of data are missing, the practice may want to create an additional form for patients to complete that requests this information.

There are a number of things to keep in mind when dealing with patients. Of course, customer service should always be your first and foremost concern, but at the same time you need to have regard for the medical office. It is important to obtain all necessary information from the patient. Remember that the primary objective of the medical biller is to minimize the amount of time between the provider's service and the complete payment of the bill.

Determining the Proper Billing Amount

Providers may be paid different amounts by different insurance companies for the same service. For example, if the patient is covered by Medicare, there are limits to the amount that Medicare will cover and to the amount that may be collected on the overall bill. However, in many states the physician is required to list the same billing charge on all insurance claims and make a write-off after the insurance has paid but before the patient is billed.

Medicare Limitations

Medicare limits the amount that may be charged by providers to patients. This limit may not always show up on the provider's initial bill.

Network Provider Limits

If the provider has signed a PPO contract, there may be limits to the amounts that the provider may collect for services. The provider must limit balance billing to the patient so that the total amount collected for the service does not exceed the contracted amount.

Before calculating any payments, it is important to determine the amount that the patient should be billed and the total amount that may be collected. This prevents overbilling the patient and having to make a refund at a later date.

If the provider has signed a contract that limits payments, the office should have a comprehensive listing of the procedures with limits and the amounts that may be charged for these procedures. Billers must first look up the appropriate CPT or HCPCS code for the services that were rendered. This description of service and code is then compared to the amount listed in the PPO contract. If there is a limit to the charge, it will be listed under the appropriate CPT or HCPCS code.

A number of situations can affect billing for patient services.

Follow-up Days

When billing for surgical services, the total surgical care is included in the charge for the surgery. Total surgical care includes the initial visit with the patient before surgery, the surgical procedure, and the routine follow-up care. If visits are related to a prior surgical episode, you cannot bill separately for them. For further information on this issue, see Chapter 13 on CPT coding.

Maternity Bundling

All maternity procedures are usually bundled together. This includes one visit per month in the months leading up to the delivery, as well as the actual delivery service itself. In addition, some carriers consider certain tests to be included in the overall maternity care (e.g., urinalysis tests).

Be sure to determine the exact services that are considered part of maternity care. Any procedures that are not routinely part of this care may be billed separately.

Unbundling

Codes for individual lab tests include the taking of a specimen for each test. If a single blood specimen is collected and a number of lab tests run from that single specimen, a panel test code should be chosen to report the procedure. Panel test codes report multiple tests run from a single specimen.

If you are billing for several laboratory tests together, make sure you use the appropriate code and charge for the combined test.

Unbundling is discussed more fully in Chapter 13 on CPT coding.

Diagnosis Related Groups

Some diseases or conditions are covered under a Diagnosis Related Group (DRG) billing. DRG billings lump under one payment all charges for hospital treatment of a specific diagnosis. For example, if a hospital treats a patient for one of these conditions, the facility will be paid a lump sum charge that will cover all treatment. If the hospital's charges are higher than the amount provided in the lump sum payment, it must write off any charges above the payment. It is not allowed to balance bill the patient for this amount. However, if the hospital's charges are less than the lump sum payment, the same amount will be paid and the hospital may keep the extra money. DRGs are only for hospital treatment.

Ambulatory Patient Classifications

An Ambulatory Patient Classification is similar to a DRG except that it is for outpatient treatment (treatment for which an overnight hospital stay is not needed).

Special Services

Providers may bill charges for other than medical services. Some medical offices charge for completing insurance or claim forms, late charges on past due amounts, charges for missed appointments, and charges for phone calls or e-mails to or from patients. These services are usually not covered by insurance carriers and are the sole responsibility of the patient.

When a provider renders medical services to another professional, such as a provider, pharmacist, or nurse, or to a relative and extends what is called **professional courtesy**, the billing procedures vary from not charging the patient to charging a percentage of the provider's usual charges for these services. You should familiarize yourself with the provider's billing procedures before billing for these services.

PRACTICE **PITFALLS**

These information tips are useful in helping to streamline the practice's billing process:

1. Be sure to understand the policies of the office regarding the completion of forms and payment of bills. This way you can explain it accurately to the patient.
2. Ask the patient to fill out all the forms required for the patient file. Give the patient sufficient time to fill out the forms and check that all of the forms have been filled out completely before accepting them. Many offices mail the forms to the patient before a visit to ensure completeness or put the forms on their Web site, where the patient can complete them electronically and at the patient's leisure.
3. Use the office forms consistently and accurately so that the tracking of information proceeds smoothly, regardless of who enters the information.
4. Look over the completed forms as soon as they are completed and returned by the patient. If any information is incomplete or illegible, ask the patient to clarify it.
5. Secure all the details of the insurance. If the patient or insured has a card, make a copy of it for the patient file. Make sure the information contains the subscriber's name, the policy number, the effective date, the company that holds the policy or the name of the policy, and the insurance carrier's address.
6. Make sure the patient understands the provider's policy regarding any amounts that the insurance carrier does not pay or does not cover.
7. Complete all insurance forms accurately and completely. This will ensure the prompt payment of claims by the insurance carrier. Also, use the forms preferred by the insurance carrier. Use of other forms can result in a delay in the processing of the claim.
8. Give the patient leaving the medical office a copy of the bill. This can be a superbill, a copy (not the original) of the CMS-1500, or a listing of the charges incurred during the current visit.
9. If an Assignment of Benefits Form is not on file or if the patient's insurance carrier requires it, have the patient sign the Assignment of Benefits box on the claim form before leaving the office.
10. Make sure the claims and all necessary papers have been signed by the provider, nurse, and anyone else who is required to do so.

Claims Submission Process

Once the provider has seen the patient and the proper billing forms have been completed, it is time to prepare a claim and submit it for payment. A number of items must be considered before submitting claims. These include whether or not the claims are considered clean claims, whether the claims are to be submitted on paper or electronically, and whether or not there are any claim submission time limits.

The first step is to prepare all claim files and print out the claims that will be submitted on paper. After the claims are printed, check over each one to make sure that it fits the definition of a clean claim and that it meets all the requirements for optical character recognition (OCR).

Submission Time Limits

Many payers require that claims be submitted within a specified period from the date that the services were rendered. If claims are not submitted within the time limits, payment may be reduced or denied.

The provider's office should have a chart indicating the time limits for submission of claims. In addition, it is best to set a standard of submitting all claims within ten days of the date services were rendered. This keeps claims billings within the time limits set by most carriers, and it also ensures that payment for the services is received as soon as possible.

Claim Attachments

A **claim attachment** is any document providing additional medical information to the claims payer that cannot be accommodated within the standard billing form. These attachments assist in claim adjudication. Claim attachments should have the patient's name and policy identification number on them and should be submitted with the claim.

Common attachments include operative reports, pathology reports, treatment plans, medical necessity reports, progress notes, consultation reports, additional ambulance information, procedure reports, medical history, a prescription for DME, and a copy of an EOB. They are sent to the insurance payer with the original claim or in response to a request for information from the payer.

These attachments and documentation provide the claims processor or medical reviewer with information to determine coverage, medical necessity, and which payer is primary. This is needed to determine the benefit due. Some information is also used to check for fraud and abuse.

The U.S. Department of Health and Human Services in 2007 published a final proposed rule to establish national standards for electronic claims attachments. The rulemaking is authorized under the HIPAA Administrative Simplification and Compliance Act (ASCA) provisions. The department proposed standards for six types of electronic attachments: ambulance services, emergency department, rehabilitation services, clinical reports, laboratory results, and medications. As of 2011, these rules have not been finalized. Once the final rule is passed, most health care providers will have two years to meet the claims attachment standards, and small health plans will have three years.

Optical Scanning Guidelines

All information should be typed or machine printed. Most insurance carriers' claims are processed using **Optical Character Recognition (OCR)** equipment. OCR is an automated scanning process that reads the information on claim forms. With OCR, claims processing is faster and more accurate than it is when processed manually.

Use the official CMS-1500 red ink version for claims submissions. The red ink used to print the CMS-1500 is a specific type of red that "drops out" or is invisible to OCR equipment. This red typically cannot be duplicated by your PC printer. If you attempt to print red ink versions of the CMS-1500 from your printer, the insurance company will not be able to process the claim.

Electronic Claims Submission

Many claims are routinely submitted electronically to insurance carriers. As of January 2012 most claims will have to be submitted electronically. These types of claims are called **electronic** claims. **Electronic claims submission** is a process whereby insurance claims are submitted via computerized data (either by CD or modem) directly from the provider to the insurance company. When claims are submitted electronically, the claims data are entered directly via a secure Internet connection. The ASCA requires claims to be submitted to Medicare electronically, with some exceptions.

Claims submitted electronically usually contain fewer errors because they eliminate the need for data entry personnel to reenter the information. Payment is also generated more quickly. In addition, insurance carriers reduce their management and overhead costs by allowing electronic claims submission. Many payers also process electronic claims faster than paper claim submissions.

Generally, electronic claims submission is performed on a weekly basis. Once a week, the medical biller logs onto the insurance carrier's server and uploads the information.

An acknowledgment report is generated by the insurance carrier and returned to the practice's office. The report confirms that the file was received and provides a list of the claims that were accepted or rejected. The medical biller should review this report carefully. If claims were rejected, an error number and message are included on the audit report to help explain the reason for rejection. The biller can make necessary corrections to the rejected claim(s) and resubmit them.

It is important to have the proper equipment and forms before attempting to submit claims electronically. The format of the claim form must be approved by the carrier, and an agreement also must be in place between the provider and the insurance carrier. This agreement contains the basics regarding the means of submitting data and the correct procedure coding system. Because electronic claims submission does not allow the opportunity for the provider to sign the claims, a provider's signature on the agreement will be accepted in lieu of a signature on the claim form. It is also imperative to have a patient signature on file for Authorization to Release Information and Assignment of Benefits.

In January everyone will be using the same system to do all of this electronic work. Data transmission problems can arise. For this reason, always keep a backup copy of the information transmitted until the claim has been processed. Also, try to submit claims to the insurance carrier early in the morning or late at night. In this way, you may miss the peak times during which your transmission may be interrupted.

As discussed in Chapter 11 on transitioning from ICD-9-CM to ICD-10-CM, the ICD-10-CM code format has required many changes to computer systems that produce and receive electronic claims and other electronic transactions.

Clean Claims

It is important to be sure that the claims you submit to an insurance carrier are clean claims. Clean claims contain all the information needed to process them quickly for benefits.

Before submitting a claim for processing, be sure to check it and make sure that all necessary information is filled in. If a claim is submitted for payment with incomplete information, many insurance carriers, including Medicare, often will reject it. Electronic systems will not let you send a claim without all needed information, but it is important to avoid spelling and coding errors that the electronic system won't notice.

Coordination of Benefits

Coordination of Benefits (COB) is a process that occurs when two or more group plans provide coverage on the same person (see "Definitions" below). Coordination between the two plans is necessary to allow for payment of 100 percent of the allowable expenses, but no more.

This process was developed in response to the growing problem of overinsurance. **Overinsurance** occurs when a person is covered under two or more policies and is eligible to collect an accumulation of benefits that will actually exceed the amount charged by the provider. The purpose of COB is to allow coverage and usually payment of 100 percent of allowable expenses without allowing the covered member(s) to make money over and above the total costs for care.

Before standardized coordination rules were adopted by the benefits industry, a person covered under two policies could collect full benefits from both. Thus, the individual would make a profit by being sick. In response to the diversity of handling procedures used by various carriers and administrators in coordinating coverages, the National Association of Insurance Commissioners (NAIC) developed a standardized model for COB administration, called the Order of Benefit Determination. The majority of benefit plans follow this model.

> ## PRACTICE **PITFALLS**
>
> 1. Batch Medicare, Medicaid, HMO, and PPO claims in separate groups before sending them electronically. This way, each of these types of forms will be processed at one time and you will have a separate batch total for each type.
> 2. Maintain a copy of all paperwork and claims submitted to the insurance carrier. Also compile and keep an insurance claims register with information on the date of submission of the claim to the insurance carrier.
> 3. Make sure that the forms that the medical office or the computer service generates are compatible with the required submission format for the insurance carrier.
> 4. If the practice is considering a new form, send a copy to all the insurance carriers you submit claims to and ask for a written approval of the form. Requesting the approval in writing can solve problems later. It may take six weeks or more to receive form approval.

Definitions

Words commonly found in COB provisions are defined as follows:

Allowable expense. Any necessary, reasonable, and customary item of medical or dental expense, at least partly covered under at least one of the plans covering the patient. Items excluded by the secondary plan, such as dental services and vision care services, would not be considered allowable. Conversely, amounts limited under the secondary plan would be considered allowable (the entire charge). For example:

1. Each plan provides a limit of $35 per visit for outpatient psychiatric care. The psychiatrist charges $50 per visit. As long as the $50 is within the usual, customary, and reasonable (UCR) guidelines of one of the two plans, the entire $50 would be considered an allowable expense under COB.
2. Based on the primary plan's UCR guidelines, the amount allowed for a surgery is $1,200. The secondary plan's UCR for the same surgery is $1,000. When coordinating benefits, the secondary plan would allow the greatest amount allowed by at least one of the plans. Therefore, the allowable amount when coordinating would be $1,200.

Claim determination period. Usually means a calendar year. It does not include any part of a year before the effective date of duplicate coverage under the secondary plan.

Explanation of Benefits (EOB). A form from a payer showing how a member's benefits have been applied in response to the submission of a claim. The EOB indicates deductibles, coinsurance amounts, nonallowed amounts, UCR limitations, and other variable items. An EOB showing the disposition of the claim (how it was paid, denied, or pended for additional information) is required by law to be generated on each claim submission.

Group plan. A form of coverage with which coordination of benefits is allowed. A plan may include:

- Group, blanket, or franchise insurance policy or plan if not individually underwritten
- Health maintenance organization or hospital or medical service prepayment policy available through an employer, union, or association
- Trustee policy or plan, union welfare policy or plan, multiple employer policy or plan, or employee benefit policy or plan
- Governmental programs (Medicare) or policies or plans required by a statute, except Medicaid
- "No fault" auto policy or plan (Applies to some plans only. The plan must specify whether or not this is applicable.)

Primary plan. Benefit plan that determines and pays its benefits first without regard to the existence of any other coverage.

Secondary plan. Plan that pays after the primary plan has paid its benefits. The benefits of the secondary plan take into consideration the benefits of the primary plan and may reduce its payment so that only 100 percent of allowable expenses is paid.

Right of Recovery

If the amount of the payments made by the plan is more than should have been paid under the COB provision, the plan may recover the excess from one or more of the following:

- The person(s) it has paid or the person(s) on whose behalf it has paid
- Other insurers/plans
- Other organizations

The "amount of the payments made" includes the reasonable cash value of any benefits provided in the form of services.

When billing for patients who have dual coverage, determine the primary carrier to be billed first. Normally the plan in which the patient is the insured is primary. For example, if a husband and wife each have group insurance through employment, the wife's plan is primary for her expenses and the husband's plan is secondary. However, the husband's plan is primary for his personal medical expenses and the wife's plan is secondary. Primary and secondary plans for children are generally determined by the birthday rule, discussed in Chapter 4. After payment is received from the primary carrier, post the payment to the patient's ledger card to determine the balance. When billing the secondary carrier, always attach a copy of the primary carrier's explanation of benefits to the claim being submitted. The secondary carrier will not process the claim without this information. On receipt of the secondary carrier's payment, post the payment to the patient's ledger card. Any balance remaining after all adjustments have been made should be billed to the patient.

COB with Health Maintenance Organizations

As explained in Chapter 7, a health maintenance organization (HMO) is a type of prepayment plan in which providers agree to charge members for their services in accordance with a fixed schedule of rates. The HMO insured may pay a specified copayment at the time that the service is rendered or may not be required to pay anything. The patient and the provider do not have to complete claim forms for payment but may need to complete them for statistical and tracking purposes. Instead, the HMO is billed directly or the HMO pays a monthly retainer fee to the provider for membership plus other specified fees. If the required medical services are available through the HMO but the insured does not go to an HMO provider for the treatment, he or she may be held entirely responsible for all of the expenses.

Prepayment plans are included in the definition of the type of policies to which COB provisions apply. However, many HMOs do not have COB provisions, although more are now starting to incorporate this concept because the spiraling costs of medical care are affecting them as well.

An example of an HMO is Kaiser Permanente. Kaiser provides a prepayment policy for hospital and professional medical services at no cost or at a small fee, as long as the member goes to a Kaiser facility. Subsequently, the Kaiser HMO provides the member with a "reasonable cost statement," which represents what would have been charged to a nonmember. If the HMO does not have a COB provision, it would be considered the primary payer. To coordinate benefits, a request must be made for receipts or statements showing the actual out-of-pocket expense. The secondary plan would pay no more than the amount that would be considered the allowable expense. If the HMO does have a COB provision, the regular OBD determination rules should be applied (see Chapter 4).

Collecting the Patient Portion

Many medical offices collect the estimated amount due from the patient at the time services are rendered. This estimated amount is based on the patient's portion of the coinsurance amount and any deductible that has not yet been satisfied. This practice requires that medical billers contact the patient's insurance company before treatment is rendered (usually within 24 hours of the scheduled appointment). The biller should confirm that the patient is covered by the insurance and then determine the correct coinsurance amount, any special circumstances that may apply to the treatment, and any deductible that has not yet been met by the patient. Once this information has been obtained, the biller should determine the estimated amount that is the patient's responsibility.

PRACTICE **PITFALLS**

Barney Bumpkiss is scheduled for a high-complexity office visit for the treatment of diabetes ($130). The provider is expected to perform a glucose monitoring of the patient ($30) and a CBC ($30).

Upon calling the insurance carrier, you determine that Barney is currently covered by insurance that has a $125 deductible. Barney has received prior treatment, satisfying $75 of his deductible. The remaining services are covered at 80 percent for medical services and 70 percent for laboratory services.

The patient's estimated amount should be determined as follows:

	Charges
Office visit	$130
Glucose monitoring	$30
CBC	$30
Total	$190

	Deductible to Be Satisfied
Amount of deductible	$125
Deductible paid	$75
Deductible remaining	$50

Office visit ($130) − deductible remaining ($50) = $80

$80 × 20 percent (patient's coinsurance) = $16

Lab charges ($60) × 30 percent (patient's coinsurance) = $18

Total patient portion ($16 + $18) = $34

+ Unmet deductible of $50 = $84 Estimated patient payment due

Be sure to inform the patient that this is an estimated amount, based on your charges. The insurance carrier may allow a smaller amount, which may result in a higher estimated patient payment.

Collecting from Medicare Patients

If the patient is enrolled in the Medicare program, it is important not to overcollect on the patient's portion of the payment. Because Medicare limits the amount that a provider can collect, it is important to determine the appropriate Medicare-allowed amount before calculating the patient's portion of the payment.

Many medical offices will have a list of their most commonly rendered services and the Medicare-allowed amount for these services. It may be necessary to either contact the Medicare Administrative Contractor (MAC) and ask what the allowed amount is, or to go back through past Medicare payments (especially those for this patient, if this treatment is for an ongoing condition) to determine the allowed amount.

If an office does not have a listing of approved amounts, the MAC may have a list it can distribute. If not, the biller should consider creating a list and adding in the Medicare-approved amount from each Medicare Notice that it receives.

In addition, if Medicare determines that the services are not medically necessary, you must refund all monies paid to the patient, even if you are appealing the decision and are waiting for a final determination.

Remember that any amount collected that is more than the Medicare-allowed amount for the procedure will need to be refunded to the patient. This can prevent ill feelings on the part of the patient, especially Medicare patients who are on a fixed income.

ACTIVITY #2

Collecting Fees

Directions: Use the following scenarios to determine the correct amount to be collected from the patient before rendering services.

Yellow Insurance covers 90 percent of all procedures except anesthesia, which is covered at 80 percent. It has a $125 annual deductible.

1. Yvonne Yang is scheduled to receive drainage of a cyst in the mouth ($340), an x-ray of the mouth and throat ($85), and an esophagotomy ($624). She has not met any portion of her deductible.
   Amount to be collected: _____

2. Yasmin Yarrow is scheduled to receive a straightforward office visit, new patient ($100). She has met $10 of her deductible.
   Amount to be collected: _____

Brown Insurance covers patients at 80 percent for medical services. The carrier requires a deductible of $150 annually.

3. Betty Boston is scheduled to have a straightforward office visit ($85) to have a skin lesion examined. She has met all of her deductible.
   Amount to be collected: _____

4. Betsy Bryman is scheduled to receive the removal of a 2.1 cm lesion on her arm ($560). She has met $30.50 of her deductible.
   Amount to be collected: _____

5. Barry Barker is scheduled to receive a moderate-complexity office visit ($110) and an X-ray of his arm ($65). He has met $5 of his deductible.
   Amount to be collected: _____

TRICARE

TRICARE is the medical program for military personnel. TRICARE, formerly known as the Civilian Health and Medical Program for the Uniformed Services (CHAMPUS), provides a comprehensive program of health care benefits for active duty and retired services personnel, their dependents, and the dependents of deceased military personnel. Persons eligible for TRICARE are enrolled in the **Defense Enrollment Eligibility Reporting System (DEERS),** which is a computer database used to verify TRICARE eligibility. Military personnel are automatically registered in DEERS, where they are known as the sponsor. The sponsor then enrolls his or her spouse or dependents. The valid Uniformed Services ID card serves as proof of eligibility for TRICARE coverage. The patient is responsible for appropriate copays, cost shares, and deductibles.

TRICARE is secondary to all other insurance or health policies except Medicaid and TRICARE supplemental insurance. However, most military personnel will be treated free of charge or for a minimal fee at Veterans Health Administration clinics and facilities. Because of this, many medical billers will never have to bill TRICARE.

Several different health care programs are included under the TRICARE banner:

TRICARE Prime. A managed care option similar to an HMO. All active-duty personnel are required to be enrolled in this option. Their spouses and dependents also are encouraged to enroll, although it is not mandatory for them.

- If a network provider is used, the provider must file the claim.
- If a nonnetwork provider is used or if emergent/urgent care outside the patient's region is required, the provider may file claims on the patient's behalf or the provider may require the patient to pay out of pocket and file a paper claim for reimbursement.

TRICARE Extra. A preferred provider organization. Patients who seek treatment from a network provider are covered at 85 percent of the allowed amount, whereas those who seek treatment from a nonnetwork provider are covered at 80 percent of the allowed amount.

- When a network provider is used, the provider must file the claim.

TRICARE Standard. A similar benefit to the original CHAMPUS program that provides coverage on a fee-for-service basis.

- The provider may file claims on behalf of the patient or require the patient to pay out of pocket and file a paper claim for reimbursement.

TRICARE For Life is a Medigap insurance that covers those who are age sixty-five or older and covered by Medicare.

Non-Availability Statement

If an individual has TRICARE but the military treatment facility (MTF) cannot provide a specific health care service or procedure, the individual must ask for a non-availability statement (NAS). An NAS is a certification from a military hospital that states it cannot provide care. If the member of TRICARE does not get an NAS before receiving inpatient care from a civilian source, then TRICARE may not share the costs.

If a member lives around an MTF, the only time the individual does not need an NAS for nonemergency inpatient care is when the individual carries other non–TRICARE Standard major medical insurance that pays first on the bills for TRICARE Standard–covered care, or when a true medical emergency is occurring.

Although outpatient NASs are not required for outpatient procedures, it is important for the member to obtain advance authorization to have any procedures done.

Balance Billing

According to the U.S. Department of Defense Appropriations Act of 1993, providers who do not accept assignment can bill TRICARE patients no more than 115 percent of the TRICARE maximum allowable charge. Billing a patient more than 115 percent of the TRICARE maximum allowable charge is considered balance billing and can result in exclusion from TRICARE and other government health care programs.

Accepting Assignment on Claims

By accepting assignment, a provider agrees to accept the TRICARE maximum allowable charge as payment in full and to write off the difference between the TRICARE maximum allowable charge and the billed charges. Providers who accept assignment also agree to file claims for the beneficiary.

The difference between the TRICARE maximum allowable charge and the amount TRICARE paid is the patient's responsibility. However, when the patient's other health insurance pays more than the TRICARE maximum allowable charge, the billed item is considered paid in full.

TRICARE as Secondary Payer

TRICARE is always the secondary payer if the patient has other insurance (including Medicare). The only exceptions are Medicaid and TRICARE supplemental policies.

TRICARE-Certified and TRICARE-Contracted Providers

A **TRICARE-certified (authorized) provider** is a facility, provider, or other health care professional who meets the licensing and certification requirements of TRICARE regulations and practices for that area of health care.

TRICARE-certified (authorized) providers may or may not agree to accept assignment—that is, accept the TRICARE maximum allowable charge as payment in full for services. If providers do not agree, then they are considered certified (authorized), nonparticipating providers. They may elect to accept assignment on a claim-by-claim basis. These also are known as TRICARE-certified (authorized), nonnetwork providers. Just because a provider is TRICARE-certified (authorized) does not mean that the provider is contracted with TRICARE.

A **TRICARE-contracted provider** is a TRICARE-certified (authorized) provider who has a contract agreement with a TRICARE Prime contractor. This provider agrees to accept the TRICARE maximum allowable charge as payment in full and to submit claim forms for beneficiaries. A TRICARE-contracted provider is also a certified (authorized), participating provider or a network provider.

Participating providers agree to accept TRICARE payment and any cost share as payment in full. Nonparticipating providers do not agree to accept the TRICARE-determined allowable charge as the total charge for services; they can bill patients up to 15 percent more than the TRI-CARE allowable charge. TRICARE will send reimbursement to the patient and the patient, in turn, will pay the provider.

PRACTICE **PITFALLS**

There are many reasons why claims are delayed or denied when they could have been processed if the correct information had been submitted initially. Here are some helpful billing tips to facilitate prompt claim payments.

1. Make sure the DEERS information is correct and current. When treating TRICARE patients, be sure to list the name, rank, station, and ID number from the enrollment card on the patient's chart. Also copy the card and place it in the chart.
2. TRICARE claims can be submitted on a CMS-1500. Complete the CMS-1500 and submit it to the fiscal intermediary or, if required, submit claims electronically.
3. When filing a TRICARE claim, be sure to indicate if someone else may be responsible for payment, such as automobile insurance or possible workers' compensation.
4. If there is other health insurance, file the claim with the other health insurance carrier before filing with TRICARE.
5. If the patient is a dual eligible beneficiary (those who are eligible for Medicare and TRICARE benefits), submit claims in the usual manner to Medicare first. Claims will automatically be transmitted from Medicare to TRICARE for secondary claims processing.
6. Keep copies of everything submitted to claims processors.
7. Be sure to send the claim to the correct address to avoid processing delays.
8. Submit claims as soon as possible. Submitting claims quickly will ensure timely reimbursement.
9. Claims must be filed within one year of the date of service to be considered for reimbursement.

Billing Reports

A number of reports can help you manage claims that have been submitted or are in various stages of the process. By generating or running these reports on a daily basis, you can be sure that all services are being billed and all claims are proceeding properly.

The most common of these reports are listed here. Some computer programs have the capacity to generate these reports. If the program does not have a report that specifically covers the information desired, some programs will allow you to create a custom report. If this is not possible, a manual report can be created.

Following are various reports, information regarding their purpose, and the information generally included in the report.

Transaction Reports

Many medical billing programs allow you to print a transaction report of the claims that were entered or completed on a given day. By printing out this report, you can compare it to the appointment book to ensure that all services that were completed during the day have been billed.

Acknowledgment Reports

Acknowledgment reports are generated by an insurance carrier. They indicate the claims that were received electronically. By comparing this report to the information in your daily journal, you can determine if all services that were performed have been billed.

Because claims may be submitted to different insurance carriers, there should be an acknowledgment report from each different insurance carrier.

Insurance Claims Register

An **insurance claims register** (Figure 14-7 ●) lists all claims that have been fully completed and are being submitted to the insurance carrier by the provider's office. This report can be compared to the acknowledgment report to ensure that all claims were received by the appropriate carriers.

PAUL PROVIDER, M.D.
5858 Peppermint Place
Anytown, USA 12345
(765) 555-6768

Insurance Claims Register

Page No. _____

Date Claims Filed	Patient Name	Name of Insurance Policy	Place Claim Sent	Claim Amount	Follow-up Date	Paid Amount	Remaining Balance

FIGURE 14-7

Insurance claims register

Claims Register

A **claims register** is a database that lists all claims created by a practice. This database can usually be sorted by date, provider, or patient name.

Prompt Payment Laws

Payment delays from insurance companies can be a significant problem for a medical practice. Because of this, many states have enacted **prompt payment laws,** also known as fair claims practice regulations. Prompt payment laws dictate how quickly (often within thirty days) an insurance company must pay a clean claim once it is received. In some states, the law only applies to non-contracted providers. This response can be payment of the claim, a denial of the claim, or a request for further information. Each time the insurance company contacts the provider for additional information, the prompt payment period starts over. For example, if the prompt payment period is thirty days, the insurance company can contact you at the end of the thirty days with a denial or request for more information. After it receives your response, a new thirty-day window begins, and by the end of this period the insurer needs to pay, issue a denial, or request additional information that results in the cycle being repeated. Therefore, it is very important to respond to insurance company inquiries or denials promptly so that reimbursement is not further delayed.

Tracer Claims/Delinquent Claims

If payment for a claim is not received within the prompt payment window, the biller should contact the carrier to determine the reason for the delay. Often the proper forms have not been received. If such is the case, ask which form is missing and who is responsible for sending it.

The insurance carrier also may state that it has not received the claim. In such a case, ask if you can fax a copy of the claim to speed up the process. This may be allowed, or some carriers will request that you remail the claim. So you have specific information to track and follow up on, ask for the name of a specific person to whom to send the duplicate claim. If the claim was sent electronically, a copy of your electronic claims submission report or the insurance carrier's acknowledgment report may be helpful in locating the missing claim. If the carrier is still unable to locate the claim, you can resubmit an electronic claim or remail a paper copy.

When speaking with the insurance carrier, try to determine when the claim will be paid. Remember that you should attempt to collect payment on services as soon as possible. The patient record also should be documented to indicate all communications with insurance carriers regarding claim payments.

Denied or Rejected Claims

Claims may be accepted as filed by Medicare systems but may be rejected or denied. Denials are subject to appeal, since a denial is a payment determination. Rejections may be corrected and resubmitted but are not subject to appeal. When a claim is denied or rejected, it is important to determine the reason. Reasons for a claim to be denied include the following:

1. Patient identifier information is incorrect.
2. Coverage has been terminated.
3. Prior authorization or precertification is required.
4. Services are not covered.
5. Medical records must be requested to obtain further information.
6. Coordination of benefits must occur.
7. Liability carrier must be billed.
8. CPT or HCPCS codes are missing or are invalid.
9. Deadline for filing was exceeded.
10. No required referral was obtained and/or documented.

If the claim was denied or rejected due to incorrect or incomplete information on the part of the provider's office, resubmit the claim using the procedures in the next section of this chapter. It is important to correct and resubmit the claim as soon as possible.

If the claim is denied for other reasons, first identify the reason and then determine the solution needed to fix the problem. If the insurance carrier says that it does not insure the patient, ask what information it used to check for coverage. This is often the insured's name, ID number, and policy name or number. If any of these items differ from what is in the insurance carrier's records, it can cause the claim to be denied.

Try to determine which piece of information is incorrect. If the information matches what is shown on the forms the patient originally filled out, check the insurance card (you should have made a copy of the insurance card at the time of the patient's first visit). Match the information on the insurance card with that on the claim. If any information is missing or incorrect, correct it in the computer and then resubmit the claim.

If the carrier denies the services as not covered, ask where specifically in the contract the services are excluded. Be sure to update your files to reflect this information.

Resubmission of Claims

If the claim was denied because of incorrect or incomplete information on the part of the provider's office, it is important to correct the problem and resubmit the claim as soon as possible. Some insurance carriers require that you get approval to resubmit a claim before doing so. This is because many insurance carriers' claims processing programs are designed to search for duplicate bills. Thus, the program will log the patient information, the date of services, and the services that were rendered. If a claim is sent in with data that match these items, the computer will automatically flag the claim as a duplicate claim, and the claim may be denied again.

To prevent this from happening, be sure to contact the insurance carrier. Make sure that the information that you are correcting on the claim includes the information that caused it to be rejected. There is no reason to resubmit a claim if the required information is not included in the resubmission.

Also be sure to ask if an approval number is needed to resubmit the claim. If so, get the number and be sure to include it in the appropriate place on the form. This will prompt the computer or the claims examiner to know that the claim needs to be reprocessed, not just flagged as duplicate.

Adjusted Claims

Sometimes the insurance carrier will adjust information on your claim. It may bundle together several services or downcode services it determines were billed inappropriately.

When an adjustment needs to be made to a claim, it is important to perform it as soon as possible. There are several ways of making adjustments:

Recreate the claim. A new claim can be created that shows only the adjusted information, not the information originally submitted. Because this may cause a discrepancy between what the medical record indicates was done and what the patient was billed for, the medical record will need to be updated. This can be done by adding in the corrected or changed information and indicating that there is an adjustment on the claim. The medical record should indicate exactly what changes were made, and why.

When this type of adjustment is made, you may need to adjust the codes on the original claim and the amounts for the codes. The patient's ledger or statement information or the medical office's accounting records also may need to be revised.

Make an adjustment to the patient account. This second method is more commonly used and is preferred for tracking and accounting reasons. Rather than recreate any documents, an adjustment is simply added to the patient's account. This adjustment should list the items being adjusted and the reason for the adjustment.

Because this type of adjustment shows up as an adjustment on the medical office's accounting records, there is no need to rerun any accounting reports for previous periods.

Appeals

If you disagree with the denial or adjustment of a claim, you have the right to appeal the decision. Most insurance carriers have a specific process to be used for appeals. This often includes submitting a copy of the claim along with a letter stating the reason you disagree with their decision.

When writing an appeal letter, it is important to be specific regarding why you think the claim payment, or lack of payment, is incorrect. Simply stating that you do not think the insurance carrier paid enough on the claim is not enough. You need to state why the payment is incorrect.

If the claim was downcoded to a lower-valued procedure, double-check your records. If you agree with the downcoding, change it in your records (including the patient's computerized records). If you disagree with the downcoding, submit the claim for appeal. Be sure to attach a copy of the medical records and a letter explaining why you believe that the higher code should be allowed.

Balance Billing Patients for Downcoded or Denied Claims

Before balance billing patients on claims that have been denied or downcoded, you need to assess the situation. You may need to adjust the original bill to reflect the downcoded amount. In some cases, you may need to remove services from the bill if they have been denied by the insurance carrier. This is especially true in the case of Medicare or Medicaid claims.

If a Medicare or Medicaid claim is denied as not medically necessary, you are not allowed to bill the patient for these services unless the patient was informed before services were rendered that Medicare or Medicaid may not cover the services. If the patient was informed, a Medicare Advance Beneficiary Notice must have been completed before the rendering of services and the services billed with the appropriate modifier. (This was discussed in Chapter 5 on Medicare.) If this notice was not signed before services were rendered, you are not allowed to bill the patient and any denied services must be written off.

If Medicare has downcoded a claim or service, you also must downcode the claim or service on the bill sent to the patient. For example, if you charged the patient for a high-complexity visit and Medicare downcoded the visit to one of moderate complexity, you must downcode the procedure on all billing reports or claims. You are only allowed to collect from the patient the amount that would be due from them for the lower-coded visit.

State Insurance Commissioner

Each state has a **state insurance commissioner**. This person is responsible for overseeing the insurance companies and their practices within the state and protecting consumers (patients). A biller who has a repeated problem regarding an insurance carrier not properly paying claims in a timely manner may file a report with the state insurance commissioner on behalf of the patient. It is important to involve the patient in the process and have them sign the letter, if possible, because insurance commissioners may be more responsive to patient complaints than provider complaints.

The state insurance commissioner will assign an investigator to the case if he or she believes that an investigation is warranted. If the insurance carrier is found not to be adhering to state mandates and laws, the commissioner can impose sanctions or fines on the carrier.

Because reporting an insurance carrier to the state insurance commissioner is a serious situation, you should make all attempts to resolve a situation with the claims examiner or the claims supervisor first. Then discuss the situation with the provider, and allow the provider to make the determination of whether or not to file a report. However, letting an insurance company know that you are prepared to contact the insurance commissioner if necessary can provide the needed motivation for an insurance company to respond to your inquiry.

Maximum Reimbursement Guidelines

Following are a few guidelines that will allow you to receive the maximum reimbursement possible on each claim.

1. Be sure that the claim form is filled out completely and accurately.
2. Be sure that each procedure is linked to its appropriate diagnosis and that the diagnosis substantiates the need for the procedure.
3. Check the contract provisions (or contact the insurance carrier to request information regarding contract provisions). Follow all provisions carefully, including precertifying procedures, preauthorization of hospitalizations, need for second surgical opinions, and so on.
4. Be sure that any benefits that are reimbursed at a higher benefit amount are clearly indicated. This can include outpatient surgery being paid at a higher percentage than inpatient surgery, preadmit testing paid at a higher percentage than inpatient testing, accident provisions, and so on.
5. If a common accident provision applies, send in the claim for the patient who has previously paid the most toward his or her deductible first.

6. Make a notation at the top of the filed copy of the claim regarding the benefit level you expect this claim to be paid at and why (e.g., 100 percent accident benefit). When the claim is paid, double-check the EOB to ensure that the claim was paid at the expected benefit level. If not, contact the insurance carrier for an explanation.

7. Double-check all EOBs to ensure that all procedures were paid or accounted for. In cases of paper claims, it is easy for a single procedure to be omitted.

8. Appeal all decisions that you do not agree with, especially in cases of downcoding or denials because of medical necessity. Be sure to include appropriate information as to why the services should be allowed at the level indicated. Simply adding a modifier is not enough. Provide lab tests, operative reports, or other written data that substantiate your point of view.

CHAPTER REVIEW

Summary

- The CMS-1500 is the most widely accepted form for billing professional services. It is vital that the correct information be inserted in each item to allow the claim to be processed without delay. Although the completion may seem simple, it takes practice to be able to properly fill out the form in the correct manner.

- Properly handling the billing of claims is the prime responsibility of the medical biller. If the proper general guidelines and procedures are not maintained, it can cause a delay in the reimbursement for services.

- If a provider's office has incomplete data on a patient, it is important to obtain that data as quickly as possible. Missing or incorrect data often can cause delays or denials on claim payments. An incomplete data master list can assist in keeping track of incomplete data if the medical biller is unable to obtain the data immediately.

- Two types of billing require special handling: TRICARE and Coordination of Benefits. It is important for the medical biller to understand the basic benefits provided by TRICARE and to know how to coordinate benefits when more than one payer may cover payment for a patient. This will allow the provider to recover the maximum amount possible from the various payers, leaving a smaller balance for the patient to pay or for the provider to write off.

- Electronic claim submission not only cuts down on errors but also dramatically decreases the time needed for payment of the claim and prevents loss of claims through the mail or other courier service.

- It is important for the medical biller to properly submit clean claims. This can be done on paper or via electronic (computer) submission. Regardless of which method used, it is important to follow the guidelines for that method to ensure that the claim can be processed quickly and easily.

- Many insurance carriers have time limits for submitting claims. Because of this, it is important for the medical biller to submit claims in a timely manner, preferably as soon as services are completed.

- If a claim is downcoded or denied, it is important for the medical biller to assess the situation and decide whether to accept the decision and create an adjustment, resubmit the claim with additional information, or file an appeal with the insurance carrier.

Review Questions

Directions: Answer the following questions without looking back at the material just covered. Write your answers in the space provided.

1. What is the CMS-1500 claim form used for?

_____

_____

2. If the provider of service is an individual, what should be placed in the box entitled Federal Tax ID number? _____

_____

3. Which box denotes that workers' compensation is involved in the claim?

_____

4. How would you indicate that the place where services were rendered was an office?

_____

5. What are the boxes at the top of the CMS-1500 form, labeled "Medicare, Medicaid, TRI-CARE, CHAMPVA, FECA Black Lung, and Other," for?

_____

6. What does the term *assignment of benefits* mean?

_____

7. On the CMS-1500, what is item 24I "EMG" for?

_____

8. On the CMS-1500, what does item 24J "COB" stand for, and what does the term mean?

_____

9. (True or False?) When a provider or provider of service signs a medical billing form, he or she is legally stating that the service(s) that they are seeking payment for have actually been performed. _____

10. What does COB stand for?

_____

11. What is the purpose of COB?

_____

12. The _____ is the benefit plan that determines and pays its benefits first without regard to the existence of any other coverage.

13. The _____ is the plan that pays after the primary plan has paid its benefits.

14. List and describe the two ways of making an adjustment.

    a. _____

    b. _____

If you are unable to answer any of these questions, refer back to that section in the chapter, and then fill in the answers.

Activity #3: Completing a Superbill and CMS-1500 Form

Directions: Complete a superbill/charge slip and a CMS-1500 form for the following scenarios. The provider of services is Paul Provider, M.D. All services are performed at his office. Amounts in parentheses are the amounts the provider is billing for the procedure. Refer to the Patient Data Table and Provider Data Table in Appendix A for information.

Upon completion of the CMS-1500, use an insurance claims register (located in Appendix A) and list all claims that have been fully prepared and are ready for submission to the insurance carrier for payment. Enter the date that you created the CMS-1500 in the Date Claim Filed column.

1. On 3/4/CCYY Abby Addison comes in to visit the provider. She has a bad case of the flu and receives a problem-focused office visit ($95) and a therapeutic injection (vitamin B_{12}) ($30).

2. On 3/3/CCYY Bobby Brumble visits the provider for treatment of a superficial abscess on his neck. The provider performs an incision and drainage of the abscess ($95).

3. On 3/4/CCYY Cathy Crenshaw visits the provider for treatment of a cut on her arm. She cut her arm on a broken window at home on 3/4/CCYY. The provider performs a moderate-complexity office visit with five stitches ($110) and a tetanus injection ($30). On 3/15/CCYY Cathy comes in to have her stitches removed.

4. On 3/3/CCYY Daisy Doolittle visits the provider for a refill of her contraceptive prescription. The provider performs a problem-focused exam and writes her a new prescription ($95).

5. On 3/3/CCYY Edward Edmunds visits the provider for pain and swelling in his shoulder. The provider does a moderate-complexity office visit ($110) and a urinalysis ($30). The final diagnosis is tendonitis. On 3/10/CCYY the provider operates to remove the calcium deposits. The operation was performed inpatient at Provider Medical Center.

Activity #4: Defining the Terms

Directions: Match the following terms with the proper definition by writing the letter of the correct definition in the space next to the term.

1. _____ CMS-1500

   a. This person is responsible for overseeing the insurance companies and their practices within the state

2. _____ Electronic claim submission

   b. Lists all claims that have been fully completed and are being submitted to the insurance carrier by the provider's office

3. _____ Incomplete data master list

   c. The 13 rules determining the order of insurance benefit payment

4. _____ Optical Character Recognition

   d. A standardized form for use as a "universal" form for billing professional services

5. _____ Order of Benefit Determination

   e. An automated scanning process that reads the information on claim forms

6. _____ Insurance claims register

   f. A complete listing of patients whose charts have not been properly filled out or who have not completed patient forms

7. _____ State insurance commissioner

   g. A process whereby insurance claims are submitted via computerized data (either by data diskette or modem) directly from the provider to the insurance company

Key Words and Concepts you will learn in this chapter:

Admission codes

Admission kit

Ambulatory patient classifications
(APCs)

Ambulatory surgical centers
(surgicenters)

Bar code

Chargemaster Description List (CDL)

Condition codes

Grouper

Interim billing

Itemized bill

Occurrence codes

Occurrence span codes

Outpatient Prospective Payment
System (OPPS)

Personal items

Revenue codes

Value codes

After completion of this chapter you should be able to:

Describe the purpose of the UB-04.

Properly code the type of bill.

Properly identify condition codes, occurrence codes, and occurrence span codes.

Properly complete the UB-04 billing form.

Identify hospital revenue codes.

Choose the proper form for billing various types of hospital services.

Describe what personal items are and give examples.

Describe what APCs are and how they affect payment.

Explain what DRGs are and how they affect payment on a hospital claim.

Explain the purpose of a chargemaster description list and the information contained on it.

▌Describe the common methods used for entering hospital charges on a patient's bill.

▌Discuss the importance of precertification, preauthorization, and utilization review.

▌Discuss how billing can affect other departments in a hospital.

▌Describe what an ambulatory surgical center does.

The UB-04 form is to be used by hospitals or other hospital-type facilities such as long-term care and rehab facilities for inpatient and outpatient billing (Figure 15-1 ●). The data elements and the design of the form were determined by the National Uniform Billing Committee (NUBC). This form was designed to provide the basic data needed by most payers to determine a large majority of their claims. The objective was to accommodate a wide range of needs while eliminating the need for attachments. The NUBC is responsible for the design of the UB-04 form and plays a major role in maintaining the integrity of the UB-04 data set.

Field Locator and Name/Description

The UB-04 form requires specific information entry in the various fields. The following list will assist in explaining the uses of the various fields on the UB-04 form. It contains the field locator number along with the name of the item and a brief description of the information required. The word *same* refers to a description that is the same as the title of the item.

Patient Information: Form Locators 1–41

1 Provider Name, Address, and Telephone Number. Name, address, and telephone number of hospital or clinic where services were rendered.

2 Pay to Name. Name of the facility where payment should be made if different from the provider information placed in field 1.

3 Patient Control Number. Patient's account number. Line a: Enter patient account number. Line b: Enter medical record number. Unnecessary field for Medicare patients.

4 Type of Bill. Three-digit code providing information regarding what type of bill is being submitted. Medicare requires four digits. Add 0 to beginning of the code.

5 Federal Tax Number. Provider's Tax Identification number or Social Security number.

6 Date of Service. The date(s) of service that this billing statement represents. Date(s) should match dates on the itemized billing statement. For services rendered on the same day, both dates should be the same.

8a Patient's ID. Same. Not required by Medicare.

8b Patient Name. Last, first, and middle initial.

9 Patient's Address. Street address or P.O. Box, City, State, Zip Code, Country code (if applicable).

10 Birth Date. Patient's date of birth (MMDDCCYY).

11 Sex. Patient's sex. Codes are "M" for male, "F" for female, "U" for unknown.

12 Date of Admission. Date patient was admitted to hospital (MMDDYY).

13 Hour of Admission. Hour patient admitted to hospital. Not required by Medicare. See Table 15-1 ● for codes.

14 Type of Admission. Numerical code denoting the priority of this admission. See Table 15-2 ● for examples of **admission codes**.

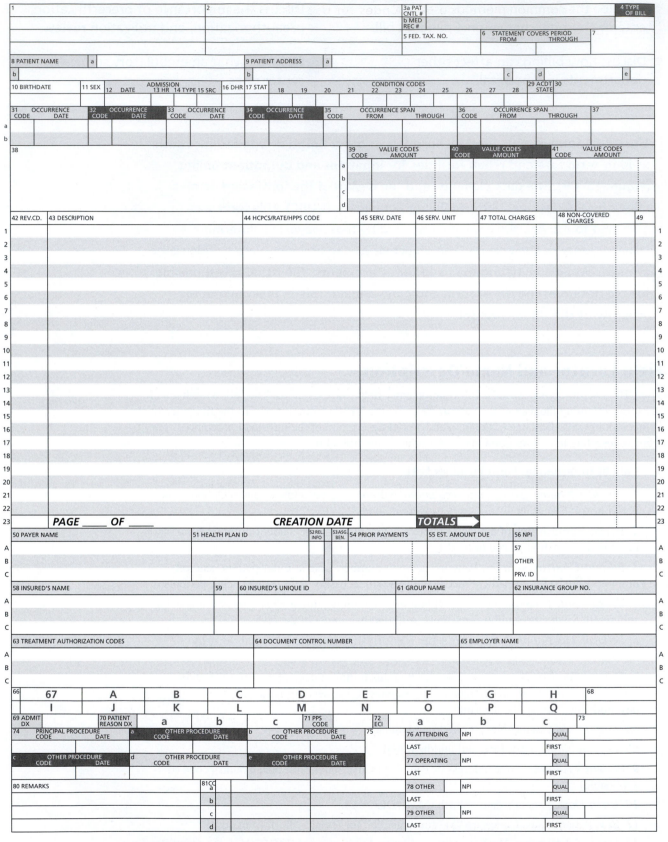

FIGURE 15-1

Sample UB-04

TABLE 15-1 Admission/Discharge Hour Codes for Use with Form Locators 13 and 16

Code	Time (A.M.)	Code	Time (P.M.)
00	12:00–12:59 Midnight	12	12:00–12:59 Noon
01	01:00–01:59	13	01:00–01:59
02	02:00–02:59	14	02:00–02:59
03	03:00–03:59	15	03:00–03:59
04	04:00–04:59	16	04:00–04:59
05	05:00–05:59	17	05:00–06:59
06	06:00–06:59	18	06:00–07:59
07	07:00–07:59	19	07:00–07:59
08	08:00–08:59	20	08:00–08:59
09	09:00–09:59	21	09:00–09:59
10	10:00–10:59	22	10:00–10:59
11	11:00–11:59	23	11:00–11:59
		99	Hour Unknown

TABLE 15-2 Admission Type Code Examples for Use with Form Locator 14

Code	Definition	Explanation
1	Emergency	The patient requires immediate medical intervention as a severe, life-threatening, or potentially disabling conditions.
2	Urgent	The patient requires immediate attention for the care and treatment of a physical or mental disorder.
3	Elective	The patient's condition permits adequate time to schedule the service.

TABLE 15-3 Discharge Status Code Examples for Use with Form Locator 17

Code	Definition
01	Discharged to home or self-care (routine discharge)
02	Discharged/transferred to a short-term general hospital for inpatient care
03	Discharged/transferred to an SNF with Medicare certification in anticipation of covered skilled care
05	Discharged/transferred to a Designated Cancer Center or Children's Hospital
06	Discharged/transferred to home under care of an organized home health service organization in anticipation of covered skilled care
07	Left against medical advice or discontinued care

15 Source of Admission. Numerical code denoting the source of this admission.

16 Discharge Hour. Time patient was discharged from inpatient care. Time should be written according to a 24-hour clock. 99 = unknown. This element is not necessary for outpatient care and not required by Medicare. See Table 15-1 for codes.

17 Discharge Status. Numerical code denoting the patient's discharge status. See Table 15-3 ● for code examples.

TABLE 15-4 Condition Code Examples for Use with Form Locators 18 through 28

Code	Description	Definition
01	Military Service Related	Medical condition incurred during military service.
02	Employment Related	Condition is employment related.
03	Ins Coverage Not Listed	Indicates that patient/patient representative has stated that coverage may exist beyond that reflected on this bill.
04	HMO Enrollee	Indicates bill is submitted for information only and the Medicare beneficiary is enrolled in a risk-based HMO and the provider expected to receive payment form the HMO.

18–28 Condition Codes. Codes used to identify conditions relating to the claim that may affect payer processing (see the next section of this chapter for further information). No specific date is associated with this code. See Table 15-4 ● for code examples.

29 Accident State. State abbreviation where accident occurred, if applicable.

31a–34b Occurrence Codes. The code and associated date defining a significant event relating to this bill that may affect payer processing. See Table 15-5 ● for codes.

35–36 Occurrence Span Codes. The code and the related dates that identify an event that relates to the payment of the claim. These codes identify occurrences that happened over a span of time. Enter the code and the dates from/through MMDDYY.

39–41 Value Codes and Amounts. Codes and the related dollar amount that identify data of a monetary nature that are necessary for the processing of this claim.

Billing Information: Form Locators 42–49 and Claim Line 23

42 Revenue Codes. Revenue code referencing the type of services provided. See Table 15-6 ● for code examples.

43 Revenue Description. A description of the services provided. Abbreviations may be used. This field is not required by Medicare.

TABLE 15-5 Occurrence Codes for Use with Form Locators 31 through 34

Code	Description	Definition
01	Auto Accident	Code indicating the date of an auto accident.
02	No-Fault Insurance Involved (Including Auto Accident/Other)	Code indicating the date of an accident including auto or other where state has applicable no-fault liability laws (i.e., legal basis for settlement without admission or proof of guilt).
03	Accident/Tort Liability	Code indicating the date of an accident resulting from a third party's action that may involve a civil court process in an attempt to require payment by the third party, other than no-fault liability.
04	Accident/Employment Related	Code indicating the date of an accident allegedly relating to the patient's employment.
11	Onset of Illness	Code indicating the date patient first became aware of symptoms/illness.
18	Date of retirement for patient/beneficiary	
24	Insurance denied	Date insurance was denied.

TABLE 15-6 Revenue Code Examples for Use with Form Locator 42

Code	Definition
0100	All-inclusive Ancillary General
0110	Room and Board - Private
0190	Subacute Care
0200	Intensive Care
0210	Coronary Care

44 HCPCS/Rates. The accommodation rate for inpatient bills, or the CPT or HCPCS code for ancillary or outpatient services.

45 Service Date. The date the service was provided. Enter the service date in MMDDYY format.

46 Units of Service. Quantitative measure of services, days, miles, pints of blood, units, or treatments (e.g., if a patient was hospitalized for three days, a "3" would be placed here).

47 Total Charges. Total charges for that line of services.

48 Noncovered Charges. The amount per line of service that is not covered by the primary payer.

23 Claim Line. End of revenue codes. Page X of X. Creation date: MMDDYY. Totals: $$$.$$

Payer Information: Form Locators 50–65

50 Payer Identification. Name of insurer(s) covered by the patient who may be responsible for payment on this bill. Insurers should be listed in order of Primary Payer, Secondary Payer, and Tertiary Payer(s). If required, numbers identifying each payer organization should be listed.

51A Health Plan ID. Health plan provider number.

51B Secondary Health Plan. List the NPI if available.

51C Tertiary Health Plan. List the NPI if available.

52A–C Release Information. A Y (yes) or N (no) designation stating whether or not patient's signature is on file authorizing the release of information. An I indicates that informed consent has been given when a signature has not been obtained.

53A–C Assignment of Benefits. A Y (yes) or N (no) designation stating whether or not patient's signature is on file authorizing the insurer to pay the provider of service directly instead of the patient. If a Y is placed in this item, you must have an assignment of benefits signed by the insured on file in your office. Medicare does not require this field.

54A Prior Payments. The amount that has been paid toward this bill before the current billing date. This can include payments by the patient, other payers, and so on. Payments, other than payments for inpatients, should be reported in this field. These can be listed as primary, secondary, and tertiary payments

55 Estimated Amount Due. The amount estimated by the provider to be due from the indicated payer. This is usually the total amount due minus any previous payments. This can be listed as a primary, secondary, or tertiary payment.

56 National Provider Identifier. Valid NPI number of the servicing provider. This is a ten-digit number.

57A–C Other Provider's ID. Legacy provider numbers for other carriers.

58A–C Insured's Name. Name of the person listed on the insurance information forms (subscriber's name). This may be a spouse or parent of the patient. There may be multiple listings for primary, secondary, and tertiary insurance with a different insured for each policy,

TABLE 15-7 Patient Relationship Code Examples for Use with Form Locator 59

Code	Definition
01	Spouse
18	Patient Is Insured
53	Life Partner
19	Child
20	Employee

Source: Copyright 2005 by the National Uniform Billing Committee (NUBC). All rights reserved.

59A–C Patient's Relationship to Insured. Numerical code designation indicating the relationship between the patient and the insured. See Table 15-7 ● for code examples.

60A–C Health Insurance Claim Identification Number. The policy number under which the insured is covered if it is an individual policy. If the insured is covered under a group policy (such as one offered by his or her employer), often the insured's Social Security number is used as the subscriber number.

61A–C Insured Group Name. The name of the group or company that holds the insured's policy. Often this is the employer of the insured. This information is required by Medicare when Medicare is not the primary payer.

62A–C Insurance Group Number. The group number denoting the group policy or plan under which the insured is covered.

63A–C Treatment Authorization Code. A number indicating that the treatment described by this bill has been authorized by the payer.

64A–C Document Control Number. The control number assigned to the original bill by the health plan.

65A–C Employer Name. Name of the employer of the insured person.

Payer Information: Form Locators 66–81

66 Diagnosis Qualifier. Edition of the ICD that was used. Currently the accepted version is ICD-9.

67 Principal Diagnosis Code. ICD-9 code for the diagnosis of the patient's condition. The diagnosis shown should reflect the information contained in the patient's medical record for the dates indicated in item 6 even if the diagnosis is changed at a later date. One of the five present on admission (POA) indicators will be listed here. (Y, N, U or W or 1 or 0. You must use 1 or blank if the service is exempt from POA reporting (it is considered the 5th indicator). Each listed diagnosis must have a POA indicator attached. The definitions of the 5 indicators are as follows:

    Y = yes (Present at the time of inpatient admission)

    N = no (Not present at the time of inpatient admission)

    U = unknown (Documentation is insufficient to determine whether condition was present at the time of admission.)

    W = clinically undetermined (Provider is unable to clinically determine whether condition was POA.)

67A–67Q Other Diagnosis Codes. ICD-9, V, and E Codes for any additional diagnosis of the patient's condition. Not required by Medicare. Additional POA indicators will be listed here.

69 Admitting Diagnosis. The ICD-9 code provided at the time of admission.

70A–C Patient's Reason for Visit. Patient's reason for visit. Required for all unscheduled outpatient visits.

71 Prospective Payment System (PPS) Code.

72A–C External Cause of Injury Code (E Code). The ICD-9 code for an external cause of injury, poisoning, or adverse effect. Not required by Medicare. (More boxes are allowed for E codes.

74 Principal Procedure Codes and Date. CPT code for principal procedure rendered and the date that procedure was rendered. Required on inpatient claims when a procedure was performed and on outpatient surgeries. Medicare does not require for outpatient claims.

74A–E Other Procedure Codes and Dates. CPT code for additional procedures rendered and the dates of those procedures. Required on inpatient claims when additional procedures are performed. Not used on outpatient claims.

76 Attending Physician ID/NPI. Name and license number of the physician who is primarily responsible for the patient.

77 Operating Physician ID/NPI. Name and license number of secondary physician, assistant surgeon, and so on.

78–79 Other Provider ID/NPI Type Qualifier Codes.

80 Remarks. Pertinent data for which there is no other specific place on the form. Often this space is used to record the nature of an accident (e.g., fell and hit head on concrete, 06/09/XX). For Medicaid, required for abortion certification when the attending physician is an employee of the hospital and does not submit a separate bill. Also, multiple visits to the ER on the same day should be recorded.

81 Code List Qualifiers:

A1—Condition codes (FL 18–28)

A2—Occurrence codes (FL 31–34,)

A3—Occurrence span codes (FL35–36)

A4—Value codes (FL 35–36)

B3—Health care provider taxonomy codes (HPTC)

ACTIVITY #1

About the UB-04 Form

Directions: Answer the following questions without looking back at the material just covered. Write your answer in the space provided.

1. Where on the UB-04 should the patient control number be placed?

   _____

2. What information should field locator 11 include? _____

   _____

3. Where on the UB-04 should you place the service date? _____

   _____

4. What information should field locator 50 include? _____

   _____

5. Where should you record pertinent data for which there is no other specific place on the form?

   _____

Item 53: Assignment of Benefits

This assignment of benefits will not allow you to release information regarding the patient. A written authorization to release information, signed by the patient or patient representative, is needed (item 53). Please note the certification procedure on the back of the UB-04 before completing this item.

Although the UB-04 eliminates the need to send an assignment of benefits to accident and health insurers, hospitals may wish to be extremely careful in the way they handle claims involving property and casualty insurers. Property and casualty insurers may not be familiar with the UB-04 and may not be aware that the wording on the back of the UB-04 is sufficient notification of assignment of benefits. Hospitals may wish to send a copy of the assignment on auto accident and similar nonhealth-oriented insurance carrier claims.

Most of us have been in a hospital at least once in our lives. At the end of a hospital stay, a bill for services is usually received. Hospital billing can be confusing if you do not understand how the process works. However, with basic knowledge and training, competently billing for hospital services should be easily accomplished.

Two main forms are used for billing insurance carriers: the CMS-1500 and the UB-04. Both claim forms are used in a hospital setting.

UB-04 Billing

Services rendered by a hospital, hospital-employed personnel, or an ambulatory surgery center may be billed on the UB-04. This may include all room and board, medications, operating room charges, supplies used by the patient, and x-ray fees (for the equipment, supplies, and room, although not necessarily for the radiologist, etc.).

Many hospitals use bar-coded stickers to assist in billing. A **bar code** is a number that is assigned to a specific item. This number is often represented by a series of thin and fat vertical lines.

In the hospital setting, items will often have a peel-off bar code affixed to them when they are received by the hospital. The bar code is different for each item.

When a patient uses an item, the item is removed from the supply area. The bar code is then either scanned or peeled off and placed on a special billing page of the patient's chart. If the patient uses two items, two separate bar codes are peeled off and affixed to the patient chart. If the bar code is scanned at the time the supply is used, the peel-and-place step is eliminated.

When billing is performed, the item numbers from each bar code are entered into the computer. This often is done using a bar-code scanner like the ones seen in many retail and grocery stores. Each number that is entered generates a line item charge on the patient's bill.

Sometimes it can be difficult to determine which charges to put on which form. Some hospitals will even combine the charges and place them on a single form. For example, the hospital may generate one all-inclusive charge for an x-ray. This charge will include not only the equipment, supplies, and the room but also the services of the radiologist.

When bills with all-inclusive charges are submitted to the insurance carrier for payment, the insurance carrier may insist that the charges be itemized according to charges for the facility (equipment, supplies, and room) and charges for professional services (the provider).

Itemized Bills

Many hospitals provide their patients with an **itemized bill**. This type of bill lists each item, service, or supply on an individual line and shows the cost for that one item. Many patients prefer to receive an itemized bill so that they can understand exactly what they are being billed for. In addition, facilities in many states are required to provide an itemized bill to any patient who requests one.

Some hospitals will routinely include an itemized bill when billing patients. The markup (the difference between what the hospital pays for an item and what it charges the patient for that same item) can be very high. It is not uncommon for a hospital to charge a patient $10 for a single aspirin.

The increased charge helps to cover the cost of the nurse speaking with the doctor, getting approval for the drug, notating the patient's chart, going to the pharmacy or drug cabinet, placing the required dosage into a paper cup, and then dispensing it to the patient. Other charges may be included, such as shipping and handling, charges for labeling and inventorying the item, the time it takes for someone to put the information into the computer system, and also the amount of time needed to bill for the item.

Some insurance carriers also will request itemized billings. This allows them to be sure that there are no noncovered services or items included in the bill.

Personal Items

Personal items are those items that are primarily for the comfort of the patient and are not medically necessary. These items are and are not usually covered by an insurance plan. These charges may need to be coded separately, or they may be combined with other ancillary charges. However, patients should be warned at the time they request such items that they are not usually covered by an insurance carrier.

Most hospitals automatically issue an admission kit to incoming patients. An **admission kit** usually includes an emesis basin, carafe, cup, lotion, tissue, and mouthwash. Some plans administratively allow for one kit. Additional kits are usually not covered. This type of kit also may be called a hygiene kit, patient comfort kit, maternity kit, OB-GYN kit, or similar name.

PRACTICE **PITFALLS**

Some personal items are not considered medically necessary and are often excluded by the insurance carrier. These include

- Barber expenses
- Personal hygiene kit
- Videotaping of birth
- Birth certificate, photos
- Cot rental
- Room transfer requested
- Lotion

- Television
- Telephone
- Toothbrush, toothpaste
- Guest trays
- Mouthwash
- Gift shop expenses
- Slippers

Diagnosis Related Groups (DRGs)

In the early days of health insurance, providers were reimbursed for each procedure they performed. There was no incentive to limit the number of procedures.

DRGs were developed by the Centers for Medicare & Medicaid Services (CMS) as a means of controlling Medicare expenses. Private insurance companies adapted DRGs a few years later. The idea was to encourage hospitals to help limit some of the costs associated with certain illnesses.

DRGs are a group of clinically similar conditions with a similar pattern of resource intensity. DRGs are assigned by a **grouper**, a coding application that uses algorithms to assign DRGs, taking into consideration the patient's principal diagnosis, secondary diagnosis, primary procedures, gender, age, discharge disposition, and the presence or absence of a complication/comorbidity (CC) or major complication/comorbidity (MCC). When the medical coder enters this information into the software, the grouper assigns a DRG. Thus, two patients being treated for the same diagnosis can group to different DRGs due to the underlying cause of the principal diagnosis.

Under a DRG, the insurance carrier (including the Medicare insurance carrier) will pay a set amount for the total care for the treatment. Even if the hospital costs are above this amount, they will only receive this set amount. They cannot balance bill the patient for any amount that is not covered by the DRG set amount. However, if the hospital's charges are less than the set amount, they will still receive the set amount from the carrier and are allowed to keep the full amount.

It is important for the hospital to note those illnesses that are covered under DRGs. Although this notation should not drastically alter patient care, it may remind doctors not to order services or procedures that are questionable.

Ambulatory Patient Classifications

Ambulatory patient classifications (APCs) are similar to DRGs but are for patients who receive services on an outpatient basis. As with DRGs, a set amount is allowed for the procedure, all ancillary services, and any necessary follow-up care.

APCs are used as part of the Medicare **Outpatient Prospective Payment System (OPPS)**. This system pays hospitals under APCs rather than on a fee-for-service basis.

It is important for billers to realize that the services provided by a hospital may cover more than one APC, and multiple APCs may be included on a single claim. In addition, many of the services covered under Medicare Part B are grouped under APCs. These include radiation therapy, clinic visits, ER visits, diagnostic tests and services, surgical pathology, cancer chemotherapy, and so on.

When billing using APCs, it is important to remember that the single APC code covers all facility charges and services. However, the professional services of physicians are paid as a separate expense. These providers should continue to bill using a separate CMS-1500 form.

Excluded Services

Certain services are excluded from APC grouping. These services include ambulance, physical and occupational therapy, speech–language pathology, clinical diagnostic laboratory, durable medical equipment, and nonimplantable prosthetic and orthotic devices. These services will be reimbursed at the separate fee-for-service rate.

In addition, physicians and nonphysician practitioners continue to be reimbursed under the fee-for-service basis. Nonphysician practitioners include physician's assistants, nurse practitioners, certified nurse midwives, and psychologists.

APCs are used only for outpatient care. Thus, services that require the patient to be admitted to the hospital are not covered under the OPPS system.

Most hospitals are automatically included in the OPPS system. This includes rural hospitals with fewer than a hundred beds, certain cancer hospitals, and children's hospitals. However, these types of hospitals may be exempt from some reductions in their Medicare payments.

Chargemaster Descriptions

In previous years, patients were not expected to understand all the items included on their hospital bill. Many of the items were listed by code number, supply number, or by a medical term that was difficult for patients to understand.

Legislation mandates that the information contained on a hospital billing be written in everyday language. This allows patients to double-check their bill and to reconcile the statement they receive from the hospital with the Explanation of Benefits received from their insurance carrier. Consequently, hospital billing departments are now required to include descriptions on their line-item bills that are written in easily understood language. All patients must be charged uniformly for the same service delivered in the same setting.

To comply with this new regulation, each provider is required to have a **chargemaster description list (CDL)**. The chargemaster is a list that includes all hospital procedures, services, supplies, and drugs that are billed on the UB-04. A complete service listing includes each of the following components:

Department Name. The name of the department in which the charge originated. Each department should have an abbreviated code that designates the department where the code originates from. For example, the Cardiac Intensive Care Unit might be designated CICU.

Department Number. Each department should be assigned its own number. This allows for quick verification of the department where the charges originated.

Charge Description Number. Each charge should be given its own individual reference number. This is a unique number assigned by the provider. Charges that originate in a single department often receive similar numbers.

Revenue Code. This is the code that normally appears on the UB-04.

Description. A description of the charge or service. This description should be specific enough to allow the patient to understand the charge for the service or item received.

CPT Code. If the service has an appropriate CPT code associated with it, that code should be listed in this field.

HCPCS Code. If the service or item has an appropriate HCPCS code associated with it, that code should be listed in this field.

Charge. The charge for the service. This should be the normal fee that the provider charges for this service.

Descriptions, codes, and other parts of the CDL should be checked on a regular basis to ensure that they are still accurate and complete. In addition, the medical biller should become aware of any charges for which the insurance-allowed amount is greater than the billed amount. This may indicate a need to perform a periodic review of the clinic's charges in order to receive optimal reimbursement from insurance carriers on future charges. This information will be included on an Explanation of Benefits (EOB), which is provided by the insurance carrier on reimbursement of the claim. It is often attached to the check and indicates how the insurance carrier determined the appropriate payment amount.

Providers also need to create an itemized billing form that lists these items. This will allow the patient to see exactly what they are being charged for and what the cost is.

As a medical biller, you may be responsible for choosing the right charge description for billing the patient and for creating itemized patient statements for those patients that request them. You may even be responsible for entering new charge descriptions into the master list.

It is important to watch the CDL as you are using it so that you can spot any errors or items that might seem to be overbilled or underbilled. These errors should be brought to your supervisor's attention immediately.

Entering Charges

There are many people who deal with a patient in a hospital setting. Each of these people may be providing goods or services that need to be billed to the patient. For example, a patient may request pain medication from a nurse. The nurse will contact the doctor with the request. The doctor will prescribe the drugs, and often will be the one to make a note on the patient's chart. The health unit coordinator may be responsible for ordering the dosage of medication from the pharmacy. However, a nurse may be responsible for actually handing the drug to the patient.

In these cases, there must be a specific policy for the recording of information in the patient's chart. If you are responsible for hospital or facility billing, it is important to understand and follow the guidelines for billing patients. Without such a policy, there is a chance that many of the drugs or other items dispensed will not be charged to the patient.

There are several common methods for ensuring that patients are billed for the services and supplies they use:

Bar coding. Some hospitals place bar codes on every item that they receive into inventory (if the item does not already have a bar code attached). This bar code contains a unique number, and each type of item will receive a different bar code number. A computer billing and inventory system is set up that contains the information to correspond with that bar code number. For example, one number will be used to designate an admit kit and the common charge of $25 for that kit.

When a patient requests or is prescribed an item, the bar code for that item will be scanned into his or her account. The charge will then appear on the account record in the same way that scanning a bar code rings up charges in a supermarket.

Some items are too small to receive a bar code (e.g., individual capsules or pills). In these cases, the bar code is placed on the outside of the bottle or on a set of labels nearby. When medicine is dispensed, the appropriate bar code is scanned and the information is entered into the patient's account.

Some hospitals choose to use peel-off bar codes. When an item is dispensed, the bar code will be peeled off the item and placed on the patient's chart. Then, at a later date, all of the items in the patient chart will be scanned in at the same time. After this is done, the page will be replaced with a new blank page. This prevents scanning an item twice and potentially double-billing the patient. In some hospitals, the job of scanning items will fall to the health unit coordinator or a nurse. In other hospitals, it may be the job of the billing department.

Coding from charts. Some hospitals have billers create claims from the information contained in the patient chart. This information can be in the form of triage reports, operative reports, patient history reports, and the day-to-day treatment reports for the patient. It is the responsibility of the hospital biller to obtain the information from the chart regarding the goods and services that were provided.

Combined bar code and chart method. Some hospitals will have some items handled by bar code; other items will need to be obtained from the patient chart. For example, the goods delivered to the patient may be covered by the bar coding method, but other items such as room and board charges will need to be entered by the biller.

Other methods. Although these situations cover many facilities, other facilities may have their own methods for keeping track of goods and services used by the patient. Therefore, it is important to verify the proper billing procedures with your supervisor before billing hospital claims.

Regardless of the type of billing method used, it is the job of the biller to bill claims in a timely manner. This usually means billing patients as soon as their hospital stay is completed. If a patient is receiving extended care, interim billings may need to be created.

Interim Billings

An **interim billing** is a periodic billing for services before the patient is discharged from the hospital. When creating interim billings, it is important to include all charges through a specified date of service on a single claim form. Subsequent claim forms should cover dates after the closing date of the earlier interim bill. It is important to include all charges in order to reduce the possibility of confusion for an insurance carrier. If the carrier receives more than one bill with the same date of service, some or all of the charges may be denied as duplicate. For example, if a patient received the same medication at two different times during the day, but each medication is billed on a separate claim, the insurance carrier may determine that the second medication charge is merely a duplicate billing of the first one.

How Billing Affects Other Departments

It is important for billers to realize that the information that they enter for patient charges will affect many other hospital departments as well. Each year, hospitals will determine their budgets based on the services and billing of the year before. If billing has been done improperly, a department might have a lower budget than it needs to maintain proficiency.

In addition, staffing is often allocated based on the amount of services provided and revenues generated by a specific department. Incorrect billing might cause a specific department to be over- or understaffed for the upcoming year.

Supplies also are ordered based on billing charts. Many computer programs have inventory programs tied to them. These programs will indicate when a certain supply is low and may need to be reordered. If items are billed incorrectly, it is possible that the facility may run out of an item needed for patient care. This can lead to extra charges incurred from having to rush-order the items or even lead to a lower level of patient care.

Because of these factors, it is vitally important that billers pay close attention to the details of the items being billed. Be sure you are choosing the correct code for the service or item provided.

Preauthorizations, Precertifications, and Utilization Reviews

One of the most common jobs of the biller is to handle the preauthorization and precertification of services. Many insurance carriers require the hospital to precertify services before or within a certain period of receiving the services. Without the proper precertification or preauthorization, the insurance carrier may reduce benefits on a claim or refuse to pay for the services altogether.

For more information on completing precertification and preauthorization, see Chapter 7 on managed care. However, you should be aware that managed care insurers are not the only plans that may require preauthorization, precertification, or utilization review.

Ambulatory Surgical Centers

Ambulatory surgical centers (surgicenters) are centers equipped to allow for the performance of surgery on an outpatient basis. These centers may be freestanding or affiliated with a major acute care facility. Surgicenters provide financial savings by eliminating the need for admission into an inpatient facility. An ambulatory surgical facility is a specialized facility that meets all eight of the professionally recognized standards:

1. Provides a setting for outpatient surgeries
2. Does not provide services or accommodations for overnight stays
3. Has at least two operating rooms and one recovery room; all the medical equipment needed to support the surgery being performed; x-ray and laboratory diagnostic facilities; and emergency equipment, trays, and supplies for use in life-threatening events
4. Has a medical staff that is supervised full time by a physician and a registered nurse when patients are in the facility
5. Maintains a medical record for each patient

6. Has a written agreement with a local acute care facility for the immediate transfer of patients who require greater care than can be provided on an outpatient basis
7. Complies with all state and federal licensing and other legal requirements
8. Is not an office or clinic for any physician

Usually plans provide benefits on a global basis, covering the facility room usage charge and supplies (e.g., anesthesia gases, medications, trays) on the same basis as inpatient hospital services.

CHAPTER REVIEW

Summary

- The UB-04 is the claim form used when billing for hospital services. It was created by the National Uniform Billing Committee to allow for the necessary information to be inserted on a single form, thus eliminating the need for attachments.
- You should familiarize yourself with the form and know the necessary information. Completely and accurately filling out the UB-04 will help to ensure proper claim payments without unnecessary delays.
- Billing in a hospital setting is different in several ways from billing in a medical office. Although medical offices often bill using only a CMS-1500, hospitals may use a CMS-1500 for professional services and a UB-04 for facility charges. In addition, an itemized bill may be used to provide patients with a list of all goods and services received.
- Hospitals often will charge for each individual item received by a patient. Billing is done using a bar code method, using information from a patient chart, a combination of these two methods, or by some other method. Regardless of the method used, it is important for the biller to ensure that all items used and all services received by the patient are billed.
- In an effort to manage costs, Medicare and other insurance carriers are implementing payment by DRGs and APCs. Payments made under DRG or APC provisions reimburse the hospital a set amount for the total cost of treatment for a specified condition rather than paying for each individual item or service.

Review Questions

Directions: Answer the following questions without looking back at the material just covered. Write your answers in the space provided.

1. For what is the UB-04 billing form used? _____

   _____

2. What does item 17 indicate? _____

   _____

3. What are occurrence codes and occurrence span codes, and what is the difference between them? _____

   _____

   _____

4. What would the code 1 indicate in Item 17 on the UB-04? _____

   _____

5. What would the code 32 indicate in Item 59 on the UB-04? _____

   _____

6. What do Revenue Codes reference? _____

   _____

7. On the UB-04 what code would be used to indicate each of the following times?

    1. 9:55 a.m. _____   6. 2:48 p.m. _____

    2. 10:25 p.m. _____   7. 5:56 p.m. _____

    3. 1:18 a.m. _____   8. Noon _____

    4. 8:01 p.m. _____   9. Midnight _____

    5. 12:23 a.m. _____   10. 6:06 p.m. _____

8. What does a Y in the Release Information item denote? _____
_____

9. A patient entered the hospital on 12/01/CCYY with chest pains. He was diagnosed as having a heart attack and admitted. On 12/05/CCYY the patient developed pneumonia. On 12/10/CCYY the patient expired because of causes associated with pneumonia. On 12/12/CCYY you bill the insurance company for services rendered through 12/04/CCYY. What is the proper diagnosis for the patient? _____

10. Admission code 1 indicates what type of admission? _____

11. What types of services are not covered under the OPPS system? _____
_____
_____

12. What is a DRG, and how does it work? _____
_____
_____

13. What is the most common claim form used to bill for hospital services? _____
_____

14. What is an APC, and to what type of facility does it apply? _____
_____
_____

If you are unable to answer any of these questions, refer back to that section in the chapter, and then fill in the answers.

Activity #2: Completing a UB-04 Form

Directions: Complete a UB-04 form for each of the following scenarios. In all cases, the hospital is Provider Medical Center. Refer to the Patient Data Table and Provider Data Table in Appendix A for information.

Upon completion of the UB-04, use an insurance claims register (located in Appendix A) and list all claims that have been fully prepared and are ready for submission to the insurance carrier for payment. Enter the date that you created the UB-04 in the Date Claim Filed column.

1. Abby Addison was brought into the ER on 3/7/CCYY after losing consciousness at home. Her condition has progressed from influenza to pneumonia. Annette Adams, M.D., was the attending physician. Dr. Adams's UPIN number is A00720.

    Additional information is as follows:

Patient Control #:	PMC97917
Medical Record #:	BA4907
Admit Time:	9:00 a.m.
Discharge Time:	4:20 p.m.
Discharged To:	Home

The following hospital charges were incurred:

Item	# Days or Units	Cost	Total Charge
Room and Board	3	$395.00	$1185.00
Pharmacy	23		845.00
IV Therapy	21		386.15
Med-Surg Supplies	18		224.25
Laboratory	36		727.00
Respiratory Services	3		269.35
EKG/ECG	1		161.53
SUBTOTAL			**$3,798.28**
PAYMENTS/ADJUSTMENTS			**$ 0.00**
BALANCE DUE			**$3,798.28**

2. Bobby Brumble entered the hospital on 3/30/CCYY with a ruptured appendix. Brett Barron, M.D., was the attending physician. Dr. Barron's UPIN number is B47041.

Additional information is as follows:

Patient Control #:	PMC71721
Medical Record #:	OB4263
Admit Time:	10:30 a.m.
Discharge Time:	3:45 p.m.
Discharged To:	Home
Procedure Performed:	Appendectomy
Date Procedure Performed:	3/30/CCYY

The following hospital charges were incurred:

Item	# Days or Units	Cost	Total Charge
Room and Board	4	$395.00	$1,580.00
Pharmacy	42		1,567.50
Laboratory	23		983.30
IV Therapy	14		561.50
Med-Surg Supplies	39		1,937.25
Pathology Lab	10		110.50
Dx X-Ray	12		898.90
OR Services	8		977.50
Anesthesia	1		882.25
Respiratory Services	2		74.75
Recovery Room	1		241.45
SUBTOTAL			**$9,814.90**
PAYMENTS/ADJUSTMENTS			**$ 500.00**
BALANCE DUE			**$9,314.90**

3. Cathy Crenshaw entered the hospital emergency room on 4/1/CCYY for treatment of a fractured arm. Cathy fractured her arm when she fell from a stool at home. Carol Carpenter, M.D., was the attending physician. Dr. Carpenter's UPIN number is C12761.

Additional information is as follows:

Patient Control #:   PMC69623

Medical Record #:   AC1616

Procedure Performed: Closed treatment of ulnar shaft fracture without manipulation

Date Procedure Performed: 4/1/CCYY

The following hospital charges were incurred:

Item	# Days or Units	Cost	Total Charge
ER	1		$250.00
Pharmacy	2		75.25
X-Ray	4		147.50
SUBTOTAL			**$472.75**
PAYMENTS/ADJUSTMENTS			**$ 0.00**
BALANCE DUE			**$472.75**

4. Daisy Doolittle entered the hospital for treatment of acute pelvic inflammatory disease on 4/1/CCYY. Deborah Davidson, M.D., was attending physician. Dr. Davidson's UPIN number is D70007.

Additional information is as follows:

Patient Control #:   PMC47898

Medical Record #:   AD7431

Admit Time: 12:15 p.m.

Discharge Time: 9:30 a.m.

Discharged To: Home

The following hospital charges were incurred:

Item	# Days or Units	Cost	Total Charge
Room and Board	3	$395.00	$1,185.00
Pharmacy	31		321.50
Laboratory	9		314.25
Med-Surg Supplies	19		783.15
Path Lab	11		652.70
IV Therapy	4		89.60
Ultrasound	2		685.20
SUBTOTAL			**$4,031.40**
PAYMENTS/ADJUSTMENTS			**$ 0.00**
BALANCE DUE			**$4,031.40**

5. Edward Edmunds entered the hospital for surgery on his shoulder on 3/10/CCYY. Edward had tendonitis with calcium deposits on his shoulder that restricted movement. Dr. Paul Provider was the attending physician.

Additional information is as follows:

Patient Control #:   PMC56962

Medical Record #:   DE9804

Admit Time: 6:40 a.m.

Discharge Time: 10:20 a.m.

Discharged To: Home

Procedure Performed: Removal of subdeltoid calcareous deposits, open

Date Procedure Performed: 3/10/CCYY

The following hospital charges were incurred:

Item	# Days or Units	Cost	Total Charge
Room and Board	2	$395.00	$790.00
Pharmacy	12		567.50
Laboratory	6		483.30
IV Therapy	3		361.50
Med-Surg Supplies	37		937.25
Pathology Lab	7		95.50
Dx X-Ray	6		298.40
OR Services	1		048.50
Anesthesia	1		875.25
Respiratory Services	4		74.75
Recovery Room	1		236.45
SUBTOTAL			**$5,648.40**
PAYMENTS/ADJUSTMENTS			**$ 0.00**
BALANCE DUE			**$5,648.40**

Activity #3: Defining Terms

Directions: Match the following terms with the proper definition by writing the letter of the correct definition in the space next to the term.

1. _____ Uniform Bill-1904

2. _____ Value code

3. _____ Occurrence span code

4. _____ Revenue code

5. _____ Occurrence code

6. _____ Condition code

a. A two-digit code used to identify conditions relating to this bill that may affect payer processing

b. A code that identifies a specific accommodation, ancillary service, or billing calculation

c. A code and associated date defining a significant event relating to this bill that may affect payer processing

d. A form used by hospitals or other hospital-type facilities for inpatient and outpatient billing

e. Code and related dates that identify an event that happened over a span of time relating to the payment of the claim

f. A code and the related dollar amount that identifies data of a monetary nature that is necessary for processing the claim

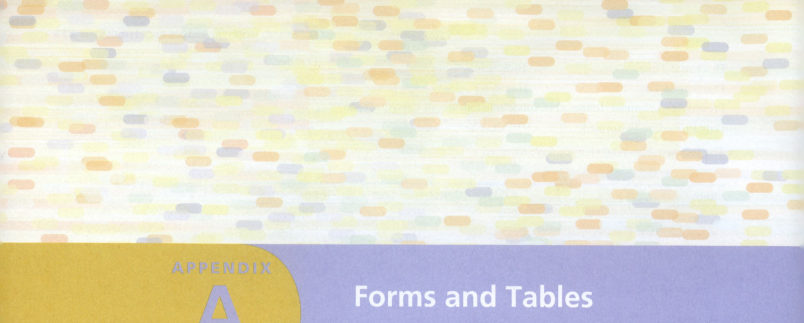

Forms and Tables

Table of Contents

Forms and Information

Tables

BALL INSURANCE CARRIERS

3895 Bubble Blvd. Ste. 283, Boxwood, CO 85931 (970) 555-5432

INSURANCE CONTACT: Betty Bell **PHONE NUMBER:** (970) 555-9876

Policy: Blue Corporation, 9817 Bobcat Blvd., Bastion, CO 81319

Insurance Group # and Suffix: 98135/BLUE

BASIC/MAJOR MEDICAL PLAN **Effective 09/1/93**

ELIGIBILITY—EMPLOYEE: Must work a minimum of 30 hours per week. Is eligible for coverage the first of the month following three consecutive months of continuous employment.

DEPENDENTS: Coverage is available to enrollees' adult children under age 26, even if the adult children no longer live with their parents, are not dependents on their parent's tax return, or are no longer students.

EFFECTIVE DATE—EMPLOYEE: If written application is made prior to eligibility date, coverage becomes effective the first of the month following three months of continuous employment.

DEPENDENTS: The date acquired by the covered employee becomes the effective date if written application is made within 31 days of eligibility date. If confined in a hospital on date of eligibility, coverage will not start until the first of the month following the date the confinement ends. Newborns are automatically covered for the first 30 days following birth. Coverage will be terminated after 30 days unless written application for coverage is submitted by the employee within 31 days of birth.

TERMINATION OF COVERAGE—EMPLOYEE: Coverage terminates the last day of the month following termination of employment, or when the employee ceases to qualify as an eligible employee, or following request for termination of coverage.

DEPENDENTS: Coverage terminates the date the employee's coverage terminates or the last day of the month during which the dependent no longer qualifies as an eligible dependent.

BASIC BENEFITS

PREADMISSION TESTING—Outpatient diagnostic tests performed prior to inpatient admissions; paid at 100% of UCR.

SUPPLEMENTAL ACCIDENT EXPENSE—100% of the first $300 for services incurred within 90 days of accident.

INPATIENT HOSPITAL EXPENSE
DEDUCTIBLE: $50.
ROOM AND BOARD: 100% Up to semi-private room charge. ICU up to $600 per day.
MISCELLANEOUS FEES: 100% Unlimited.
MAXIMUM PERIOD: Ten days per period of disability.

SURGERY
CONVERSION FACTOR: $8.50.
CALENDAR YEAR MAXIMUM: $1,600 per person.
REMARKS: Voluntary sterilizations covered.

ASSISTANT SURGERY
CONVERSION FACTOR: $8.50.
CALENDAR YEAR MAXIMUM ALLOWANCE: $320 per person. Maximum of 20% of surgeon's allowance or billed charge, whichever is less.
REMARKS: Voluntary sterilizations covered for women only.

IN-HOSPITAL PHYSICIANS
DAILY MAXIMUM: $21 for the first day; $8 per day thereafter.
MAXIMUM PERIOD: Ten days per period of disability.
REMARKS: Only one doctor can be paid per day.

(Continued)

ANESTHESIA
CONVERSION FACTOR: $7.50.
CALENDAR YEAR MAXIMUM: $300 per person.
REMARKS: Voluntary sterilizations covered.

OUTPATIENT PHYSICIANS VISITS
CONVERSION FACTOR: $7.50.
CALENDAR YEAR MAXIMUM: $300 per person.
REMARKS: Chiropractors, M.D.s, D.O.s, and acupuncturists allowed.

X-RAY AND LABORATORY
CONVERSION FACTOR: $7.
CALENDAR YEAR MAXIMUM: $200 per person.
REMARKS: Professional component charges covered at 40% of UCR allowance for procedure. Routine procedures are not covered.

MAJOR MEDICAL EXPENSES

INDIVIDUAL CALENDAR YEAR DEDUCTIBLE—$125; three-month carryover provision.

FAMILY MAXIMUM DEDUCTIBLE—Two family members must satisfy their individual calendar year deductible in order to satisfy the family deductible.

STANDARD COINSURANCE—80%.

COINSURANCE LIMIT: $400 out-of-pocket per individual; $800 out-of-pocket per family (not to include deductible); aggregate.

APPLICATION OF COINSURANCE LIMIT—Coinsurance limit applies in the calendar year in which the limit is met and the following calendar year.

OUTPATIENT MENTAL/NERVOUS EXPENSE—50% coinsurance while not a hospital inpatient.

LIFETIME MAXIMUM—$1,000,000 per person.

ROOM LIMIT—Semi-private room rate.

HOSPITAL DEDUCTIBLE—Not covered.

HOME HEALTH CARE—120 visits per calendar year. Prior hospital confinement required.

PRE-EXISTING LIMITATION—If treatment received within six months prior to effective date, $2,000 maximum payment until patient has been covered continuously under the plan for 12 months.

ANESTHESIA—Calculated using actual time.

MEDICARE
TYPE: Coordination of Benefits.
REMARKS: Assume all Medicare benefits whether or not individual actually enrolled. Subject to all other plan provisions.

EXCLUSIONS

1. Expenses resulting from self-inflicted injuries.
2. Work-related injuries or illnesses.
3. Services for which there is no charge in the absence of insurance.
4. Charges or services in excess of UCR or not medically necessary.
5. Charges for completion of claim forms and failure to keep appointments.
6. Routine or preventative or experimental services.
7. Eye refractions; contacts or glasses; orthotics (eye exercises); radial keratotomy or other procedures for surgical correction of refractive errors.
8. Custodial care.
9. Cosmetic surgery unless for repair of an injury or surgery incurred while covered or result of mastectomy.

(Continued)

10. Dental care of teeth, gums, or alveolar process (TMJ) except: a) reduction of fractures of the jaw or facial bones; b) surgical correction of harelip, cleft palate, or prognathism; c) removal of salivary duct stones; d) removal of bony cysts of jaw, torus palatinus, leukoplakia, or malignant tissues.

11. Reversal of voluntary sterilization.

12. Diagnosis or treatment of infertility, including artificial insemination, in vitro fertilization, etc.

13. Contraceptive materials or devices.

14. Non-therapeutic abortions except where the life of the mother is endangered.

15. Expenses for obesity, weight reduction, or diet control unless at least 100 lbs. overweight.

16. Vitamins, food supplements, and/or protein supplements.

17. Sex-altering treatments or surgeries, or related studies.

18. Orthopedic shoes or other devices for support or treatment of feet except as medically necessary following foot surgery.

19. Biofeedback-related services or treatment.

20. Experimental transplants.

21. EDTA chelation therapy.

COMPREHENSIVE DENTAL BENEFITS

DEDUCTIBLE—$50.

FAMILY DEDUCTIBLE LIMIT—$150; non-aggregate. COINSURANCE: 80%.

MAXIMUM—No lifetime maximum. $1,000-per-calendar-year maximum.

SPACE MAINTAINER ELIGIBILITY—Employees and dependents.

FLUORIDE ELIGIBILITY—Dependents up to age 18 only.

ORTHODONTIA—No coverage.

CLAIM COST CONTROL—Predetermination of benefits and alternate course of treatment based on customarily employed methods.

PROSTHETIC REPLACEMENTS—Five-year replacement rule applies to replacements of any previously installed prosthetics.

ORDERED AND UNDELIVERED—Excludes expenses for any devices installed or delivered after 30 days following termination of insurance.

ORAL SURGERY—Covered at regular coinsurance rate, subject to calendar year maximum.

EXTENSION OF BENEFITS—12 months.

MISSING AND UNREPLACED—Applies.

ROVER INSURERS INC.

5931 ROLLING ROAD, RONSON, CO 81369   (970) 555-1369

INSURANCE CONTACT: Ravyn Ranger   **PHONE NUMBER:** (970) 555-0863

POLICY: RED CORPORATION, 1234 Nockout Road, Newton, NM 88012   **Effective** 01/01/01

INSURANCE GROUP # AND SUFFIX: 41935/RED

ELIGIBILITY—EMPLOYEES must work a minimum of 30 hours per week. They are eligible for coverage the first of the month following one consecutive month of continuous employment.
DEPENDENTS: Coverage is available to enrollees' adult children under age 26, even if the adult children no longer live with their parents, are not dependents on their parent's tax return, or are no longer students.

EFFECTIVE DATE—EMPLOYEE becomes effective, if written application is made prior to eligibility date, on the first of the month following 30 days of continuous employment. If employee is absent from work due to disability on the date of eligibility, coverage will not start until the first of the month following the date of return to active work.
DEPENDENTS become effective on the date the covered employee becomes effective, if written application is made within 31 days of eligibility date. If confined in a hospital on the date of eligibility, coverage will not start until the first of the month following the date the confinement ends. Newborns are automatically covered for the first 14 days following birth. Coverage terminates after 14 days unless written application for coverage is submitted by the employee within 31 days of birth.

TERMINATION OF COVERAGE—EMPLOYEE'S coverage terminates the last day of the month following termination of employment or when the employee ceases to qualify as an eligible employee, or following request for termination of coverage.
DEPENDENTS' coverage terminates the date the employee's coverage terminates, or the last day of the month during which the dependent no longer qualifies as an eligible dependent.

EXTENSION OF BENEFITS—If covered under the plan when disabled, may continue coverage in accordance with COBRA. No other extension available.

COMPREHENSIVE MEDICAL BENEFITS

PREADMISSION TESTING—Outpatient diagnostic tests performed prior to inpatient admissions are paid at 100% whether through a network provider or not.

PRECERTIFICATION—Voluntary, non-emergency inpatient admissions must be approved at least five days prior to admission. Emergency admissions must be precertified within 48 hrs. of admission. Benefits are reduced to 50% if not performed as required.

SECOND SURGICAL OPINION—The SSO is paid at 100% of UCR. It is required for the following: bunionectomy, cataract extraction, chemonucleolysis, cholecystectomy, coronary bypass, hemorrhoidectomy, hysterectomy, inguinal herniorrhaphy, laparotomy, laminectomy, mastectomy, meniscectomy, oophorectomy, prostatectomy, salpingectomy, submucous resection, total joint replacement (hip or knee), tenotomy, varicose veins (all procedures). **IF SSO NOT PERFORMED, ALL RELATED EXPENSES PAYABLE AT 50%.**

SUPPLEMENTAL ACCIDENT EXPENSE—100% is paid on the first $500 for services incurred within 90 days of the date of accident. Subject to $20 copayment. After $500, payments are subject to calendar year deductible. Provider does not have to be a network member to receive 100% benefit. Common accident provision applies.

OUTPATIENT FACILITY CHARGES PAYABLE AT 100%—Network outpatient facility expenses for following procedures paid 100%. Does not include professional charges: arthroscopy, breast biopsy, cataract removal, bronchoscopy, deviated nasal septum, pilonidal cyst, myringotomy w/tubes, esophagoscopy, colonoscopy, herniorrhaphy (umbilical, to five years old), skin and subsequent lesions, benign and malignant (2cms+).

INDIVIDUAL CALENDAR YEAR DEDUCTIBLE—$150; three-month carryover provision. All plan services subject to deductible unless otherwise indicated.

FAMILY MAXIMUM DEDUCTIBLE—$300, non-aggregate. Two family members must meet individual deductible limit.

(Continued)

STANDARD COINSURANCE—80% for network providers; 60% for non-network providers.

COINSURANCE LIMIT—$1,250 out-of-pocket per individual; $2,500 out-of-pocket per family. Two individuals must meet their individual out-of-pocket limit to satisfy the family limit. Limits not to include deductible, surgery expenses reduced because SSO not performed, or hospital benefits reduced because precertification not performed. 100% of allowed amount paid thereafter for network providers; 80% for non-network providers.

LIFETIME MAXIMUM—$1,000,000 per person.

PRE-EXISTING LIMITATION—If treatment is received within 90 days prior to effective date, no coverage on that condition for six months from the effective date (continuously covered for six consecutive months) unless treatment-free for three consecutive months which ends after the effective date of coverage.

INPATIENT HOSPITAL EXPENSE IF NO PRECERTIFICATION, ADMISSION PAID AT 50%

DEDUCTIBLE—$200, waived for network facilities, applies to non-network. Inpatient hospital expenses not subject to regular Major Medical deductible.

ROOM AND BOARD—Network providers: 80% of semi-private/ICU; non-network providers: 60% of semi-private/ICU.

MISCELLANEOUS FEES—Network: 80%; non-network: 60%.

EXCLUSIONS—Well baby care. Automatic coverage for first seven days if baby is ill. Otherwise, no coverage.

MENTAL/NERVOUS/PSYCHONEUROTIC—Includes substance abuse and alcoholism.

OUTPATIENT MENTAL AND NERVOUS TREATMENT
PAYABLE: $60 per visit for first 5 visits; $30 per visit for next 21 visits.
COINSURANCE: 80% for first 5 visits (maximum payable: $60 per visit), 50% per visit for next 21 visits (maximum payable: $30 per visit).
CALENDAR YEAR MAXIMUM: 26 visits.

INPATIENT MENTAL AND NERVOUS TREATMENT
PHYSICIAN SERVICES: 70% applies to network and non-network providers.
HOSPITAL SERVICES: 70% network and non-network providers.

MAMMOGRAMS
COINSURANCE: 80% network providers; 60% non-network providers.
REQUIREMENTS: Baseline mammogram for women age 35–39; for ages 40–49, one allowed every two years; for ages 50+, one allowed every year.

X-RAY AND LABORATORY—PROFESSIONAL COMPONENTS: Professional charges paid at 25% of UCR.

DURABLE MEDICAL EQUIPMENT
COINSURANCE: 50%.
REQUIREMENTS: Prescribed by M.D.; must not be primarily necessary for exercise, environmental control, convenience, comfort, or hygiene. Must be an article useful only for the prescribed patient. Covered up to purchase price only.
ANESTHESIA: Use actual time.

MEDICARE
TYPE: Maintenance of benefits.
REMARKS: Assume all Medicare benefits whether or not individual actually enrolled. Subject to all other plan provisions.

EXCLUSIONS

1. Expenses resulting from self-inflicted injuries.
2. Work-related injuries or illnesses.
3. Services for which there is no charge in the absence of insurance.
4. Charges or services in excess of UCR or not medically necessary.
5. Pre-existing conditions.
6. Charges for completion of claim forms and failure to keep appointments.
7. Routine or preventative or experimental services.

(Continued)

8. Eye refractions; contacts or glasses; orthotics (eye exercises); radial keratotomy or other procedures for surgical correction of refractive errors.

9. Custodial care.

10. Cosmetic surgery unless for repair of an injury or surgery incurred while covered or result of mastectomy.

11. Biofeedback-related services or treatment.

12. Dental care of teeth, gums, or alveolar process (TMJ) except: a) reduction of fractures of the jaw or facial bones; b) surgical correction of harelip, cleft palate, or prognathism; c) removal of salivary duct stones; d) removal of bony cysts of jaw, torus palatinus, leukoplakia, or malignant tissues.

13. Reversal of voluntary sterilization.

14. Diagnosis or treatment of infertility, including artificial insemination, in vitro fertilization, etc.

15. Contraceptive materials or devices.

16. Pregnancy; pregnancy-related expenses of dependent children for the delivery, including Caesarian section. Related illnesses may be covered such as pre-eclampsia, vaginal bleeding, etc.

17. Non-therapeutic abortions except where the life of the mother is endangered.

18. Vitamins.

CREATIVE CREATIONS CORP.

1234 Creature Lane, Crevice, CT 06192, (919) 555-5631   EFFECTIVE DATE: 06/01/02

INSURANCE CONTACT: Wilma Williams   **PHONE NUMBER:** (970) 555-1234

INSURANCE GROUP # and SUFFIX: 54321/CRC

ELIGIBILITY—EMPLOYEE: Must work a minimum of 35 hours per week. Is eligible for coverage the first of the month following 60 consecutive days of continuous employment.
DEPENDENTS: Coverage is available to enrollees' adult children under age 26, even if the adult children no longer live with their parents, are not dependents on their parent's tax return, or are no longer students.

EFFECTIVE DATE—EMPLOYEE: If written application is made prior to the eligibility date, coverage becomes effective the first of the month following 60 days of employment.
DEPENDENTS: The date acquired by the covered employee becomes the effective date if written application is made within 31 days of the eligibility date. Newborns are automatically covered for the first seven days following birth; well baby charges excluded. Coverage will terminate after seven days unless written application for coverage is submitted by the employee within 31 days of birth.

TERMINATION OF COVERAGE—EMPLOYEE: Coverage terminates the last day of the month following termination of employment or when the employee ceases to qualify as an eligible employee, or following request for termination of coverage.
DEPENDENTS: Coverage terminates the date the employee's coverage terminates, or the last day of the month during which the dependent no longer qualifies as an eligible dependent.

EXTENSION OF BENEFITS—If covered under the plan when disabled, employee may continue coverage for 12 months following the date of termination or until no longer disabled, whichever is less.

COMPREHENSIVE MEDICAL BENEFITS

SUPPLEMENTAL ACCIDENT EXPENSE—100% of first $300 for services incurred within 120 days of date of accident. Not subject to deductible.

PLAN BENEFITS
INDIVIDUAL CALENDAR YEAR DEDUCTIBLE: $100; three-month carryover provision.
FAMILY MAXIMUM DEDUCTIBLE: $200, aggregate.
STANDARD COINSURANCE: 90% except 100% of hospital room and board expenses for 365 days per lifetime.
COINSURANCE LIMIT: $750 out-of-pocket per individual; $1,500 out-of-pocket per family. Two separate members must satisfy the individual limit, not to include deductible. Applies only in the calendar year in which the limit is met.
LIFETIME MAXIMUM: $300,000 per person.
PRE-EXISTING LIMITATION: On 6/1/99 no restriction. After 6/1/99, if treatment received within 90 days prior to effective date, no coverage for that condition for 12 months from the effective date (continuously covered for 12 months) unless treatment-free for three consecutive months ending after the effective date of coverage.

X-RAY AND LABORATORY—REMARKS: Professional component charges covered at 40% of UCR allowance for procedure. Routine procedures are not covered.

INPATIENT HOSPITAL EXPENSE—Room and board payable at 100% of semi-private room rate. Miscellaneous expenses covered at 90%. Non-medically necessary, well baby care, and cosmetic services excluded. Personal comfort items not covered.

MENTAL/NERVOUS/PSYCHONEUROTIC—INCLUDES SUBSTANCE ABUSE AND ALCOHOLISM.

OUTPATIENT MENTAL/NERVOUS TREATMENT
COINSURANCE: 50% while not hospital-confined.
CALENDAR YEAR MAXIMUM: None.

(Continued)

INPATIENT MENTAL/NERVOUS TREATMENT

PHYSICIAN SERVICES: Covered at 90%.

HOSPITAL SERVICES: Covered at 90%.

ALLOWED PROVIDERS: Psychiatrists and clinical psychologists. Marriage and Family Child Counselor and Licensed Clinical Social Worker allowed with referral from M.D.

EXTENDED CARE FACILITY

LIFETIME MAXIMUM: 60 days.

HOSPITAL SERVICES: 80% of billed room and board charge.

REQUIREMENTS: Stay must begin within 14 days of acute hospital stay of at least three days. Extended care must be due to same disability that caused hospitalization and continued hospital care would otherwise be required.

DURABLE MEDICAL EQUIPMENT

COINSURANCE: Covered at 90%.

REQUIREMENTS: Must be prescribed by M.D. Must not be primarily necessary for exercise, environmental control, convenience, comfort, or hygiene. Must be useful only for the prescribed patient. Covered up to purchase price only.

ANESTHESIA—Computed using block time.

REMARKS—Covered expenses include charges for the initial set of contact lenses necessary due to cataract surgery. Handicapped children are limited to a $15,000 lifetime maximum after attainment of age 19. Coordination of Benefits according to National Association of Insurance Carriers (NAIC) guidelines. Subject to Third Party Liability and subrogation.

MEDICARE INTEGRATION TYPE—Nonduplication of benefits applies.

REMARKS: Assume all Medicare benefits whether or not individual actually enrolled.

EXCLUSIONS

1. Expenses resulting from self-inflicted injuries, work-related injuries, or illnesses.

2. Charges or services: in excess of UCR, not medically necessary, for completion of claim forms, for failure to keep appointments; for routine, preventative, or experimental services.

3. Eye refractions; contacts or glasses; orthotics (eye exercises); radial keratotomy or other procedures for surgical correction of refractive errors.

4. Custodial care and/or convalescent facility coverage.

5. Cosmetic surgery unless for repair of an injury or surgery incurred while covered or result of mastectomy.

6. Diagnosis or treatment of infertility, including artificial insemination, in vitro fertilization, etc., contraceptive materials or devices, non-therapeutic abortions except where the life of the mother is endangered, reversal of voluntary sterilization.

7. Pregnancy-related expenses for dependent children.

8. Expenses for obesity, weight reduction, or diet control unless at least 100 lbs. overweight.

9. Vitamins, food supplements, and/or protein supplements.

10. Sex-altering treatments or surgeries, or related studies.

11. Orthopedic shoes or other devices for support or treatment of feet except as medically necessary following foot surgery.

12. Biofeedback-related services or treatment, EDTA chelation therapy.

COMPREHENSIVE DENTAL BENEFITS

INTEGRATED—Deductible provisions, lifetime maximum and coinsurance limit combined with comprehensive Major Medical.

CALENDAR YEAR DEDUCTIBLE—$100.

DEDUCTIBLE CARRYOVER—No carryover.

FAMILY DEDUCTIBLE LIMIT—$200, aggregate.

COINSURANCE—90%.

(Continued)

COINSURANCE LIMIT—$500 (Patient responsibility, not to include disallowed amounts or the deductible.)

APPLICATION OF COINSURANCE LIMIT—Applies only in the calendar year in which the limit is met.

FAMILY COINSURANCE LIMIT—$1,000.

MAXIMUM—$300,000 lifetime.

MAXIMUM PER CALENDAR YEAR—$1,500.

ORTHODONTIA ELIGIBILITY—Dependents only.

SPACE MAINTAINER ELIGIBILITY—Dependents only.

FLUORIDE ELIGIBILITY—Employees and dependents.

ORTHODONTIC—90% coinsurance.

ORTHODONTIC MAXIMUM—$800 lifetime; not subject to the $1,500 calendar year maximum.

CLAIM COST CONTROL OPTIONS—Predetermination of benefits required on claims over $500; alternate course of treatment based on customarily employed method. Benefits cut to 50% if no predetermination done.

PROSTHETIC REPLACEMENTS—Five-year rule applies to replacement of any previously installed prosthetics.

ORDERED AND UNDELIVERED—Excludes expenses for any devices installed or delivered after 30 days following termination date of insurance.

MISSING AND UNREPLACED EXCLUSION—Applies.

REMARKS—Orthodontic benefits are payable as incurred, rather than amortized over the period of time during which work is performed.

CMS-1500 Claim Form Matrix

Header—Top of Form Purpose: Directs the claim to the appropriate payer.

HEALTH INSURANCE CLAIM FORM

APPROVED MOB-0938-0008

PICA □□□

PLEASE
DO NOT
STAPLE
IN THIS
AREA
□□□ PICA

ROVER INSURERS INC
5931 ROLLING ROAD
RONSON CO 81369

Information to Enter	Commercial/Private	Medicare	Medicaid	Workers' Compensation
Enter the name and address of the payer(s) to whom this claim is being sent. Use spaces to separate names. Enter address information as follows: 1st line=Name; 2nd line=First line of address; 3rd line=Second line of address, if necessary; and 4th line=city, state (2 digits) and zip code. Do not use punctuation except "#" and "-." If an attention line is needed place it in the second line.	Required.	Required.	Required.	Required.

Block 1—Insurance Coverage Information Purpose: Shows the type of health insurance coverage applicable to this claim.

1. MEDICARE   MEDICAID   CHAMPUS   CHAMPVA   GROUP HEALTH PLAN   FECA BLK LUNG   OTHER

□ (Medicare #) □ (Medicaid #) □ (Sponsor's SSN) □ (VA File #) ⊠ (SSN or ID) □ (SSN) □ (ID)

Information to Enter	Commercial/Private	Medicare	Medicaid	Workers' Compensation
Enter an X in the applicable box.	For an Individual Plan place an X in "OTHER." For a Group Plan place an X in "GROUP."	Enter an X in the "MEDICARE" box.	Enter an X in the "MEDICAID" box.	Enter an X in "OTHER," unless diagnosis is for "FECA BLK LUNG." If FECA, place an X in that box.

Block 1a—Insured's Identification, Policy or Certificate Number and Group Number Purpose: Identifies the patient to the payer.

1a INSURED'S I.D NUMBER (FOR PROGRAM IN ITEM 1)

001 00 RED

Information to Enter	Commercial/Private	Medicare	Medicaid	Workers' Compensation
Enter the insured's identification number as shown on the insured's health	Required.	Enter the patient's	Enter the	Enter the patient's WC

Table AD–1 CMS-1500 Claim Form Matrix

Information to Enter	Commercial/Private	Medicare	Medicaid	Workers' Compensation
insurance card for the payer to whom the claim is being submitted. Do not use punctuation.		Medicare HICN.	patient's Medicaid ID number, complete with any prefixes and suffixes.	claim number if available. If not, enter employer's policy number, or patient's SSN. If a SSN is not available, a driver's license number and jurisdiction, a green card number, a visa number, or passport number can be used.

Block 2—Patient's Name   Purpose: Identifies the patient.

2. PATIENT'S NAME (Last, First, Middle Initial).
ADDISON ABBY

Information to Enter	Commercial/Private	Medicare	Medicaid	Workers' Compensation
Enter the patient's full last name, first name, and middle initial. Use spaces to separate names. If the patient uses a last name suffix (i.e., Jr, Sr) enter it after the last name and before the first name. Do not use punctuation except a "-", which may be used for hyphenated names.	Required.	Required.	Required.	Required.

Block 3—Patient's Birth Date   Purpose: Identifies the patient; distinguishes persons with similar names.

3. PATIENT'S BIRTH DATE
MM DD YY   SEX
12 12 1968   M☐ F☒

Information to Enter	Commercial/Private	Medicare	Medicaid	Workers' Compensation
Enter the patient's date of birth. Use the eight-digit numeric date (MM DD CCYY). Use spaces to separate parts of the field. Enter an X in the correct box to indicate the sex of the patient.	Required.	Required.	Required.	Required.

Block 4—Insured's Name   Purpose: Identifies the patient's source of insurance.

4. INSURED'S NAME (Last, First, Middle Initial)
SAME

Information to Enter	Commercial/Private	Medicare	Medicaid	Workers' Compensation
Enter the insured's full last name, first name, and middle initial. If the insured uses a last name suffix (i.e., Jr, Sr) enter it after the last name and before the first name. Do not use punctuation except a "-"; which may be used for hyphenated names. If the patient and insured are the same enter "SAME."	Required.	If Medicare is the primary carrier, leave empty. If not, list name.	If insured is also the patient, leave empty. If not, list name.	Enter the name of the patient's employer.

Block 5—Patient's Address — Purpose: Further identifies patient; allows contact for questions.

5. PATIENT'S ADDRESS (No., Street)
5678 ANY AVENUE

CITY		STATE
ANYTOWN		USA

ZIP CODE	TELEPHONE (Include Area Code)
12345	(765) 555 4321

Information to Enter	Commercial/Private	Medicare	Medicaid	Workers' Compensation
Enter the patient's mailing address and telephone number. Do not use punctuation except "#" and "-". Use the two-digit state code and if available nine-digit zip code.	Required.	Required.	Required.	Required.

Block 6—Patient's Relationship to Insured — Purpose: Identifies patient's source of insurance; also distinguishes patient from insured.

6. PATIENT'S RELATIONSHIP TO INSURED
Self ☒   Spouse ☐   Child ☐   Other ☐

Information to Enter	Commercial/Private	Medicare	Medicaid	Workers' Compensation
Enter an X in the correct box to indicate the patient's relationship to the insured. For unmarried domestic partner check the "OTHER" box.	Required.	Use only if block 4 is completed.	Leave empty, unless there is other coverage.	Enter an X in the "OTHER" box.

Block 7—Insured's Address — Purpose: Further identifies insured; allows contact for questions.

7. INSURED'S ADDRESS (No., Street)
SAME

CITY		STATE

ZIP CODE	TELEPHONE (INCLUDE AREA CODE)

Information to Enter	Commercial/Private	Medicare	Medicaid	Workers' Compensation
Enter the insured's address and telephone number. Do not use punctuation except "#" and "-". Use the two-digit state code and if available nine-digit zip code. Enter "SAME" if block 4 is completed and the address is the same as block 5.	Required.	Complete only if block 4 is completed.	Complete only if block 4 is completed.	Enter the address and telephone number of the patient's employer.

Block 8—Patient Status   Purpose: Allows determination of liability and COB.

8. PATIENT STATUS

Single ☐   Married ☐   Other ☒
Employed ☒   Full-Time ☐   Part-Time ☐
Student   Student

Information to Enter	Commercial/Private	Medicare	Medicaid	Workers' Compensation
Enter an X in the box for the patient's marital status and for the patient's employment or student status. If widowed or divorced select the "Single" box. Use "Other" for domestic partner.	Required.	Required.	Not required.	Enter an X in the "Employed" box.

Block 9—Other Insured's Name   Purpose: Identifies other sources of insurance.

9. OTHER INSURED'S NAME (Last, First, Middle Initial)

Information to Enter	Commercial/Private	Medicare	Medicaid	Workers' Compensation
If item 11d is marked, complete fields 9–9-d, otherwise leave blank. Enter the name of the holder of a secondary or other policy that may cover the patient. Enter the other insured's full last name, first name, and middle initial of the enrollee in another health plan. Use spaces to separate names. Do not use punctuation except a "-"; which may be used for hyphenated names. If the patient and insured are the same enter "SAME."	Required.	If Medicare is the primary insurer leave 9–9d empty. If not, enter info.	If Medicaid is the primary insurer leave 9–9d empty. If not, enter info.	Not required unless claim has not been declared WC.

Block 9a—Other Insured's Policy or Group Number   Purpose: Identifies other sources of insurance.

a. OTHER INSURED'S POLICY OR GROUP NUMBER

Information to Enter	Commercial/Private	Medicare	Medicaid	Workers' Compensation
Enter the policy or group number of the other insured as indicated in block 9. Copy the number from the health identification card. Complete only if block 9 is completed.	Required.	Indicate "Medigap" if Medigap insurance is listed.	Required.	Not required unless claim has not been declared WC.

Block 9b—Other Insured's Date of Birth Purpose: Identifies other insurance source. Also used to determine the primary source of insurance.

b. OTHER INSURED'S DATE OF BIRTH
MM | DD | YY   SEX
M ☐   F ☐

Information to Enter	Commercial/Private	Medicare	Medicaid	Workers' Compensation
Enter the date of birth and sex of the other insured as indicated in block 9. Enter an X in the correct box to indicate the sex of the other insured. Use the eight-digit numeric date (MM DD CCYY). Use spaces to separate parts of the field. Complete only if block 9 is completed.	Required.	Required.	Required.	Not required unless claim has not been declared WC.

Block 9c—Employer's Name or School Name Purpose: Identifies other sources of insurance.

c. EMPLOYER'S NAME OR SCHOOL NAME

Information to Enter	Commercial/Private	Medicare	Medicaid	Workers' Compensation
Enter the name of the other insured's employer or school as indicated in block 9. Complete only if block 9 completed.	Required.	Required.	Required.	Not required unless claim has not been declared WC.

Block 9d—Insurance Plan Name or Program Name Purpose: Identifies other sources of insurance.

d. INSURANCE PLAN NAME OR PROGRAM NAME

Information to Enter	Commercial/Private	Medicare	Medicaid	Workers' Compensation
Enter the other insured's insurance plan or program name. Complete only if block 9 completed.	Required.	Required.	Required.	Not required unless claim has not been declared WC.

Block 10a–10c—Is Patient's Condition Related to Employment? Purpose: Identifies primary liability for condition.

10. IS PATIENT'S CONDITION RELATED TO:

a. EMPLOYMENT? (CURRENT OR PREVIOUS)
☐ YES ☒ NO

b. AUTO ACCIDENT?   PLACE (State)
☐ YES ☒ NO ☐

c. OTHER ACCIDENT?
☐ YES ☒ NO

Information to Enter	Commercial/Private	Medicare	Medicaid	Workers' Compensation

Enter an X in the correct box to indicate whether one or more of the services described in Item 24 are for a condition or injury that occurred on-the-job or as a result of an automobile or other accident. The state postal code must be shown if "YES" is checked in 10b for "Auto Accident." Any item marked "Yes" indicates that there may be other applicable insurance coverage that would be primary, such as automobile liability insurance.

Required.	Enter an X in the "No" box. If "Yes," the other payer should be billed as primary, before billing Medicare.	Enter an X in the "No" box. If "Yes," the other payer should be billed as primary, before billing Medicaid.	Enter an X in the "Yes" box for 10a.

Block 10d—Reserved for Local Use?   Purpose: To be determined by local payer.

10d.   RESERVED FOR LOCAL USE

Information to Enter
Refer to the most current instructions from the applicable public or private payer regarding the use of this field.

Commercial/Private	Medicare	Medicaid	Workers' Compensation
Per payer specifications; otherwise leave empty.	Per payer specifications; otherwise leave empty.	Enter the share of cost collected from patient.	Per payer specifications; otherwise leave empty.

Block 11—Insured's Policy Group or FECA Number   Purpose: Identifies insured's policy or group number.

11.   INSURED'S POLICY GROUP OR FECA NUMBER:
41935

Information to Enter
Enter the insured's policy or group number as it appears on the insured's health care identification card. The FECA number is a 9-digit alphanumeric identifier assigned to a patient claiming work-related conditions under FECA.

Commercial/Private	Medicare	Medicaid	Workers' Compensation
Required.	If Medicare is the primary insurance carrier, list "NONE" and proceed to block 12. If there is a terminating event with regard to insurance (e.g., insured retired) enter "NONE" and proceed to block 11b.	Not required.	Not required.

Block 11a—Insured's Date of Birth   Purpose: Identifies other sources of insurance. Used to determine the primary source of insurance.

a. INSURED'S DATE OF BIRTH
MM   DD   YY
12   12   1968   SEX   M☐   F☒

Information to Enter

Commercial/Private	Medicare	Medicaid	Workers' Compensation

Enter the insured's date of birth (this refers to the insured indicated in block 1a). Enter an X in the correct box to indicate the sex of the insured. Use the eight-digit numeric date (MM DD CCYY). Use spaces to separate parts of the field.

Required.	Not required.	Not required.	Not required.

Block 11b—Employer's Name or School Name   Purpose: Identifies other sources of insurance.

b. EMPLOYER'S NAME OR SCHOOL NAME
RED CORPORATION

Commercial/Private	**Medicare**	**Medicaid**	**Workers' Compensation**
Information to Enter Enter the name of the insured's employer or school.			
Required.	If a change in the insured's insurance status has occurred enter the reason (e.g., RETIRED).	Not required.	Not required.

Block 11c—Insurance Plan Name or Program Name   Purpose: Identifies other sources of insurance.

c. INSURANCE PLAN NAME OR PROGRAM NAME
ROVER INSURERS INC

Commercial/Private	**Medicare**	**Medicaid**	**Workers' Compensation**
Information to Enter Enter the name of the insured's insurance plan or program name.			
Required.	Not Required.	Not required.	Not required.

Block 11d—Is There Another Health Benefit Plan?   Purpose: Identifies other sources of insurance.

d. IS THERE ANOTHER HEALTH BENEFIT PLAN?
[ ] YES [X] NO   *If yes, return to and complete item 9 a–d*

Commercial/Private	**Medicare**	**Medicaid**	**Workers' Compensation**
Information to Enter When appropriate enter an X in the correct box, if there is another health benefit plan other than the plan indicated in block 1. If marked "YES" complete blocks 9–9d.			
Required.	Required.	Required.	Not required, unless claim has not been declared WC, then enter an X in the "Yes" box and complete 9–9d.

Block 12—Authorization for Release of Medical Information   Purpose: Gives permission to release any medical or other information necessary to process and/or adjudicate the claim.

READ BACK OF FORM BEFORE COMPLETING & SIGNING THIS FORM

12. PATIENT'S OR AUTHORIZED PERSON'S SIGNATURE I authorize the release of any medical or other information necessary to process this claim. I also request payment of government benefits either to myself or to the party who accepts assignment below.

SIGNED __SIGNATURE ON FILE__   DATE _____

Information to Enter	Commercial/Private	Medicare	Medicaid	Workers' Compensation
Enter "Signature on File", "SOF" or legal signature. When a legal signature is provided, enter date signed in the six-digit format (MMDDYY) or eight-digit (MMDDCCYY) format. If there is no signature on file, leave blank or enter "No Signature on File."	Required.	Required.	Not required.	Not required.

Block 13—Authorization for Assignment of Benefits to Provider   Purpose: Gives permission authorizing payment of benefits to the provider of services.

13. INSURED'S OR AUTHORIZED PERSON'S SIGNATURE I authorize payment of medical benefits to the undersigned physician or supplier for services described below.

SIGNED __SIGNATURE ON FILE__

Information to Enter	Commercial/Private	Medicare	Medicaid	Workers' Compensation
Enter "Signature on File", "SOF" or legal signature. If there is no signature on file, leave blank or enter "No Signature on File."	Required.	Required.	Not required.	Not required.

Block 14—Date of Illness, Injury, or Pregnancy   Purpose: Helps payers identify benefits.

14. DATE OF CURRENT: ILLNESS (1st symptom)
MM | DD | YY   INJURY (Accident)
                    PREGNANCY (LMP)

Information to Enter	Commercial/Private	Medicare	Medicaid	Workers' Compensation
Enter the first date of the present illness, injury, or pregnancy. Use the six-digit format (MM DD YY). Use spaces to separate parts of the field. For pregnancy, use the date of the last menstrual period.	Required.	Required.	Not required.	Requires a specific date for the on-the-job illness or injury. The date should be the same as that indicated on the Doctor's First Report.

397

Block 15—If Patient Has Had Same or Similar Illness, Give First Date   Purpose: Allows determination of liability and COB.

15. IF PATIENT HAS HAD SAME OR SIMILAR ILLNESS,
    GIVE FIRST DATE   MM | DD | YY

Commercial/Private	Medicare	Medicaid	Workers' Compensation
Required.	Not required.	Not required.	Not required.

Information to Enter

Enter the first date that the patient had the same or a similar illness. Use the six-digit numeric date (MM DD YY). Use spaces to separate parts of the field.

Block 16—Patient Disability Dates for Current Occupation   Purpose: Identifies dates of disability.

16. DATES PATIENT UNABLE TO WORK IN CURRENT OCCUPATION
    MM | DD | YY   MM | DD | YY
    FROM   TO

Commercial/Private	Medicare	Medicaid	Workers' Compensation
Required.	Required.	Not required.	Required.

Information to Enter

If the patient is employed and is unable to work in current occupation, an eight-digit numeric date (MMDDCCYY) must be shown for the "from-to" dates that the patient is unable to work. An entry in this field may indicate employment-related insurance coverage.

Block 17—Name of Referring Physician or Other Source   Purpose: Identifies referral source.

17. NAME OF REFERRING PHYSICIAN OR OTHER SOURCE

DOROTHY DOCTOR MD

Commercial/Private	Medicare	Medicaid	Workers' Compensation
Required.	Required.	Required.	Enter the SSN or EIN of the employer.

Information to Enter

Enter the name (First Name, Middle Initial, Last Name) and credentials of the professional who referred or ordered the service(s) or supply(s) on the claim. Use spaces to separate names. Do not use punctuation except a "-" which may be used for hyphenated names. For services billed by an assistant surgeon or anesthesiologist enter the name and credential of the primary surgeon. For DME claims enter the name of the prescribing provider.

Block 17a—I.D. Number of Referring Physician   Purpose: Identifies referral source.

17a. I.D. NUMBER OF REFERRING PHYSICIAN

D45678

Information to Enter	Commercial/Private	Medicare	Medicaid	Workers' Compensation
Enter the identifying number (i.e., NPI, UPIN, MHCP ID numbers) of the referring or ordering physician, or other source. Required when block 17 is completed.	Enter a UPIN, PIN or NPI number.	Enter a UPIN, PIN or NPI number.	Enter a UPIN, PIN or NPI number.	Enter a SSN or EIN number.

Block 18—Hospitalization Dates   Purpose: Identifies services related to an inpatient stay.

18. HOSPITALIZATION DATES RELATED TO CURRENT SERVICES

FROM   MM | DD | YY   TO   MM | DD | YY

Information to Enter	Commercial/Private	Medicare	Medicaid	Workers' Compensation
Enter the inpatient hospital admission date followed by the discharge date (if discharge has occurred). If not discharged, leave discharge date blank. Use the eight-digit numeric date (MM DD CCYY). Use spaces to separate parts of the field. This date is when a medical service is furnished as a result of, or subsequent to, a related hospitalization.	Required.	Required.	Required.	Required.

Block 19—Reserved for Local Use   Purpose: Provides additional information.

19. RESERVED FOR LOCAL USE

Information to Enter	Commercial/Private	Medicare	Medicaid	Workers' Compensation
Refer to the most current instructions from the applicable public or private payer regarding the use of this field.	Per payer specifications; otherwise leave empty.	Per payer specifications; otherwise leave empty.	Per payer specifications; otherwise leave empty.	Per payer specifications; otherwise leave empty.

Block 20—Outside Lab $Charges   Purpose: Identifies purchased laboratory, pathology, or radiology services.

20. OUTSIDE LAB? $ CHARGES
☐ YES ☒ NO

Information to Enter	Commercial/Private	Medicare	Medicaid	Workers' Compensation
Complete this field when billing for purchased services. Enter an X in the "Yes" box if the reported service(s) were performed by an outside laboratory. If "Yes", enter the purchase price. Do not use a dollar sign. Use	Required.	Required.	Enter an X in the "No" box as outside	Required.

a space to divide the dollars and cents. Enter an X in the "No" box if outside laboratory service(s) are not included on the claim. When "YES" is marked, enter the independent provider's name and address in Block 32.

| | | | | | laboratories must bill Medicaid directly. |

Block 21—Diagnosis or Nature of Illness or Injury   Purpose: Supports the reason for the service(s) and provides information necessary to process the claim. The diagnosis must relate to the service(s) performed.

21. DIAGNOSIS OR NATURE OF ILLNESS OR INJURY, (RELATE ITEMS 1,2,3, OR 4 TO ITEM 24E BY LINE)

1. | 401 . |
2. | . |
3. | . |
4. | . |

Information to Enter

Enter the patient's diagnosis/condition. Enter up to four ICD-9CM diagnosis codes. Relate lines 1,2,3,4 to the lines of service in 24E by line number. Use the highest level of specificity. Do not use punctuation.

Commercial/Private	Medicare	Medicaid	Workers' Compensation
Required.	Required.	Required.	Required.

Block 22—Medicaid Resubmission   Purpose: Use to identify a resubmission of an incorrectly processed Medicaid claim.

22. MEDICAID RESUBMISSION CODE | ORIGINAL REF. NO.

Information to Enter

List the original reference number for resubmitted claims. Refer to the most current instructions from the applicable public or private payer regarding the use of this field. Leave empty for all payers except Medicaid.

Commercial/Private	Medicare	Medicaid	Workers' Compensation
Not required.	Not required.	Enter the correct Medicaid Transaction Control Number.	Not required.

Block 23—Prior Authorization Number   Purpose: Determines eligibility of the current service(s).

23. PRIOR AUTHORIZATION NUMBER

Information to Enter

Enter any of the following: prior authorization or precertification number; referral number; or CLIA number; as assigned by the payer for the current service when applicable. Notations such as "Prescription on File" can be noted for DME or pharmacy claims; or "SSO Performed" can be noted for claims which require an SSO to be performed.

Commercial/Private	Medicare	Medicaid	Workers' Compensation
Required.	Required.	Required.	Not required.

Block 24A—Date(s) of Service [lines 1-6]   Purpose: Informs the payer of the date(s) of service(s).

24.	A						
	DATE(S) OF SERVICE						
	From			To			
MM	DD	YY	MM	DD	YY		
01	26	YY	01	26	YY		

Information to Enter	Commercial/Private	Medicare	Medicaid	Workers' Compensation
Enter date(s) of service, from and to: If one date of service only, enter the date under "From." Leave "To" blank or re-enter "From" date. If grouping services, the place of service, type of service, procedure code, charges, and individual provider for each line must be identical for that service line. The number of days must correspond to the number of units in 24G. Use the six-digit numeric date (MM DD YY). Use spaces to separate parts of the field.	Required.	Required.	Leave "To" date empty. No date ranging allowed.	Required.

Block 24B—Place of Service [lines 1-6]   Purpose: Informs the payer as to where the service(s) were performed.

B			
Place of Service			
11			

Information to Enter	Commercial/Private	Medicare	Medicaid	Workers' Compensation
Enter the two-digit code for the "Place of Service" for each item used or service performed. Refer to the Place of Service list in Appendix C.	Required.	Required.	Required.	Required.

Block 24C—Type of Service [lines 1-6]   Purpose: No longer used.

C
Type of Service

Information to Enter
Leave empty.

Commercial/Private	Medicare	Medicaid	Workers' Compensation
Not required.	Not required.	Not required.	Not required.

Block 24D—Procedures, Services, or Supplies [lines 1-6]   Purpose: Informs payer as to what services were performed.

D
PROCEDURES, SERVICES, OR SUPPLIES (Explain Unusual Circumstances)
CPT/HCPS | MODIFIER
99212

Information to Enter
Enter the CPT® or HCPCS codes and modifier(s) (if applicable) from the appropriate code set in effect on the date of service. Use spaces to separate parts of field. Do not use hyphens for modifiers.

Commercial/Private	Medicare	Medicaid	Workers' Compensation
Required.	Required.	Required.	Required.

Block 24E—Diagnosis Code [lines 1-6]   Purpose: Informs the payer which diagnosis relates to each procedure.

E
DIAGNOSIS CODE
1

	Commercial/Private	Medicare	Medicaid	Workers' Compensation
Information to Enter	Required.	Required.	Required.	Required.

Enter the diagnosis code reference number as shown in block 21 to relate the date of service and the procedures performed to the primary diagnosis. When multiple services are performed, the primary reference number for each service should be listed first, other applicable services should follow. The reference number(s) should be a 1, or 2, or 3, or 4; or multiple numbers as applicable. Do not use punctuation or enter ICD-9-CM codes here. Use spaces to separate line numbers.

Block 24F—$ Charges [lines 1-6]   Purpose: Informs the payer of the total amount charged for each service line.

F
$ CHARGES

40 : 00

	Commercial/Private	Medicare	Medicaid	Workers' Compensation
Information to Enter	Required.	Required.	Required.	Required.

Enter the charge for each listed service. Enter numbers right justified in the dollar area of the field. If more than one date or unit is shown in 24G, the dollars shown should reflect the total of the services. Do not use dollar signs. Do not use commas as thousands marker. Use a space to separate parts of field.

Block 24G—Days or Units [lines 1-6]   Purpose: Informs the payer of the number or quantity of each service provided.

G
DAYS
OR
UNITS

1

Information to Enter	Commercial/Private	Medicare	Medicaid	Workers' Compensation
Enter the number of days or units for each service line. This field is most commonly used for multiple visits, units of supplies, anesthesia units or minutes, or oxygen volume. If only one service is performed, the number 1 must be entered. For anesthesia, enter the total minutes of anesthesia provided (convert hours to minutes).	Required.	Required.	Required.	Required.

Block 24H—EPSDT / Family Plan [lines 1-6]   Purpose: Indicates whether the services were for Early, Periodic, Screening, Diagnosis and Treatment services.

H
EPSDT
Family
Plan

Information to Enter	Commercial/Private	Medicare	Medicaid	Workers' Compensation
Leave empty unless Medicaid Claim.	Not required.	Not required.	Enter "E" for EPSDT services, or enter "F" for family planning services.	Not required.

Block 24I—EMG [lines 1-6]   Purpose: Contains the ID Qualifer

I.
ID.
QUAL.

Information to Enter	Commercial/Private	Medicare	Medicaid	Workers' Compensation

Information to Enter	Commercial/Private	Medicare	Medicaid	Workers' Compensation
Check with payer to determine if this field is required. If required, enter Y for "YES" or leave blank if "NO."	Per payer specifications; otherwise leave empty.	Per payer specifications; otherwise leave empty.	If services rendered in the ER, enter an "X"	Not required.

Block 24J—COB [lines 1-6]   Purpose: Indicates the rendering provides by the provider's NPI.

COB

Information to Enter	Commercial/Private	Medicare	Medicaid	Workers' Compensation
Check with payer to determine if this field is required. If required, enter an X if the patient has other insurance, and an EOB is attached.	Per payer specifications; otherwise leave empty.	Per payer specifications; otherwise leave empty.	Per payer specifications; otherwise leave empty.	Not required.

Block 24K—Reserved For Local Use   Purpose: Identifies the specific doctor that performed the services.

K
RESERVED FOR
LOCAL USE

Information to Enter	Commercial/Private	Medicare	Medicaid	Workers' Compensation
If a medical group is the provider listed in block 33 enter the UPIN, PIN or NPI number of the individual provider that performed the services.	Required.	Required.	Required.	Required.

Block 25—Federal Tax I.D. Number   Purpose: Identifies the billing provider.

25. FEDERAL TAX I.D. NUMBER   SSN EIN
99-1234567   ☐ ☒

Information to Enter	Commercial/Private	Medicare	Medicaid	Workers' Compensation
Enter the billing provider's federal tax identification number (include hyphen), social security, or employer identification number (include hyphen). Specify type of number by entering an X in the correct box. Use spaces to separate parts of field.	Required.	Required.	Required.	Required.

Block 26—Patient's Account Number   Purpose: Identifies the patient.

26. PATIENTS ACCOUNT NO.
GMBC5509 001

Information to Enter	Commercial/Private	Medicare	Medicaid	Workers' Compensation
Enter the patient's account number assigned by the billing provider.	Required.	Required.	Required.	Required.

Block 27—Accept Assignment?   Purpose: Indicates if the provider accepts assignment of Medicare benefits.

27. ACCEPT ASSIGNMENT?
(For govt. claims, see back)
☒ YES   ☐ NO $

Information to Enter	Commercial/Private	Medicare	Medicaid	Workers' Compensation
Enter an X in the correct box.	Required.	Required.	"Yes" box must be marked.	Not required.

Block 28—Total Charge   Purpose: Informs the payer of the total dollars charged for the billed services.

28. TOTAL CHARGE
$ 40 ¦ 00

Information to Enter	Commercial/Private	Medicare	Medicaid	Workers' Compensation
Enter the sum of the charges in column 24F [lines 1-6]. Use a space to divide the dollars and cents. Do not use dollar signs. Do not use commas as thousands marker.	Required.	Required.	Required.	Required.

Block 29—Amount Paid   Purpose: Indicates payments made by other payers or by the patient.

29. AMOUNT PAID

$ 5 | 00 $

Information to Enter	Commercial/Private	Medicare	Medicaid	Workers' Compensation
Enter the amount the patient or other payers paid on covered services only. Use a space to divide the dollars and cents. Do not use dollar signs. Do not use commas as thousands marker.	Required.	Required.	Do not enter the Medicaid copayment amount.	Required.

Block 30—Balance Due   Purpose: Indicates the balance due to be paid to the provider of services.

30. BALANCE DUE

$ 35 | 00

Information to Enter	Commercial/Private	Medicare	Medicaid	Workers' Compensation
Subtract block 29 from block 28 to arrive at the amount to be entered in this block.	Required.	Not required.	Enter the balance due if Medicaid is the secondary payer. Otherwise not required.	Required.

Block 31—Signature of Physician or Supplier Including Degrees or Credentials   Purpose: Identifies the provider of service(s) or supply(s).

31. SIGNATURE OF PHYSICIAN OR SUPPLIER
INCLUDING DEGREES OR CREDENTIALS
(I certify that the statements on the reverse
apply to this bill and are made a part thereof.)

SIGNED Paul Provider MD DATE
0126CCYY

Information to Enter	Commercial/Private	Medicare	Medicaid	Workers' Compensation
Enter the signature of the physician, supplier or representative with the degree, credentials, or title and the date signed. Use the eight-digit numeric date (MM DD CCYY).	Required.	Required.	Required.	Required.

Block 32—Name and Address of Facility Where Services Were Rendered   Purpose: Identifies where the service(s) were rendered or supplies provided. The service provider

32. NAME AND ADDRESS OF FACILITY WHERE SERVICES
    WERE RENDERED (If other than home or office)

a.

b.

Information to Enter	Commercial/Private	Medicare	Medicaid	Workers' Compensation
Enter the name and address, city, state, and zip code of the location where the services were rendered if other than box 33 or patient's home. Suppliers should enter the location where supplies were accepted. Do not use punctuation except "#" and "-." Use two-digit state code and, if available, nine-digit zip code. If block 18 is completed or block 20 contains an X in the "Yes" box enter name and address of facility here.	Required.	Required.	Required.	Required.

Block 33—Physician's/Supplier's Billing Name, Address, Zip Code and Phone Number   Purpose: Identifies the billing provider and the NPI

33. PHYSICIANS, SUPPLIERS BILLING NAME, ADDRESS, ZIP CODE &
    PHONE #

PAUL PROVIDER MD
5858 PEPPERMINT PLACE
ANYTOWN USA 12345
(765) 555 6768

a.   b.

Information to Enter	Commercial/Private	Medicare	Medicaid	Workers' Compensation
Enter the billing provider's name, address, city, state, zip code, and telephone number. Enter the PIN, NPI, or Group Number. Do not use punctuation except "#" and "-." Use the two-digit state code and, if available, the nine-digit zip code.	Required.	Required.	Enter the provider's Medicaid number in the Group # field.	Required.

PATIENT INFORMATION SHEET
(Please Print)

Date: _____

Patient's
Name: _____   DOB: _____ /_____ /_____
      First   Middle   Last   Month Day   Year

Address: _____   Phone: _____ /_____ -_____
         Street   City   State   Zip   (Area code)

Patient's SS#: _____ - _____ - _____

Method of payment (circle):   cash   check   credit card   insurance co-payment

Primary Insurance: _____

Member's ID #: _____   Group Policy #: _____

Secondary Insurance: _____

Member's ID #: _____   Group Policy #: _____

Person
Responsible
For Payment: _____   _____
        First   Middle   Last   Relationship

Address: _____   Phone: _____ /_____ -_____
         Street   City   State   Zip   (Area code)

Employer Name: _____   Dept: _____
        First   Middle   Last

Address: _____   Phone: _____ /_____ -_____
         Street   City   State   Zip   (Area code)

Emergency
Contact: _____   _____
       First   Middle   Last   Relationship

Address: _____   Phone: _____ /_____ -_____
         Street   City   State   Zip   (Area code)

How were you referred to this office?_____

_____

Statement of Financial Responsibility: I, _____
do hereby agree to pay all medical charges incurred by the above listed patient. I further understand
that these charges are my responsibility, regardless of insurance coverage.

Responsible Person's Signature: _____

Paul Provider, M.D.
5858 Peppermint Place
Anytown, USA 12345
(765) 555-6768

Insurance Coverage Form

INSURED: _____ BIRTH DATE: _____

SSN: _____ EFFECTIVE DATE: _____

INSURANCE POLICY: _____

ADDRESS: _____

ID/MEMBER #: _____ GROUP #: _____

DEPENDENT AGE LIMIT: _____

_____

INDIV. DEDUCTIBLE AMOUNT: _____ 3 MO CARRYOVER:_____

FAMILY DEDUCTIBLE: _____ AGGREGATE/NONAGGREGATE

STANDARD COINSURANCE:_____LIFETIME MAXIMUM:_____

COINSURANCE LIMIT _____

_____

BENEFITS PAID AT OTHER THAN THE STANDARD COINSURANCE % [Including benefit, coinsurance amount and special circumstances (i.e., SSO allowed at 100%, required for hysterectomy, coronary bypass, etc.)]:

_____

_____

PREAUTHORIZATION REQUIRED FOR: _____

_____

_____

ACCIDENT BENEFIT AMOUNT: _____ TREATMENT TO BE RECEIVED WITHIN _____ DAYS

OTHER NOTES/COMMENTS: _____

_____

TOTAL PAYMENTS (CCYY)

Indicate below the names of the insured and his or her dependents. When any of the following information is received, write it in pencil followed by the date. This will help you to realize when a patient's deductible has been met and if the patient is nearing any maximum benefit.

	INSURED	DEPENDENT	DEPENDENT	DEPENDENT	DEPENDENT
NAME:	_____	_____	_____	_____	_____
DEDUCTIBLE:	_____	_____	_____	_____	_____
COINS PD:	_____	_____	_____	_____	_____
LIFETIME:	_____	_____	_____	_____	_____

Paul Provider, M.D.
5858 Peppermint Place
Anytown, USA 12345
(765) 555-6768

INSURANCE TRACER

Date: _____

Dear Insurance Carrier:

    We sent a claim to you over six weeks ago and have not heard back from you.
Patient:
Insured:
Address:
SSN/Birth Date:
Group Number:
Claim Amount:
Date Billed:
Date of Services:
Date of Illness or Injury:
Diagnosis:
Employer:
Address:

    Please supply the following information on the above named claim within ten days. Payment on this claim is overdue and we would like to avoid involving the patient and the state insurance commissioner in a reimbursement complaint.

Claim pending because:_____

Payment in progress. Check will be mailed on:_____

Payment previously made. Date: _____

To whom:_____

Check #: _____ Payment Amount: _____

Claim denied. Reason: _____

Patient notified: Yes   No

Remarks: _____

Thank you for your assistance.

Completed by: _____

Encounter Form

Date:

Paul Provider, M.D.
5858 Peppermint Place ● Anytown, USA 12345 ● (765) 555-6768

Provider Information

Name:	
Address:	
City:	State:	Zip Code:
Telephone #:	
Fax #:	
Tax ID #:	
Medicaid ID #:	
Medicare ID #:	

Provider's Signature: _____ Date: _____

Patient Information

Name:	
Address:	
City:	State:	Zip Code:
Telephone #:	
Patient Account #:	
Date of Birth:	
Gender:	
Relationship to Guarantor:	
Marital Status:	
SSN #:	

Insurance Type: ☐ Private   ☐ Medicare   ☐ Medicaid   ☐ Workers' Compensation   ☐ Other _____

Appointment Information

Appt. Date:		Time:	
Request Next Appt. Date:		Time:	
Date of First Visit:			
Date of Injury:			
Referring Physician:			

Guarantor Information

Name:	
Insurance ID #:	
Insurance Plan Name:	
Insurance Plan Group #:	
Employer Name:	
Employer Address:	
City:	State:	Zip Code:
SSN #:	

Authorization

☐ Authorization to Release Information
☐ Authorization for Assignment of Benefits
☐ Authorization for Consent for Treatment
☐ I understand that my insurance will be billed as a courtesy to me but that there may be a patient responsibility remaining on account.

Signature: _____ Date: _____

Clinical Information

	Date of Service	Place of Service	CPT® Code/Description	ICD-9 Code/ Description	Fee
1.					
2.					
3.					
4.					
5.					
6.					
7.					
8.					

Billing Instructions

Notes:

Special Instructions:

Statement of Account Information

Previous Balance:	$	Payment:	$
Today's Fee:	$	Received by:	
Copay:	$	☐ Cash	
Adjustment:	$	☐ Check	
		☐ Credit Card	
New Balance:	$	☐ Other	

PAUL PROVIDER, M.D.
5858 Peppermint Place
Anytown, USA 12345

RECEIPT

Date _____   CC _____ No.

Received From _____

Address _____

Dollars $ _____

For _____

ACCOUNT			HOW PAID		
AMT OF ACCOUNT			CASH		
AMT PAID			CHECK		
BALANCE DUE			MONEY ORDER		

By _____

PAUL PROVIDER, M.D.
5858 Peppermint Place
Anytown, USA 12345

RECEIPT

Date _____   CC _____ No.

Received From _____

Address _____

Dollars $ _____

For _____

ACCOUNT			HOW PAID		
AMT OF ACCOUNT			CASH		
AMT PAID			CHECK		
BALANCE DUE			MONEY ORDER		

By _____

PAUL PROVIDER, M.D.
5858 Peppermint Place
Anytown, USA 12345

RECEIPT

Date _____   CC _____ No.

Received From _____

Address _____

Dollars $ _____

For _____

ACCOUNT			HOW PAID		
AMT OF ACCOUNT			CASH		
AMT PAID			CHECK		
BALANCE DUE			MONEY ORDER		

By _____

Paul Provider, M.D.
5858 Peppermint Place
Anytown, USA 12345
(765) 555-6768

Ledger Card/Statement of Account

RESPONSIBLE PARTY: _____

ADDRESS: _____

TELEPHONE #: _____

PATIENT NAME: _____ PATIENT ACCOUNT #: _____

SPECIAL NOTES: _____

Date	Description of Service	Charge	Payments	Adjustments	Remaining Balance

Paul Provider, M.D.
5858 Peppermint Place
Anytown, USA 12345
(765) 555-6768

Day Sheet/Daily Journal

Date	Name	Description of Service	Charge	Payments	Adjustments	Remaining Balance

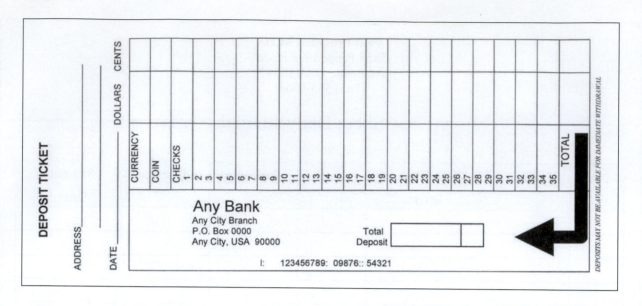

SAMPLE

1500

HEALTH INSURANCE CLAIM FORM

APPROVED BY NATIONAL UNIFORM CLAIM COMMITTEE 08/05

PICA

PICA

CARRIER

1. MEDICARE ☐ (Medicare #) MEDICAID ☐ (Medicaid #) TRICARE CHAMPUS ☐ (Sponsor's SSN) CHAMPVA ☐ (Member ID#) GROUP HEALTH PLAN ☐ (SSN or ID) FECA BLK LUNG ☐ (SSN) OTHER ☐ (ID)   1a. INSURED'S I.D. NUMBER   (For Program in Item 1)

2. PATIENT'S NAME (Last Name, First Name, Middle Initial)

3. PATIENT'S BIRTH DATE   MM | DD | YY   SEX   M ☐   F ☐

4. INSURED'S NAME (Last Name, First Name, Middle Initial)

5. PATIENT'S ADDRESS (No., Street)

6. PATIENT RELATIONSHIP TO INSURED   Self ☐   Spouse ☐   Child ☐   Other ☐

7. INSURED'S ADDRESS (No., Street)

CITY   STATE

8. PATIENT STATUS   Single ☐   Married ☐   Other ☐

CITY   STATE

ZIP CODE   TELEPHONE (Include Area Code) (   )

Employed ☐   Full-Time Student ☐   Part-Time Student ☐

ZIP CODE   TELEPHONE (Include Area Code) (   )

9. OTHER INSURED'S NAME (Last Name, First Name, Middle Initial)

10. IS PATIENT'S CONDITION RELATED TO:

11. INSURED'S POLICY GROUP OR FECA NUMBER

a. OTHER INSURED'S POLICY OR GROUP NUMBER

a. EMPLOYMENT? (Current or Previous)   YES ☐   NO ☐

a. INSURED'S DATE OF BIRTH   MM | DD | YY   SEX   M ☐   F ☐

b. OTHER INSURED'S DATE OF BIRTH   MM | DD | YY   SEX   M ☐   F ☐

b. AUTO ACCIDENT?   PLACE (State)   YES ☐   NO ☐

b. EMPLOYER'S NAME OR SCHOOL NAME

c. EMPLOYER'S NAME OR SCHOOL NAME

c. OTHER ACCIDENT?   YES ☐   NO ☐

c. INSURANCE PLAN NAME OR PROGRAM NAME

d. INSURANCE PLAN NAME OR PROGRAM NAME

10d. RESERVED FOR LOCAL USE

d. IS THERE ANOTHER HEALTH BENEFIT PLAN?   YES ☐   NO ☐   **If yes**, return to and complete item 9 a-d.

PATIENT AND INSURED INFORMATION

READ BACK OF FORM BEFORE COMPLETING & SIGNING THIS FORM.

12. PATIENT'S OR AUTHORIZED PERSON'S SIGNATURE I authorize the release of any medical or other information necessary to process this claim. I also request payment of government benefits either to myself or to the party who accepts assignment below.

SIGNED_____   DATE _____

13. INSURED'S OR AUTHORIZED PERSON'S SIGNATURE I authorize payment of medical benefits to the undersigned physician or supplier for services described below.

SIGNED_____

14. DATE OF CURRENT: MM | DD | YY   ILLNESS (First symptom) OR INJURY (Accident) OR PREGNANCY(LMP)

15. IF PATIENT HAS HAD SAME OR SIMILAR ILLNESS. GIVE FIRST DATE   MM | DD | YY

16. DATES PATIENT UNABLE TO WORK IN CURRENT OCCUPATION   FROM MM | DD | YY   TO MM | DD | YY

17. NAME OF REFERRING PROVIDER OR OTHER SOURCE

17a.
17b. NPI

18. HOSPITALIZATION DATES RELATED TO CURRENT SERVICES   FROM MM | DD | YY   TO MM | DD | YY

19. RESERVED FOR LOCAL USE

20. OUTSIDE LAB?   YES ☐   NO ☐ $ CHARGES

21. DIAGNOSIS OR NATURE OF ILLNESS OR INJURY (Relate Items 1, 2, 3 or 4 to Item 24E by Line)

1. |___.___
2. |___.___
3. |___.___
4. |___.___

22. MEDICAID RESUBMISSION CODE   ORIGINAL REF. NO.

23. PRIOR AUTHORIZATION NUMBER

24. A. DATE(S) OF SERVICE						B. PLACE OF SERVICE	C. EMG	D. PROCEDURES, SERVICES, OR SUPPLIES (Explain Unusual Circumstances)		E. DIAGNOSIS POINTER	F. $ CHARGES	G. DAYS OR UNITS	H. EPSDT Family Plan	I. ID. QUAL.	J. RENDERING PROVIDER ID. #
From			To					CPT/HCPCS	MODIFIER						
MM	DD	YY	MM	DD	YY										
1														NPI	
2														NPI	
3														NPI	
4														NPI	
5														NPI	
6														NPI	

25. FEDERAL TAX I.D. NUMBER   SSN ☐ EIN ☐

26. PATIENT'S ACCOUNT NO.

27. ACCEPT ASSIGNMENT? (For govt. claims, see back)   YES ☐   NO ☐

28. TOTAL CHARGE $

29. AMOUNT PAID $

30. BALANCE DUE $

31. SIGNATURE OF PHYSICIAN OR SUPPLIER INCLUDING DEGREES OR CREDENTIALS (I certify that the statements on the reverse apply to this bill and are made a part thereof.)

SIGNED_____   DATE _____

32. SERVICE FACILITY LOCATION INFORMATION

a. NPI   b.

33. BILLING PROVIDER INFO & PH # (   )

a. NPI   b.

PHYSICIAN OR SUPPLIER INFORMATION

NUCC Instruction Manual available at: www.nucc.org

OMB APPROVAL PENDING

Patient Claim Form

Information must be printed or typewritten. Claim form must be completed and returned to us at the indicated address.

Medicare Patients: Submit this claim to Medicare FIRST! A copy of the Medicare Explanation of Benefits must be submitted with this claim form.

TO BE COMPLETED BY MEMBER

1. Information Pertaining to Member

Name: Last, First, M.I.		Sex:	Date of Birth	Member ID #
Home Address: Street	City	State Zip		Telephone Number
Marital Status	Name of Spouse	Spouse's Date of Birth		Member ID #
Is Spouse Employed?	If Yes, Name and Address of Employer			Employer Phone Number

2. Information Pertaining to Patient

Patient Name: Last, First, M.I.		Sex	Date of Birth	Member ID #
Home Address: Street	City	State Zip		Telephone Number
Is Patient Employed? Full-Time Part Time No	Relationship to Employee?	If Dependent Child Over 19, Name of School Where Full-time Student:		

3. Information Regarding Current Treatment

Related to Illness?	Related to Pregnancy?	Related to Work?	Description of Illness or Injury
Date of Accident	Where Happened?	Describe Accident	

4. Information Regarding Insurance

Are You, Your Spouse, or Dependent Children Covered by Any Other Insurance?	Name of Insured
If Yes, Name, and Address of Insurance	Insurance Phone Number

Patient's or Guardian's Signature

I certify that the above information is true and correct and I authorize the release of any medical information necessary to process this claim.

Signed: Date:

Assignment of Benefits:

I assign payment of benefits to the following provider:

Address: Street	City	State Zip	Telephone Number

TO BE COMPLETED BY PHYSICIAN

Patient's Name: Last, First, M.I.

Home Address: Street	City	State	Zip	Telephone Number

Is Condition Due To Illness?	Injury?	Work Related?	Pregnancy?	If Yes, Date Of Last Menstrual Period

Diagnosis Or Nature Of Illness Or Injuries. Give Description And ICD-9 Code.

_____

_____

Date Of Service	Place Of Service	Description Of Medical Services Or Supplies Provided	CPT® Code	ICD-9-CM Code	Charge

Date Of First Symptoms	Date Of Accident	Date Patient First Seen		Total Charges	
Dates Patient Unable To Work From To:	If Still Disabled, Date Patient Should Return To Work			Amount Paid	
Patient Still Under Care For This Condition?	Date Of Same Or Similar Illness Or Condition		Does Patient Have Other Health Coverage?		

Under Section 6019 Of The Internal Revenue Code, Recipients Of Medical Payments Must Provide Identifying Numbers To Payors Who Must Report Such Payments To The Internal Revenue Service.   Taxpayer ID Number: _____ Social Security Number: _____

Physician's Name: _____   Signature: _____

_____

Street Address	City	State	Zip

INFORMATION REGARDING THIS CLAIM FORM

A Separate Claim Must Be Filed For Each Different Injury Or Illness.

A Claim Must Be Filed Within 90 Days of The Date Of Service Or Claim Benefits May Be Reduced.

If Patient Is Medicare Eligible, Claim Must First Be Submitted To Medicare For Payment. We Cannot Process Claim Without Information Regarding Medicare's Payment.

PAUL PROVIDER, M.D.
5858 Peppermint Place
Anytown, USA 12345
(765) 555-6768

Insurance Claims Register

Page No. _____

Date Claims Filed	Patient Name	Name of Insurance Policy	Place Claim Sent	Claim Amount	Follow-up Date	Paid Amount	Remaining Balance

Paul Provider, M.D.
5858 Peppermint Place
Anytown, USA 12345
(765) 555-6768

Superbill/Charge Slip

Date of Service: _____ Account Number: _____

Name (Last, First): _____

X	Code	Description	Fee	X	Code	Description	Fee	X	Code	Description	Fee
Initial				**Established**				**Special Procedures**			
	99202	Expanded Exam	60.00		99211	Minimal Exam	35.00				
	99203	Detailed Low Complexity	100.00		99212	Brief Straightforward Exam	40.00				
	99204	Comp Moderate Complexity Exam	140.00		99213	Expanded Low Complexity Exam	45.00				
	99205	Comp High Complexity Exam	160.00		99214	Detailed Moderate Complexity Exam	60.00				
					99215	Comp High Complexity Exam	90.00				
Consultations				**Laboratory**				**Prescriptions**			
	99244	Comprehensive	150.00		36415	Venipuncture	20.00				
					81000	Urinalysis	30.00				
					82948	Glucose Fingerstick	18.00				
					93000	EKG	55.00				

X	Code	Diagnosis	X	Code	Diagnosis	X	Code	Diagnosis
	466	Bronchitis, Acute		401	Hypertension		460	Upper Resp Tract Infection
	428	Congestive Heart Failure		414	Ischemic Heart Disease		599.0	Urinary Tract Infection
	431	CVA		724.2	Low Back Syndrome		616	Vaginitis
	250.0	Diabetes Mellitus		278.0	Obesity		490	Bronchitis
	625.3	Dysmenorrhea		715	Osteoarthritis		244	Acquired Hypothyroidism
	345	Epilepsy		462	Pharyngitis. Acute		**ICD-9-CM**	**Other Diagnosis**
	0009.0	Gastroenteritis		714	Rheumatoid Arthritis			

Remarks/Special Instructions	New Appointment	Statement of Account	
		Old Balance	
		Today's Fee	
Referring Physician	Recall	Payment	
		New Balance	

CPI® codes, descriptions, and two-digit numeric modifiers are copyrighted 2005 American Medical Association. All Rights Reserved

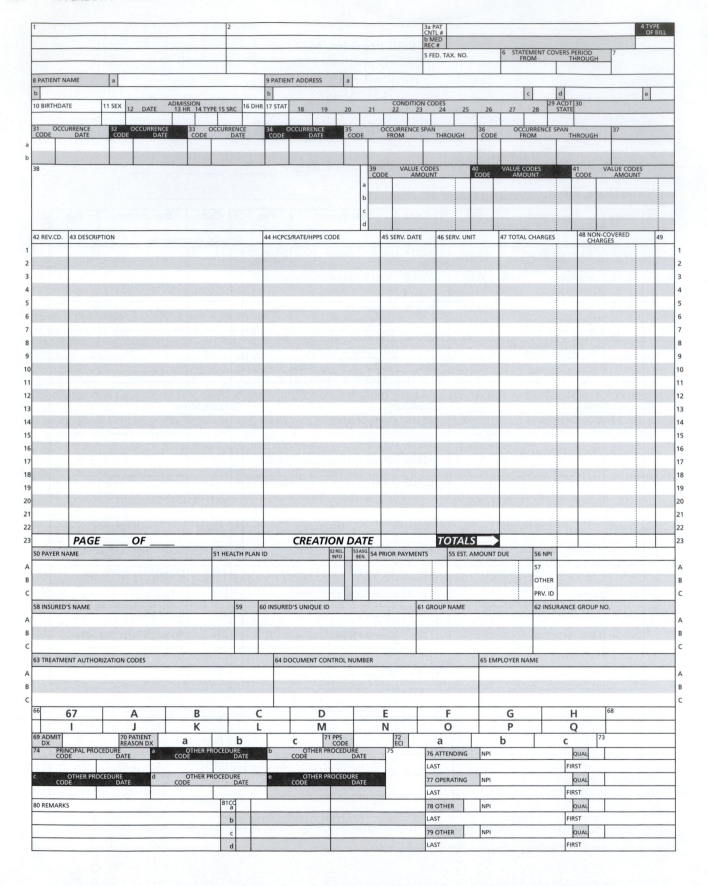

Patient Data Table

Patient Name	Abby Addison	Bobby Brumble	Cathy Crenshaw	Daisy Doolittle	Edward Edmunds
Address	5678 Any Avenue, Newton, NM 88012	93485 Bumpkiss Court Denver, CO 80128	9191 Carson Court Crabapple, CT 06192	1234 Daffy Lane Danbury, DE 19876	8888 Every Lane Evansville, CA 90012
Telephone # Home Work	(765) 555-4321 (765) 555-4567	(303) 555-4756 (303) 555-6272	(919) 555-4712 (919) 555-0101	(512) 555-4747	(323) 555-7171 (323) 555-8484
Date of Birth	12/12/1968	10/1/1963	8/12/1941	8/1/1959	1/10/27
Social Security #	001-01-0010	222-58-2342	323-83-5433	004-04-0218	508-12-3456
Marital Status/Gender	Single/Female	Married/Male	Single/Female	Married/Female	Widow/Male
Patient Account #	GMBC5509-001	GMBC5509-002	GMBC5509-003	GMBC5509-004	GMBC5509-005
Allergies/Medical Conditions	None/Hypertension	None/Diabetes	None/Chronic Bronchitis	None/Congenital Hypothyroidism	None/Coronary Artery Disease
Insurance Carrier	Rover Insurers, Inc. 5931 Rolling Road Ronson, CO 81369	Ball Ins. Carriers 3895 Bubble Blvd. Ste. 283 Boxwood, CO 85931	No Insurance (Cash patient)	Medicaid P.O. Box 0098 Danbury, DE 19342	Medicare P.O. Box 1234 Evansville, CA 90012
Member's ID #	001-01 RED	002-02 BLUE		004-04 MEDI	508-12-3456A
Group Policy #	41935	98135		Part A and B	
Policy/Employer	Red Corporation 1234 Nockout Road Newton, NM 88012 (970) 555-0863	Blue Corporation 9817 Bobcat Blvd. Bastion, CO 81319 (970) 555-5432	Creative Creations Corp. 1234 Creature Lane Crevice, CT 06192 (919) 555-5631	Retired	Retired
Workers' Comp Ins. Carrier	Red Apple Ins. 1234 Abbey Road Addison, NJ 11112	Blueberry Ins. 4662 Beach Blvd. Benton, CO 85931			
Workers' Comp Claim Number					
Assigned Provider	Paul Provider, M.D.	Paul Provider, M.D.	Paul Provider, M.D.	Paul Provider, M.D.	Paul Provider, M.D.
Referred By	Friend	Spouse	Friend	Dr. Daniel Dobby	Edith Evans
Responsible Party	Self	Self	Self	Self	Self
Person to Contact in Emergency	Alice Avery (friend) 2222 Archel Avenue Alverville, AK 99087 (765) 555-1414	Betty Brumble (spouse) 93485 Bumpkiss Court Denver, CO 80128 (303) 555-2222	Carmen Castro (friend) 6789 Cranbury Lane Crabapple, CT 06192 (919) 555-6565	David Daugherty (spouse) 1234 Daffy Lane Danbury, DE 19876 (512) 555-4748	Edgar Edmunds (brother) 7777 Every Lane Evansville, CA 90012 (323) 555-1569

Provider Data Table

Provider Name:	Paul Provider, M.D.	Laboratory Provider	Saint Mary Medical Center
Address:	5858 Peppermint Place	5859 Peppermint Place	2789 Court Street
City, State Zip	Anytown, USA 12345	Anytown, USA 12345	Anytown, USA 12345
Telephone #:	(765) 555-6768	(765) 555-6766	(765) 555-8844
Accepts Medicare Assignment	Yes	Yes	Yes
Authorization to Release Information on File	Yes	Yes	Yes
Assignment of Benefits on File	Yes	Yes	Yes
TIN:	57-1233758	99-9874343	88-1577935
UPIN:	A54321	000277	000202
PIN:	AA345678	2315845	6981423

Glossary

Abuse—When a payment for items or services is obtained when there is no legal entitlement to that payment and the provider unintentionally (or without knowledge) misrepresents the facts to obtain payment. Abuse includes any item or procedure that is inconsistent with accepted norms or practices.

Accident—An unintentional injury that has a specific time, date, and place.

Accounting control summary—A weekly or monthly report form that shows each day's charges, payments, and adjustments for the period indicated.

Accounts payable—Money the practice owes to others.

Accounts receivable—Money owed to the practice.

Accredited Standards Committee (ASC) X12N Version 4010—The electronic transaction standard that was used prior to ICD-10-CM.

Acknowledgment reports—Generated by an insurance carrier and indicate the claims that were received electronically.

Active member roster—Lists patients whose coverage has continued into the next month.

Actively-at-work provision—States that a person must be at work (or actively engaged in his or her normal activities, if a dependent) on the date coverage becomes effective.

Adjustments—Changes that can either increase or decrease the remaining balance on an account.

Admission codes—Numerical code denoting the priority of the admission.

Admission kit—Usually includes an emesis basin, carafe, cup, lotion, tissue, and mouthwash and is provided to patients who are being admitted to the hospital.

Advance Beneficiary Notice (ABN)—A written notice a provider gives a Medicare beneficiary before rendering services. This notice informs a patient that a particular procedure may not be considered medically necessary by Medicare, and that if payment is denied by Medicare, the patient will be responsible for paying for the procedure.

Aggregate deductible—Requires all major medical deductibles applied for all family members to be added together to attain the family limit.

Air ambulance—A helicopter or other flight vehicle used to transport a severely injured or ill person to a hospital.

Allowed amount—What the insurance company considers to be a reasonable charge for the procedure performed. Is often less than the amount that the provider bills.

Alphabetical filing—Filing the charts alphabetically by the first letter of the patient's last name.

Alter—Change or amend (add to) the information contained in a record or chart.

Ambulatory patient classifications (APCs)—Similar to DRGs but are for patients who receive services on an outpatient basis.

Ambulatory surgical centers (surgicenters)—Centers equipped to allow for the performance of surgery on an outpatient basis.

Assignment of Benefits Form—A request for all insurance payments to be directed to the provider holding the assignment.

Audit—A formal examination that is performed to prevent and detect fraud.

Authorized Treatment Record Form—Is used to track the usage of preauthorized services rendered by a provider's office.

Backward mapping—Lists each ICD-10-CM/PCS code, respectively, and the closest equivalent(s) in ICD-9-CM/PCS.

Balance billing—Sending an additional bill to another party for payment of any remaining amounts on a claim.

Bankruptcy—When a debtor announces that he or she no longer has the ability to pay creditors and requests relief for debts from the bankruptcy court.

Bar code—A number that is assigned to a specific item.

Base call charge—The amount automatically charged for the ambulance to respond to a call even if the patient is not subsequently transported.

Basic benefits—Those benefits usually paid at 100 percent and are paid before major medical benefits are paid.

Benefit period—Begins with the first day of admission to the hospital.

Benign—Localized growth that does not spread (metastasize) and is not usually terminal.

Bilateral procedures—Surgeries that involve a pair of similar body parts (e.g., breasts, eyes).

Biofeedback—Technique of making unconscious or involuntary bodily processes (as heartbeats or brain waves) perceptible to the senses (as by the use of an oscilloscope) in order to manipulate them by conscious mental control.

Block—In ICD-10-CM, comparable to a section in ICD-9-CM; a contiguous range of codes within a chapter.

Block procedures—Multiple surgical procedures performed during the same operative session, in the same operative area, usually on the integumentary system.

Bonding—The process by which an employer can be indemnified (insured) for the loss of money or other property sustained through dishonest acts of a "bonded" employee.

Capitation—The practice of paying a provider a set amount per month to provide treatment to managed care plan members and for performing other administrative duties.

Carryover provision—Any amounts that the patient pays in the last three months of the year toward the designated deductible will carry over and will be applied toward the next year's deductible.

Category—In ICD-10, three characters in length.

Categorically needy—Class of Medicaid recipient. These recipients usually make less than the poverty level every month, may or may not be working, and may or may not have other health insurance.

Centers for Medicare and Medicaid Services (CMS)—The organization that oversees the Medicare program.

Chargemaster Description List (CDL)—A list that includes all hospital procedures, services, supplies, and drugs that are billed on the UB-04.

Children's charts—Type of chart used in some offices for pediatric patients that may contain additional or different forms.

Claim—Also known as a bill. A form prepared to show the services rendered by a provider.

Claim attachment—Any document providing additional medical information to the claims payer that cannot be accommodated within the standard billing form.

Claims audit—An analysis of claims payments made to a health care provider to determine whether the claims were allowable and whether the provider was paid the appropriate amount for services rendered.

Claims register—A database that lists all claims created by a practice. This database can usually be sorted by date, provider, or patient name.

Clean claim—A claim that can be paid as soon as it is received because it is complete in all aspects and does not need additional investigation.

CMS-1500—A standardized form approved by both the American Medical Association and CMS for use as a "universal" form for billing professional services.

Code—The final level of subdivision.

Coinsurance—A predetermined percentage of additional annual expenses up to a preset maximum.

Combination codes—In ICD-10, codes that describe multiple conditions with one code.

Complaints—A patient's verbal expressions regarding quality of services, access to care, interpersonal communication, any other aspect of their care, or their relationship with their provider.

Concurrent care—When two providers are seeing a patient at the same time for two unrelated medical conditions.

Concurrent review—Determines whether the estimated length of time and scope of the inpatient stay are justified by the diagnosis and symptoms.

Condition codes—Used to identify conditions relating to the claim that may affect payer processing.

Consultation—Opinion provided by a specialist at the request of another provider.

Controlled drugs—Drugs that are tightly controlled by federal mandates because of their addictive, experimental, toxic, or other highly volatile properties.

Conventions—Use of symbols, typeface, and layout features.

Conversion factor—A monetary amount that is determined by the CMS.

Coordination of benefits (COB)—A process that occurs when two or more plans provide coverage on the same person.

Copayment—A fixed amount a member must pay for a covered service.

Crosswalks—Imply a one-to-one correlation between codes in two data sets.

CT (computed tomography) scan—Provides a three-dimensional picture of an area and is used to help identify tumors and cancers located in an organ.

Cumulative trial balance—Lists each patient alphabetically and shows any charges, payments, or adjustments to the patient's account.

Custodial care—Primarily for the purpose of meeting the personal daily needs of the patient and could be provided by personnel without medical care skills or training.

Daily journal—Also known as the day sheet; indicates the patient's name, the individual fee charged for the day, any payments made, and the current balance.

Day sheet—Also known as the daily journal. Form used to indicate the patient's name, the individual fee charged for the day, any payments made, and the current balance.

Death benefits—Compensation for the family of a deceased injured worker for the loss of income that the injured worker would have provided to the family.

Deductible—A predetermined portion of annual out-of-pocket medical expenses. The amount that the individual patient must pay before benefits are paid by the insurance carrier.

Default—Always "without," meaning that if the documentation does not specifically state "with" or "without," the code for "without" should be assigned

Default code—In ICD-10, represents that condition that is most commonly associated with the main term, or is the unspecified code for the condition.

Defendant—The person who is being sued.

Defense Enrollment Eligibility Reporting System (DEERS)—A computer database used to verify TRICARE eligibility.

Deposit slip—Also referred to as deposit ticket; provides an overview and balance of monies being deposited.

Deposit ticket—Also referred to as deposit slip; provides an overview and balance of monies being deposited.

Diagnosis-related group (DRG)—Method used to determine payments for inpatient hospital claims. The program is now known as MS-DRG rather than DRG.

Diagnostic x-rays—All uses of radiant energy in medical diagnosis and therapeutic procedures.

Dialysis—A maintenance procedure used for end-stage renal disease when the kidneys cease functioning.

Disenrollment—When a patient transfers care from a provider.

Doctor's First Report of Injury/Illness—Requests basic information on the date, time, and location of the injury/illness and treatment, the patient's subjective complaints and objective findings, the diagnosis and the treatment rendered.

Downcoding—Occurs when an insurance carrier changes a code to a similar code that has a lower level of service.

Dunning notice—A statement, or sentence included on the statement, reminding the recipient to make a payment on his or her account.

Durable medical equipment (DME)—Equipment that can withstand repeated use, is primarily and customarily used to serve a medical purpose, is generally not useful to a person in the absence of an illness or injury, and is appropriate for use in the home.

Durable Medical Equipment Regional Carriers (DMERCs)—Carriers that process durable medical equipment, prosthetics, orthotics, and supplies (DMEPOS) claims.

Early and Periodic Screening, Diagnosis, and Treatment (EPSDT) Program—Preventive screening program designed for the early detection and treatment of medical problems in welfare children (known in California as the Child Health and Disability Prevention [CHDP] program).

E code listing—In ICD-9-CM, a supplementary classification of external causes of injury and poisoning.

Electronic claims—Claims routinely submitted electronically to insurance carriers.

Electronic claims submission—A process whereby insurance claims are submitted via computerized data (either by data diskette or modem) directly from the provider to the insurance company.

Electronic prescriptions—Prescriptions that are entered into the provider's computer, and then electronically sent to the patient's pharmacy.

Electronic transactions—Data transmitted via computers.

Eligibility—The qualifications that make a person eligible for coverage.

Eligibility card—Shows that the individual is eligible for Medicaid.

Eligibility roster—Assists the provider in determining who is eligible for treatment; lists those patients who have chosen the provider as their primary care provider (PCP).

Emancipated minor—A minor child who has gone through the emancipation process.

Emancipation—A legal process whereby a child assumes responsibility for himself, and the child's parent or legal guardian is no longer legally responsible for the child.

Embezzlement—The fraudulent appropriation of funds entrusted to one's care.

Emergency—Exists when delay in treatment of the patient would lead to a significant increase in the threat to life or body part.

Encounter Forms—Used to record both clinical and financial information about the patient, and frequently used as billing and routing documents. These forms can be referred to as charge tickets, fee slips, and superbills in the provider's office, and as a chargemaster in the hospital.

End-stage renal disease (ESRD)—Occurs when a person's kidneys fail to function.

Enteral therapy—Involves the administration of nutritional products directly into the intestines.

Eponyms—Illnesses or conditions named after a person (e.g., Gerhardt disease).

Errors and omissions insurance—Covers damages caused by mistakes (errors) or damages caused by something an employee failed to do (omissions).

Established patient—One who has received professional services from the provider, or another provider of the same specialty who belongs to the same group practice, within the past three years.

Etiology—Causes of disease.

Evaluation and management (E/M) codes—Designate services provided in the provider's office, outpatient or ambulatory facility.

Excludes1—Indicates that the condition represented by the code and the condition excluded are mutually exclusive and should not be coded together, such as the acquired and congenital forms of the same condition.

Excludes2—Indicates that the condition excluded is not part of the condition represented by the code, but the patient may have both conditions at the same time.

Exclusions—Items that the insurance carrier does not cover.

Exclusive Provider Organization (EPO)—Basically a much smaller Physician Provider Organization (PPO) where the patient must select a primary care provider (PCP) and can use only those providers who are part of the network or who are referred by the PCP.

Explanation of Benefits (EOB)—Form created by the insurance carrier that lists the patient, the date of the service, the service performed, the amount that was allowed for the procedure, the percentage covered by insurance, and the amount that the insurance carrier will pay.

Extensions—The seventh character of a code that must appear in that position, regardless of the length of the code.

External audit—Considered to be a retrospective review because it is performed after a claim has been submitted for payment and after the claim has been processed by the insurance carrier.

External auditor—Someone hired by an insurance company or governmental organization such as Medicare or Medicaid to perform an audit.

Family deductible—A specified number of family members must satisfy their individual deductible.

Fee-for-service—Also called an indemnity insurance plan. A principle of insurance that provides medical coverage when a loss occurs, and restores the insured party to their the approximate financial condition that they he or she was in before the loss occurred.

Fee schedule—A list of predetermined charges for medical services and supplies.

First-listed diagnosis—The main reason for the services provided.

Fiscal Intermediaries—Insurance companies that are now known as Medicare Administrative Contractors (MAC).

Follow-up days—Days of service for complications or other circumstances requiring additional or unusual services concurrent with a procedure or procedures, or during the listed period of normal follow-up care; may warrant additional charges on a fee-for-service basis.

Forward mapping—Lists each ICD-9-CM/PCS code respectively and the closest equivalent(s) in ICD-10-CM/PCS.

Fraud—Intentional misrepresentation of a fact with the intent to deprive a person of property or legal rights.

General Equivalence Mappings (GEMs)—Allows users to map forward and backward between the ICD-9-CM and ICD-10-CM coding systems.

Generic drugs—Nonproprietary drugs not protected by trademark. Their name is usually descriptive of the drug's chemical structure.

Geographical Cost Practice Index (GCPI)—A numerical factor used to multiply by to arrive at a sum for billing purposes.

Glasgow Coma Scale (GCS)—Rates visual, verbal, and motor responses.

Global period—The days immediately following a surgical procedure for which a provider must monitor a patient's condition in regard to that particular procedure.

Granularity—Detail.

Grievances—Written complaints made by a member regarding quality of services, access to care, interpersonal communication, any other aspect of care, or relationship with the provider.

Grouper—A coding application that uses algorithms to assign DRGs, taking into consideration the patient's principal diagnosis, secondary diagnosis, primary procedures, gender, age, discharge disposition, and the presence or absence of a complication/comorbidity (CC) or major complication/comorbidity (MCC).

Guarantor—A person who undertakes the responsibility for payment of a debt.

Healthcare Common Procedure Coding System (HCPCS)—A listing of codes and descriptive terminology used for reporting the provision of supplies, materials, injections, and certain services and procedures.

Health Insurance Portability and Accountability Act (HIPAA)—Signed into law to set a national standard for electronic transfer of health data.

Health Maintenance Organizations (HMOs)—Groups that provide services in exchange for premiums.

Health Savings Account—A medical savings account that is available to individuals who are enrolled in high-deductible health insurance plans.

Home services—Visits performed by a provider in the patient's home.

Hospital inpatient services—Evaluation and management provided in an inpatient hospital setting for a patient who has been formally admitted to such a facility.

ICD-9-CM—*International Classification of Diseases—9th Revision Clinical Modification.*

ICD-10-PCS (Procedure Coding System) Replaces ICD-9-CM Volume 3 procedure codes for hospital inpatient coding in the United States.

Incomplete data master list—A complete listing of patients whose patient chart does not have properly filled out or completed patient forms.

Indemnity insurance plans—Also called fee-for-service. A principle of insurance that provides medical coverage when a loss occurs and restores the insured party to the approximate financial condition he or she was in before the loss occurred.

Independent Practice Association (IPA)—Sometimes called individual practice organization or IPO; a legal entity, comprised of a network of private practice providers, who have organized to negotiate contracts with insurance companies and HMOs.

In-network providers—Providers who are contracted by a preferred provider organization (PPO) to provide services.

Insurance claims register—Lists all claims that have been fully completed and are being submitted to the insurance carrier by the provider's office.

Insurance Coverage Form—A form used to verify and document insurance coverage information.

Insurance premium—The actual amount of money charged by insurance companies for active coverage.

Insurance tracer—A form or letter sent to the insurance carrier to inquire about the status of a previously submitted claim.

Interim billing—A periodic billing for services before the patient is discharged from the hospital.

Internal audit—Considered to be a prospective review because it is performed before a claim is submitted for payment.

International Classification of Diseases—9th Revision Clinical Modification (ICD-9-CM)—An indexing of diseases and conditions.

International Classification of Diseases—10th Revision, Clinical Modification (ICD-10-CM)—An update to ICD-9-CM that will go into effect on October 1, 2013.

Itemized bill—Lists each item, service, or supply on an individual line and shows the cost for that one item.

Job stress—The harmful physical and emotional responses that occur when the requirements of the job do not match the capabilities, resources, or needs of the worker.

Laboratory examinations—The analyses of body substances to determine their chemical or tissue makeup.

Laterality—Right or left side.

Legal damages—Monetary awards that a plan member may attempt to recover, which are above and beyond the benefits provided by the group plan.

Legend drugs—Drugs that can be obtained only with a prescription.

Lien—A legal document that expresses claim on the property of another for payment of a debt.

Lifetime maximum—The maximum amount of money an insurance plan will pay over the lifetime of the insured.

Limiting charge—Federal law that prohibits a doctor who does not accept assignment from charging more than 15 percent above Medicare's approved amount.

Maintaining records—Keeping the information in a chart updated and, if using a paper record, filing the chart or recording it in a manner that makes it easy to locate if needed in the future.

Main terms—Usually identify disease conditions rather than locations.

Malignant—Means that the cancer or growth is growing.

Malignant CA in situ—The malignant growth is still localized in one area and has not spread within the organ of origin.

Malignant primary—The site of the tumor is the point of origin of the neoplasm.

Malignant secondary—The site of the tumor in question is not where the disease originated; it has spread to this location from the primary site.

Managed care—A system for organizing the delivery of health services so that the cost of care is reduced and the quality of care is maintained or improved.

Management Service Organization (MSO)—A separate corporation set up to provide management services to a medical group for a fee.

Mandatory program—Requires the patient to obtain a second surgical opinion for special procedures, or there is an automatic reduction or denial of benefits.

Many-to-one—When several codes in ICD-10-CM are combined into a single equivalent code in ICD-9-CM, or vice versa.

Medicaid—A joint federal–state medical assistance program for certain categories of low-income people.

Medicaid Remittance Advice (MRA)—Issued to providers for claims submitted to Medicaid for a certain period of time. Provides information about claims that were paid, adjusted, voided, and denied.

Medical dictionary—Lists medical terms and their definitions, synonyms, illustrations, and supplemental information.

Medical–legal evaluation—Provides medical evidence for the purpose of proving or disproving medical issues in a contested workers' compensation claim.

Medically needy—Class of Medicaid recipients whose high medical expenses and inadequate health care coverage (often a result of catastrophic illnesses) have left them at risk of being indigent. Many disabled and elderly persons fall into this category.

Medically oriented equipment—Equipment primarily and customarily used for medical purposes (i.e., it is designed to fulfill a medical need).

Medical service order—A form stating the patient is being referred to the provider in regard to a work-related injury and that the employer is responsible for coverage of services.

Medicare—The Federal Health Insurance Benefit Plan for the Aged and Disabled.

Medicare abuse—Similar to Medicare fraud, except that it is not possible to establish that abusive acts were committed knowingly, willfully, and intentionally.

Medicare fraud—The intentional misrepresentation of information that could result in an unauthorized benefit.

Medicare Health Insurance Claim Number (HICN)—A unique identification number assigned to Medicare beneficiaries, which normally consists of a Social Security number followed by a letter of the alphabet and possibly another letter or number (e.g., 123–45-6789A).

Medicare HMO—An HMO that has contracted with the federal government under the Medicare Advantage program (formerly called Medicare+Choice) to provide health benefits to persons eligible for Medicare who choose to enroll in the HMO, instead of receiving their benefits and care through the traditional fee-for-service Medicare program.

Medicare Necessity Denials—Reason for denial of claims by Medicare; The most common reason is for services that are considered not medically necessary.

Medicare Part A—Covers facility charges for acute inpatient hospital care, skilled nursing, home health care, and hospice care.

Medicare Part B—Covers provider services, outpatient hospital services, home health care, outpatient speech and physical therapy, and durable medical equipment.

Medicare Part C—Medicare Advantage, includes coverage in an HMO, PPO, and so on.

Medicare Part D—Prescription drug component (effective 2006).

Medicare Redetermination Notice—The redetermination letter issued by the Appeals Department.

Medicare Remittance Notice (MRN)—Used to convey payments to providers who accept assignment for Medicare claims.

Medicare Secondary Payer (MSP)—Medicare pays secondary to other insurance such as employer-sponsored group insurance, individual policies carried by the employee, workers' compensation insurance, beneficiary entitled to Black Lung benefits, automobile or no-fault insurance, and third-party liability when an individual is covered by one of these plans.

Medicare Severity-Diagnosis Related Group (MS-DRG)—Instead of the hospital itemized billing system, a flat-rate payment is made based on complications or comorbidities (CCs) or major CCs (MCCs) that the patient may be experiencing along with the principal diagnosis.

Medicare Summary Notice (MSN)—An explanation of benefits sent to the Medicare beneficiary, detailing the processing of claims submitted for payment.

Medicare Supplemental Insurance—Also known as Medigap policies. Separate plans written exclusively for Medicare participants that pay for amounts that Medicare does not pay.

Medications—Drugs (often called pharmaceuticals) used to treat diseases, symptoms, or discomforts (e.g., pain medications).

Medigap—Policies specifically designed to supplement Medicare's benefits; regulated by federal and state law.

Mental health expenses—Include claims submitted for psychiatric services, marriage and family counseling services, and drug and alcohol treatment.

Modifiers—Two-digit codes that can be added to CPT codes to denote unusual circumstances.

Morbidity—The rate of incidence of disease.

Mortality—The number of deaths in a given time and place; the proportion of deaths to population.

Multiple coding—Using two or more codes to fully describe a condition.

Multiple procedures—More than one surgical procedure performed during the same operative session.

NCPDP Version 3.0—Medicaid pharmacy plans.

NCPDP Version D.0—Medicare Part D pharmacies and suppliers.

National Center for Health Statistics (NCHS)—Under the direction of NCHS, the United States has adapted and expanded ICD-10 for tracking and billing of both inpatient and outpatient encounters, using terminology and detail consistent with medical practice in the United States.

National Council for Prescription Drug Programs (NCPDP)—Established new formats for Medicare Part D pharmacies and suppliers (NCPDP Version D.0) and Medicaid pharmacy plans (NCPDP Version 3.0).

National Provider Identifiers (NPIs)—A provider identification system established by the Centers for Medicare and Medicaid Services (CMS).

Neoplasm—A growth (tumor) that results from abnormal cell activity.

New member roster—Shows those patients who have signed up for MCP coverage and have chosen the provider as their PCP. In addition to members who have just begun coverage, the new member roster shows those existing patients who have recently chosen this provider as their PCP.

New patient—One who has not received any professional services from the provider, or another provider of the same specialty who belongs to the same group practice, within the past three years.

Nonaggregate deductible—Requires a specified number of individual deductibles to be satisfied before the family limit is met.

Noncompliance—Not following the instructions given by the provider.

Nondisability claims—Claims for minor injuries that will not require the patient to be kept from his or her job. The.

Nonessential modifiers—The words in parentheses ( ) after the main term.

Nonlegend drugs—Drugs that can be obtained without a prescription; also known as over-the-counter drugs (OTCs).

Nonparticipating providers—Providers who treat Medicare patients but who decide whether to accept assignment on a case-by-case basis.

Notice of Noncoverage—A letter that advises Medicare HMO members of their right to an immediate professional review on a proposed discharge from an inpatient facility.

Nuclear medicine—Combines use of radioactive elements and X-rays to image an organ or body part.

Occupational therapy—Objective is to either restore normal movement, or, in the case of paralysis, to teach the patient alternative ways of dealing with his or her handicap in order to meet the demands of everyday living.

Occurrence codes—Codes and associated dates defining a significant event relating to the bill that may affect payer processing.

Occurrence span codes—Codes and related dates that identify an event that relates to the payment of the claim.

Office visits—Evaluation and management of a patient's condition in a provider's office, clinic, or hospital outpatient department; problem-oriented visits during which the provider manages an active illness or disease.

One-to-many—When a single code in ICD-9-CM has several possible equivalents in ICD-10-CM, or vice versa.

Optical Character Recognition (OCR)—An automated scanning process that reads the information on claim forms.

Order of Benefit Determinations (OBD)—The thirteen rules determining the order of payment.

Orthotics—Devices used to correct a deformity or disability.

Out-of-network provider—Provider who chooses not to contract with a preferred provider organization (PPO).

Outpatient Prospective Payment System (OPPS)—Under Medicare, pays hospitals under APCs rather than on a fee-for-service basis.

Overinsurance—Occurs when a person is covered under two or more policies and is eligible to collect an accumulation of benefits that will actually exceed the amount charged by the provider.

Over-the-counter drugs—Drugs not requiring a prescription; also known as nonlegend drugs.

Parenteral therapy—Involves administering substances to a patient via a tube inserted into a vein (e.g., medications or nutritional supplements).

Participating providers—Providers who agree to accept assignment for all bills for Medicare-eligible persons.

Patient Aging Report—Allows the medical biller to categorize a patient account's outstanding balance by the length of time the charges have been due.

Patient History Form—Helps identify previous medical history that may be important in treating the patient's present condition.

Patient Information Sheet—Sometimes called the patient registration form. Used to collect general information regarding the patient.

Patient Ledger Card—Used to indicate a chronologic record of all services rendered to a patient and record all payments and adjustments made on his or her account.

Patient Receipt—A written acknowledgment that a specific sum of money has been received.

Patient Statement—An individual summary (either by patient or by family) that lists all the services, charges, payments, adjustments, and balances due that occurred during the month.

Payer of last resort—Means that all third parties, including Medicare, TRICARE, workers' compensation, and private insurance carriers, must pay before Medicaid pays.

Pediatric charts—Charts on children.

Pended—When a claim is held for further information by the insurance carrier if there are omissions or errors on the form.

Permanent disability claims—Usually commence after temporary disability when it is determined that the patient will not be able to return to work.

Personal items—Those items that are primarily for the comfort of the patient and are not medically necessary.

Petty Cash Count Slip—Used to keep track of the amount of money kept in petty cash.

Petty cash fund—Used to make change for patients who are making cash payments and for purchasing miscellaneous small offices supplies.

Petty Cash Receipt—Used to document each time cash is removed from the petty cash fund.

Pharmaceuticals—Drugs (also known as medications) used to treat diseases, symptoms, or discomforts (e.g., pain medications).

Physical medicine and rehabilitation—Also known as physiatry or rehabilitation medicine; the manipulation and therapy associated with the nonsurgical care and treatment of the patient.

Physical therapy—The science of physical or corrective rehabilitation or treatment of abnormal conditions of the musculoskeletal system through the use of heat; light; water; electricity; sound; massage; and active, passive, or restrictive exercise.

Physicians' Desk Reference **(PDR)**—Medical reference book that provides comprehensive information about the particular use of a drug; how the drug works in the body; possible side effects; and warnings against use for the elderly, pregnant women, and for people with other health complications.

Placeholder—Used to fill the empty positions on a code less than six characters in length

Post—To list items such as payments or charges in a log.

Preadmission testing—Testing done before the patient enters the hospital for surgery.

Preauthorization—The means to gain approval for services that are to be performed, as well as to obtain an understanding of whether or not the insurance carrier will provide coverage for these services.

Precertify—Same as prospective review. To get preapproval for admission on elective, nonemergency hospitalization.

Preexisting condition—A conditions that existed before a patient was covered under a contract.

Preferred Provider Organization (PPO)—The second most common managed care alternative where the insurance carrier contracts with providers to provide services at a contracted rate.

Prescription legend—Pharmaceutical manufacturer's warning on label, which states, "Caution: Federal law prohibits dispensing without a prescription."

Preventive medicine—Routine well care provided when there is not an active illness or disease.

Primary care provider (PCP)—A specific provider chosen by the plan member for care; also called a primary care physician (PCP).

Principal diagnosis—The main reason that services were provided.

Problem-oriented medical record (POMR)—One method used to track a patient's medical progress.

Professional courtesy—When a provider renders medical services to another professional without charging the full amount of the usual charges for these services.

Prompt payment laws—Also known as fair claims practice regulations.

Proprietary drugs—Drugs that are patented or controlled by a manufacturer.

Prospective review—Same as precertification. To get preapproval for admission on elective, nonemergency hospitalization.

Prosthetic devices—Devices designed to replace a missing body part or to restore some function to a paralyzed body part.

Provider—Individuals who provide health care, including medical doctors, dentists, optometrists, chiropractors, physical therapists, and others.

Provider Hospital Organization (PHO)—An organization of providers and hospitals that band together for the purpose of obtaining contracts from payer organizations.

Provider's Current Procedure Terminology **(CPT)**—A systematic listing for coding the procedures or services performed by a provider.

Provider's Final Report—A report that the provider submits to notify the workers' compensation carrier that no further treatment is needed (or that no further treatment will significantly alter the patient's condition) and that the patient has been discharged.

Psychiatric services—Evaluation and treatment for psychotic and neurotic disorders, organic brain dysfunction, alcoholism, and chemical dependency.

Qualifying circumstances—Situations that significantly impact on the character of the anesthetic service provided.

Radiation oncology services—The use of radiation to treat a condition.

Reference book—A source of information to which a reader is referred.

Rehabilitation benefit—A benefit provided to retrain the injured worker in a physical ability that will help when seeking future employment (e.g., proper use of a wheelchair, use of the left hand when a person loses their right hand).

Reinsurance—Also known as stop-loss insurance; an insurance policy that protects the company against catastrophic medical costs levied against its plan, either by a single employee or by all employees as a whole.

Relative value scale—A scale of numeric values (relative value units) based on how difficult a procedure is to perform, the overhead involved, and the chance of incurring a malpractice lawsuit.

Relative value unit—A numeric value for a procedure.

Release of Information Form—Used to allow the provider to request additional information from other providers of service or to share information with an insurance carrier.

Request for Additional Information Form—Form designed to ask for information or records from various sources.

Resource-based relative value scale (RBRVS)—Designed to address the soaring cost of provider health care in the United States.

Respondeat superior—When an employer is liable for harms caused by an employee while that employee is acting within the scope of his or her employment.

Retrospective review—Used to determine after discharge whether the hospitalization and treatment were medically necessary and covered by the terms of the benefit program.

Revenue code—Code referencing the type of services provided.

Second surgical opinion (SSO) consultation—Performed to eliminate elective surgical procedures that are classified as unnecessary.

Self-funded plan—A company plan that insures the company and its own workers.

Self-insurance—Instead of paying monthly premiums to an insurance carrier, employers place the money in an escrow account; when an employee receives medical attention, the claim is submitted to the employer and is reimbursed according to the terms of the employer's contract.

Sequela—Late effect or delayed healing.

Share of cost—Also known as payment or fixed copayment from the patient; the amount the patient is responsible for paying for services rendered.

Short dash—When an ICD-10-CM code has a "-" following it, it signifies additional characters should be assigned; additional characters may be number or letters, depending on the code.

Signature card—Shows the person authorized to make changes, the dates of the individual's authorization period, and the scope of the changes that may be made.

Skilled nursing facility (SNF)—Primarily engaged in providing skilled nursing care and related services for residents who require medical or nursing care; or rehabilitation services for the rehabilitation of injured, disabled, or sick persons.

Skip—A person who has received services without payment and has moved and left no forwarding address.

SOAP notes—Stands for *Subjective, Objective, Assessment,* and *Plan.* A note format used to standardize medical evaluation entries made in clinical records.

Social Health Maintenance Organization (S/HMO)—Also known as a Medicare HMO; an organization that provides the full range of Medicare benefits offered by standard HMOs plus additional services.

Speech therapy—Therapy given to improve speech and verbal communication skills.

State insurance commissioner—Person responsible for overseeing the insurance companies and their practices within the state and protecting consumers (patients).

Statement of account—Also known as a patient ledger card; used to indicate a chronological record of all services rendered to a patient and to record all payments and adjustments made on the patient's account.

Statute of limitations—The maximum time that a debt can be collected from the time the debt was incurred or became due.

Stop-loss—An attempt to limit payments by an insured person, or a provider/group/IPA, in the case of a catastrophic illness or injury to a member.

Stop-loss protection—Means that if the costs to the provider exceed a specified amount, the provider will be reimbursed by the group/IPA for at least 90 percent of expenditures over that amount.

Subcategory—Either four or five characters.

Subjective findings—Those findings that cannot be discerned by anyone other than the patient (e.g., pain, discomfort).

Subpoena—A court order mandating a person to appear at a certain time and place.

Subpoena duces tecum—Also known as a subpoena for production of evidence; requires the person to produce books, records, papers, or other tangible evidence.

Subterms—Secondary classifications under a main term.

Superbills—Billing forms used by many providers of service and suppliers.

Temporary disability claims—Claims submitted when the patient is not able to perform his or her job requirements until he or she recovers from the injury involved.

Terminated member roster—Shows those members whose coverage has been terminated or who have chosen to terminate a certain provider as their PCP.

Treating providers (TP)—Used to initially establish the employee's eligibility for workers' compensation benefits.

Treatment plan—Schedule of procedures and appointments designed to restore, step by step, the health of a patient.

TRICARE—Formerly known as the Civilian Health and Medical Program for the Uniformed Services (CHAMPUS), provides a comprehensive program of health care benefits for active-duty and retired services personnel, their dependents, and the dependents of deceased military personnel.

TRICARE-certified (authorized) provider—A facility, provider, or other health care professional who meets the licensing and certification requirements of TRICARE regulations and practices for that area of health care.

TRICARE-contracted provider—A TRICARE-certified (authorized) provider who has a contract agreement with a TRICARE Prime Contractor.

TRICARE Extra—A preferred provider organization.

TRICARE For Life—A Medigap insurance that covers those who are age sixty-five or older and covered by Medicare.

TRICARE Prime—A managed care option similar to an HMO.

TRICARE Standard—A similar benefit to the original CHAMPUS program; provides coverage on a fee-for-service basis.

Ultrasonography—A radiologic technique in which deep structures of the body are visualized by recording the reflections of ultrasonic waves directed into the tissue.

Unbundling—The idea of using two or more CPT codes rather than one inclusive code; considered fraudulent behavior by CPT.

Unlisted codes—Codes that end in "99" and are used only when no other appropriate code is available.

Unnecessary surgery—Surgery that is recommended as an elective procedure when an alternative method of treatment may be preferable for a number of reasons.

Usual, Customary, and Reasonable (UCR)—Mostly used in reference to fee-for-service reimbursement. The usual fee is the fee that a provider typically charges for a specific procedure. The customary fee is the range of usual fees that providers in the same geographic area charge for the same procedure. To determine if a fee is reasonable, both the usual and customary fees are taken into account and the payment is the lesser of the two.

Utilization review—The process of monitoring the use and delivery of medical services.

Value codes—Codes and the related dollar amount that identify data of a monetary nature that is necessary for the processing of the claim.

V code listing—In ICD-9-CM, a supplementary listing of factors that affect the health status of the patient.

Version 4010—The HIPAA-mandated electronic transaction standards that preceded Version 5010.

Version 5010—The HIPAA-mandated electronic transaction standards for ICD-10-CM codes and related data that replace the previous electronic standards called Version 4010.

Voluntary program—Encourages participants to have a second surgical opinion, but there is no automatic reduction of benefits if the patient does not comply.

Withhold—A portion of the monthly capitation amount that the managed care plan (MCP) may retain to protect the Health Maintenance Organization (HMO) from inadequate patient care or financial management by the primary care provider (PCP).

Workers' compensation (WC)—A separate medical and disability reimbursement program that provides 100 percent coverage for job-related injuries, illnesses, or conditions arising out of and in the course of employment.

Index